Baby & Child
A to Z
Medical
Handbook

THE BODY PRESS/PERIGEE BOOKS

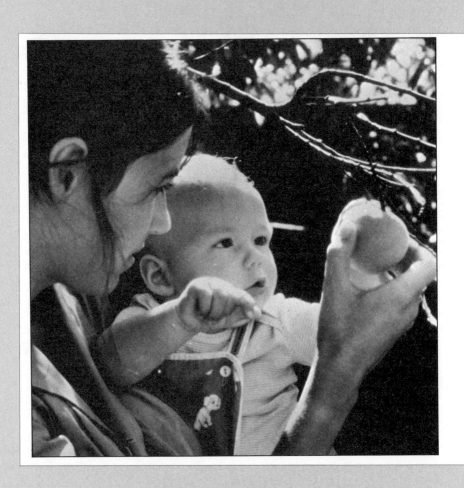

Miriam Stoppard MD MRCP

Baby & Child
A to Z
Medical
Handbook

THE BODY PRESS/PERIGEE BOOKS

For Diana and Scott

The Body Press/Perigee Books
Published by
The Berkley Publishing Group
A division of Penguin Putnam Inc.
375 Hudson Street
New York, New York 10014.

First Body Press/Perigee edition: 1992

First published in Great Britain in 1986
by Dorling Kindersley Publishers Limited,
9 Henrietta Street, London WC2E 8PS

The Penguin Putnam Inc. World Wide Web site address is
http://www.penguinputnam.com

ISBN: 0-399-51765-0

Library of Congress Catalog Card Number: 85-60486

Notice: The information in this book is true and complete to the best of our knowledge. The book is intended only as a supplementary guide to medical treatment. It is not intended as a replacement for sound medical advice from a doctor. Only a doctor can include the variables of a child's age, sex and past medical history and any other extenuating factors relating to medical symptoms and illnesses. Important decisions about treating an ill child must be made by the child's parents and the pediatrician or physician. All recommendations are made without guarantees on the part of the author, technical consultants or the publisher. The author and publisher disclaim all liability in connection with the use of this information.

Printed in the United States of America

16   17   18   19   20

This book is printed on acid-free paper.

Contents

Why I wrote this book

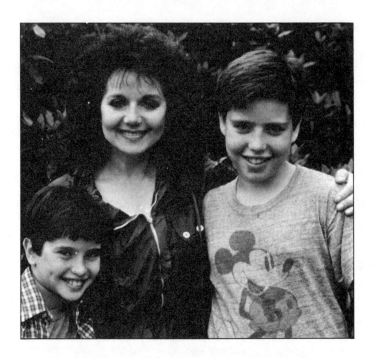

It seems strange, so few books devoted entirely to children's illnesses have been written for parents. Many baby books have a section on common childhood illnesses and problems. Some books include treatment; others approach the subject in a dictionary form, relying heavily on definitions without providing much background information and practical help. Few books treat the subject with the kind of detail, explanations and guidelines that we have come to expect from books on adult diseases. There seemed to be a gap, a need to be filled, hence this book.

The A-Z of common childhood complaints is the "meat" of this book. Information is given in simple terms that are easy to understand. You are directed to possible courses of action in a clear, logical way, and advice is given in a step-by-step format. Emphasis on speed is always made when time is of the essence and a doctor should be contacted immediately or an ambulance called.

It can be difficult to tell exactly what is wrong with your child from various symptoms—fever, pain, redness, swelling, vomiting—and on most occasions it requires a doctor for an accurate diagnosis. However, to help you narrow the possible causes of the problem, a section is devoted to the analysis of symptoms.

For some parents, having an ill child is not a transient event but one that stretches into the future. Their responsibility is to cope with a chronically ill child. I have tried to cover the most common conditions, giving information on causative factors, the expected course of the disease and how to make life easy on your child, yourself and the rest of your family. Trying to foresee the longterm outcome is always difficult, and sometimes dangerous, but I have attempted to indicate what the future might hold so that you can make plans and get some idea of what to expect over the years. I apologize for those conditions that could not be included.

The Baby and Child A-Z Medical Handbook is full of illustrations, drawings and photographs. In some chapters, the text is in the form of annotation to the illustrations. This is because one of my goals is to give information in a readily accessible form, almost at a glance. There is, of course, ample opportunity to use the book as a straightforward reference book so you gradually build your knowledge. But more than this, an anxious parent faced with a sick child in the middle of the night needs straight, uncomplicated information and advice; I have tried to arrange this in a way that I would like to see it if I found myself in that situation.

The book reflects my beliefs and I make no apologies for this. For instance, despite ongoing controversy, I hold strong views on the desirability of whooping cough immunization in the first year of an infant's life, and state them clearly. Where such an opinion is given, it is based on controlled research studies, or the lack of them, not on a purely personal basis. Throughout the book, my goal remains the same—to give you enough clear, modern information, backed by your own instincts, to know how to take care of your sick child and, on the other hand, to know when it is essential to seek medical help.

Miriam Stoppard

Note
We use the masculine pronoun "he"
when referring to the baby or child.
This is for convenience and clarity and
does not reflect a preference for
either sex.

How to use this book

When your child is ill, you need to know what to do—whether to call the doctor or whether you can safely treat your child at home yourself. You may also be unsure of what is wrong with him and need help in determining exactly what is wrong.

If your child is ill and you think you know what is wrong

Turn straight to the relevant article in the A-Z of Common Complaints, pages 52 to 262. This is an alphabetical listing of the most common complaints affecting children, from bruises to bronchitis, stings to styes. There, you will find an explanation of the illness, with a list of the symptoms most likely to appear. The circumstances under which you should call the doctor are clearly defined, followed by the probable treatment. There is also advice on what you can do to help your child (both treatment and nursing tips). There are special charts to aid diagnosis for diarrhea, fever and vomiting.

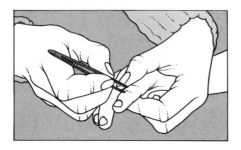

If you're not sure what is wrong

If your child has an obvious symptom, but you aren't sure which A-Z entry to look up, turn to the Visual Diagnosis Guides, pages 43 to 48. Although it is difficult to give a definitive diagnosis from only one or two symptoms, these guides should help point you in the right direction

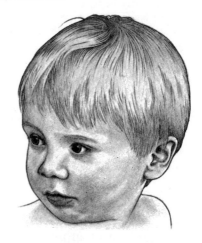

If your child has an accident

If your child has an accident, you must be prepared to deal with it. Where possible, this preparation should involve attending a first-aid course, but you should frequently remind yourself of the basic life-saving techniques by referring to the First-Aid section on pages 281 to 302.

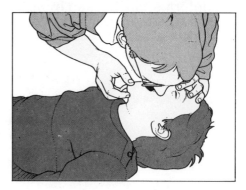

How to use this book

If you are looking after a sick child
The section on pages 24 to 40 gives tips on caring for a sick child and shows, with step-by-step illustrations, how to take a temperature and give medicines. It also provides practical advice on how to reduce fevers and make your child comfortable, how and what to feed him, how to keep him amused and, should the need arise, how to prepare him for a stay in hospital.

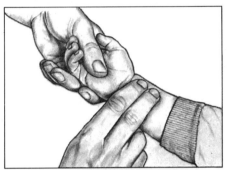

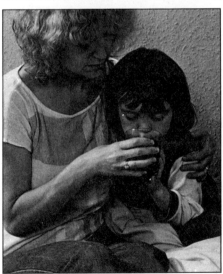

How to prevent accidents
The most sensible precautions for safeguarding your child inside and outside—at home and at play—are shown on pages 264 to 280. Road and safety precautions are also dealt with.

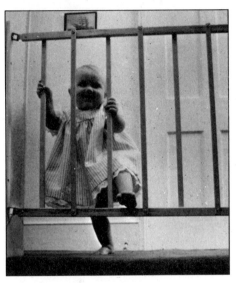

How your child's body works
An illustrated guide to the skeleton, muscles, organs and glands of your child's body is given on pages 12 to 22. This will help you to understand what parts of the body look like, where they are and how they function.

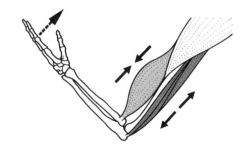

Understanding your child's body

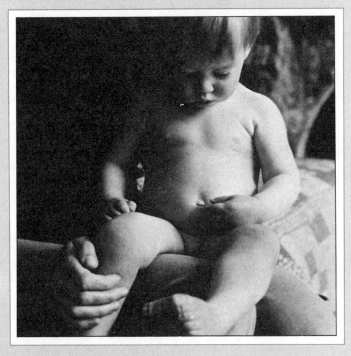

Bones

The body is built on a framework, called the skeleton, of 206 bones. These bones act as levers for muscles to pull against, thus enabling movement, and they surround and protect the vital organs of the head, chest and abdomen.

How bones develop

Bones consist of a central shaft and two shaped ends. In a mature bone, the shaft and ends are hard structures, with a soft inner core of bone marrow (see below). In newborn babies, the bones are mostly made up of a soft, bendy material called *cartilage.* As your child develops, cartilage is gradually converted to bone in a process called *ossification.* In early childhood, the shaft is bone but the ends still consist largely of soft cartilage. By the time your child reaches adolescence, the bone formed in the ends joins the bone in the shaft and growth stops. Throughout childhood, the bones are fairly soft, which is why so-called "greenstick fractures," where the bone bends rather than breaks, can occur (*see page 73*).

What happens when your child grows

Your child grows in height as his bones lengthen. This growth does not take place over the whole length of a bone, but at each end. Growth occurs gradually throughout childhood. At puberty, both girls and boys put on a rapid growth spurt. With girls, this normally begins when they are about age 11 and in boys, at about 12. Girls stop growing when they are about 18; boys continue growing for 1 or 2 years longer, which in part may account for the greater average height in boys.

Joints

The separate bones of the skeleton are connected by joints, and these joints are held together by strong bands of fibrous tissue called *ligaments.* There are several different types of joints—fixed, partly movable and freely movable. *Fixed joints* allow no movement; *partly movable joints* allow slight movement; *freely movable joints* allow movement in several directions. There are two different types— hinge joints and ball-and-socket joints.

How bone is constructed

Each bone consists of a shaft and two ends. When fully developed, the shaft consists largely of hard (compact) bone with a soft central core of bone marrow. Most of the blood cells are made in the bone marrow—particularly in large bones, such as the thigh bone. Ends are made of spongy bone and capped with cartilage to cushion them against the next bone.

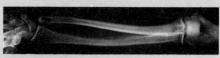

Adult's forearm

Child's forearm

Cross-section of mature bone

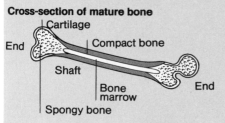

End
Cartilage
Compact bone
Shaft
Bone marrow
Spongy bone
End

Bone development The X-rays above show what happens to bones as they develop. The shape of each bone is present at birth. The bones in the child's arm are made up of areas of cartilage *(not visible on the X-ray) and bone (visible as solid white areas). As a child develops, the cartilage is converted to bone. By adolescence, this conversion is complete, and the bones are solid.*

Bones

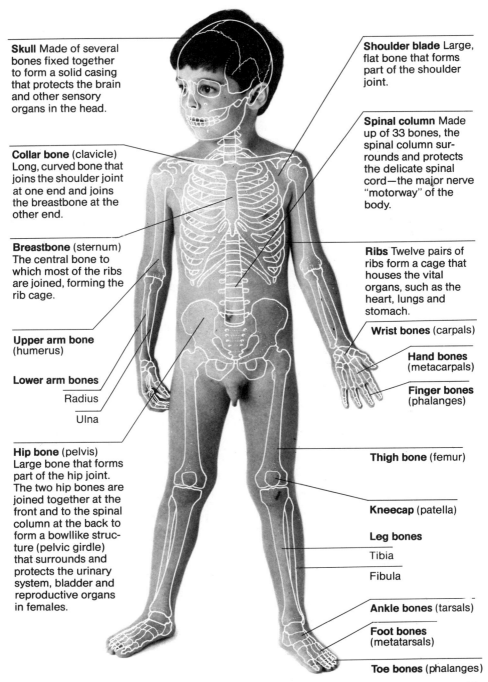

Skull Made of several bones fixed together to form a solid casing that protects the brain and other sensory organs in the head.

Collar bone (clavicle) Long, curved bone that joins the shoulder joint at one end and joins the breastbone at the other end.

Breastbone (sternum) The central bone to which most of the ribs are joined, forming the rib cage.

Upper arm bone (humerus)

Lower arm bones

Radius

Ulna

Hip bone (pelvis) Large bone that forms part of the hip joint. The two hip bones are joined together at the front and to the spinal column at the back to form a bowllike structure (pelvic girdle) that surrounds and protects the urinary system, bladder and reproductive organs in females.

Shoulder blade Large, flat bone that forms part of the shoulder joint.

Spinal column Made up of 33 bones, the spinal column surrounds and protects the delicate spinal cord—the major nerve "motorway" of the body.

Ribs Twelve pairs of ribs form a cage that houses the vital organs, such as the heart, lungs and stomach.

Wrist bones (carpals)

Hand bones (metacarpals)

Finger bones (phalanges)

Thigh bone (femur)

Kneecap (patella)

Leg bones

Tibia

Fibula

Ankle bones (tarsals)

Foot bones (metatarsals)

Toe bones (phalanges)

Muscles

Muscles are made up of long bands of closely interlocking fibers that cause movement by contracting and relaxing. There are two main types of muscle in the body—involuntary and voluntary. *Involuntary muscles* operate all the time without conscious control and include the muscles of the heart and the digestive system. *Voluntary muscles,* also called skeletal muscles, can be consciously controlled, and it is these muscles that cause visible movement of limbs.

Some muscles are designed to relax and contract quickly to make specific movements, such as lifting an arm or kicking a ball, while others, such as the spinal muscles, are designed to remain in contraction for long periods of time. There are over 600 named muscles in the body. Illustrated on the right page are some of the larger or more obvious ones.

How muscles grow

Although your baby can move quite vigorously at birth and all his muscles are present, muscles are not fully developed and will grow in length, breadth and thickness as your baby develops. The three most important factors affecting muscle development are the hormones present in the body, the child's physical activity and diet. Before adolescence, there is little difference in the bulk and strength of boys' and girls' muscles. Any difference is largely due to the tendency of some boys to spend more time on activities that require physical strength. After adolescence, male hormones are important in the development of a boy's greater bulk and strength.

To develop properly, muscles must be used; if they are not used, they will actually decrease in size. A child who is encouraged to be active and pursue physical activities requiring increasing stamina will have larger, stronger and more well-coordinated muscles than a child who is lethargic and gets little exercise. Some children have muscles that show great endurance while other children seem to tire more easily, so let your child set his own limits. Don't expect your child to continue to the point of exhaustion. On the other hand, if he is full of energy, don't try to stop him after other children have given up. Let him be the judge of his own limitations.

How muscles work

Muscles consist of a large central part, called the *belly*, which tapers at each end. The ends are attached to a bone, either directly or by means of a narrow band of fiber called a *tendon*. Most skeletal muscles work in pairs, so as one contracts, the other relaxes. To bend the elbow, the biceps muscle contracts and the triceps muscle relaxes. To straighten it, the triceps contracts and the biceps relaxes.

Muscles used to bend and straighten the elbow

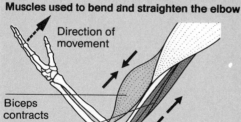

Direction of movement

Biceps contracts

Triceps relaxes

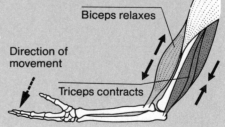

Biceps relaxes

Direction of movement

Triceps contracts

Muscles

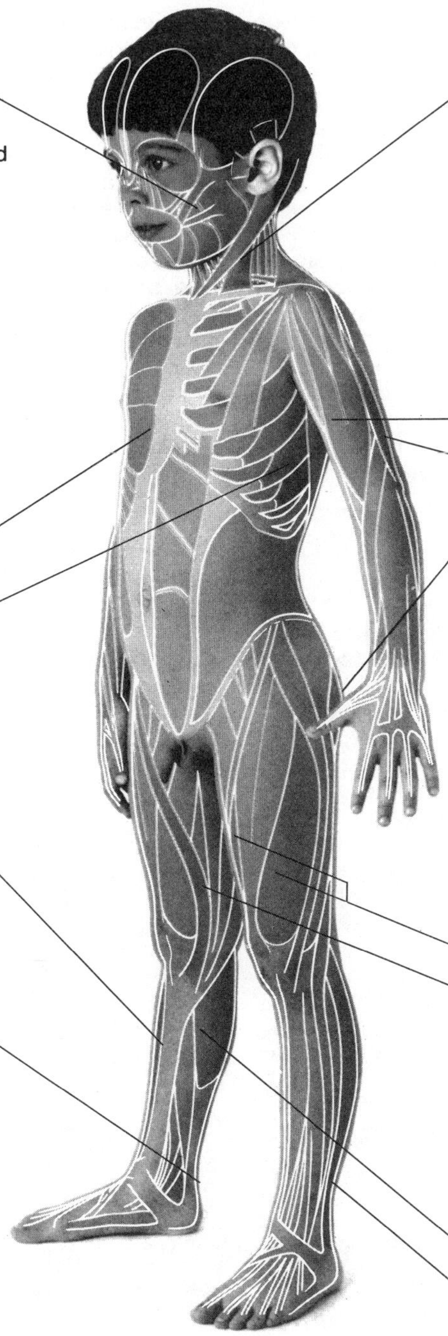

Facial muscles There are 67 different muscles in the face, and each has a different purpose. Fewer are used to smile than to frown.

Chest muscles The large muscle across the top of the chest, the *pectoralis major,* helps to move the shoulder and is involved in deep breathing. The *intercostal muscles* between the ribs also help with breathing.

Pectoralis major

Intercostal muscles

Leg muscle The *tibialis anterior* at the front of the leg assists with walking and running.

Achilles tendon This attaches the calf muscle to the heel bone and is one of the largest tendons in the body.

Neck muscles Some muscles control swallowing; others support the neck and enable the head to turn and nod.

Upper-arm muscles The *biceps* muscle in front bends the elbow; the *triceps* muscle at the back straightens the arm again.

Biceps

Triceps

Buttock muscles The *gluteus maximus* muscle of the buttocks helps with standing and climbing.

Thigh muscles The huge *hamstrings* at the back of the thighs move the hips and knees for kicking and running. The *sartorius* bends the knee, and the *quadriceps* at the front straightens it.

Quadriceps

Sartorius

Calf muscles The *gastrocnemius* and the *soleus* muscles at the back of the calf help with walking, running and standing.

Gastrocnemius

Soleus

15

The head

The brain and the most important sensory organs of the body (the eyes, ears, nose and mouth) are situated in the head. They are surrounded and protected by the skull. The skull is made of several bones that are fused together in older children and adults.

The brain

The brain is a very important, complex structure. It is the main control center of the nervous system—the system comprising the brain, spinal cord and nerves—that controls all bodily functions. The brain receives information from the outside world through the various sensory organs, including the skin, and acts on this information by sending out instruc-

tions to different parts of the body. Some parts of the body receive their instructions from nerves directly connected to the brain. Others, such as arms and legs, receive their messages via nerves branching off the spinal cord.

The brain is divided into three main parts—the *cerebral hemispheres*, the *cerebellum* and the *brain stem*. Each part controls a different body function. The brain is protected by three membranes called the *meninges*; the brain is cushioned by fluid called *cerebrospinal fluid*. This fluid, which is produced in the center of the brain, flows between the two inner membranes and surrounds the spinal cord.

Teeth

Your child's first teeth, called *baby teeth*, may begin to appear when he is about 6 or 7 months old. The full set of 20 teeth should have come through by the time your child is about 3 years old. Permanent adult teeth begin to appear when your child is about 6, but the full set of 32 teeth will not be complete until he is about 17. The first permanent teeth to come through are the first molars. Baby teeth become loose and fall out one at a time and are normally replaced immediately by permanent teeth.

Sometimes, a permanent tooth begins to come through *before* the baby tooth has fallen out. This can cause pain, and the dentist may have to extract the baby tooth.

Permanent teeth
Age of appearance

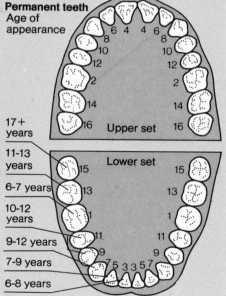

17+ years
11-13 years
6-7 years
10-12 years
9-12 years
7-9 years
6-8 years

Upper set
Lower set

Baby teeth
Age of appearance

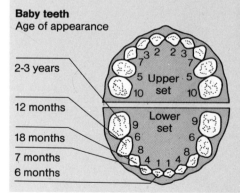

2-3 years
12 months
18 months
7 months
6 months

Upper set
Lower set

The head

Areas of control

Certain areas of the brain are responsible for controlling specific bodily functions. For example, the *occipital lobe* is for vision and *motor cortex* is for voluntary movement. Memory cannot be localized in the same way, but is thought to be dealt with by the cerebral hemispheres as a whole.

Motor cortex This part of the brain is concerned with initiating movement. Different areas are responsible for each part of the body, as follows: **A** toes, feet and legs; **B** thighs, abdomen and trunk; **C** shoulders and arms; **D** head, eyelids and cheeks; **E** jaws and lips.

Frontal lobes Emotions are controlled in this part of the brain.

Speech center Speech is controlled in a small area of the frontal lobe. If your child is right-handed, the speech center is in the left cerebral hemisphere, as shown here, and vice versa, if he is left-handed.

Sensory cortex All the sensations felt by the body are received and interpreted in this area.

Parietal lobe Involved with understanding speech, this area works with the occipital lobe to work out the size and shape of objects and to read.

Occipital lobe Vision is controlled in this part of the brain.

Temporal lobe Area responsible for controlling hearing.

Cerebellum Mainly concerned with balance and coordination of muscles and joints.

Brain stem This controls the involuntary functions of the body, such as heartbeat, breathing rate and temperature regulation.

Left cerebral hemisphere

Right cerebral hemisphere

Inside the brain

This cross section of the brain shows the right cerebral hemisphere. It is joined to the left by a band of tissue called the *corpus callosum*. Each cerebral hemisphere is made of two types of tissue: gray matter and white matter. Gray matter consists of the nerve cells, and white matter consists of the nerve fibers. The *hypothalamus* is situated at the base of the brain and controls sleep and appetite. Under the central part of the brain is the pituitary gland that controls growth and development and ensures all the hormone-producing glands (*see page 21*) are functioning properly.

Cross-section of the brain

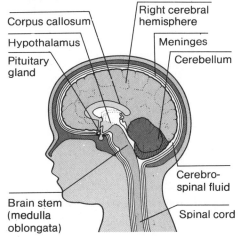

Corpus callosum

Hypothalamus

Pituitary gland

Right cerebral hemisphere

Meninges

Cerebellum

Cerebrospinal fluid

Brain stem (medulla oblongata)

Spinal cord

The head

The sense organs

The most important sense organs of the body (nose, mouth, eyes and ears) are situated in the head. Between them, they give us a great deal of information about the outside world.

The nose and mouth

The nose is the organ of smell and forms the main entrance to the respiratory system. Air is breathed in through the nose and passes down into the lungs through the windpipe (*trachea*). The nose is lined with a hair-covered membrane that filters, moistens and warms air as it is taken into the body. The nose is also linked to the sinuses, which is why nasal infections can pass into the sinuses.

The mouth forms the entrance to the digestive system (*see page 21*); it is also involved (with tongue, lips and larynx) in speech. The tongue is the organ of taste—different areas of the tongue distinguish the main types of flavor: salty, sweet, bitter and sour.

Cross section of the nose and mouth

Sinuses Hollow, air-filled tubes that make the skull light in weight and give the voice resonance.

Frontal sinuses

Sphenoidal sinus

Maxillary sinus (dotted line)

Nasal passage Main passage through which air is taken into the body.

Palate Roof of the mouth.

Teeth

Gums

Tongue Major organ of taste. It also moves food around the mouth during chewing and swallowing.

Epiglottis

Throat Area between the back of the mouth and the windpipe, made up of the *pharynx* and *larynx*.

Windpipe (trăchea) Tube that carries air to the lungs.

Olfactory bulb (in brain)

Olfactory nerves Nerves that detect smells and carry the information to the brain.

Pharynx

Larynx

Gullet (esophagus) Tube that carries food to the stomach.

The head

The eye

The eye works by focusing rays of light through a lens onto a sensitive layer in the back of the eye called the *retina*. The information is then sent to the brain through the optic nerve to be interpreted.

Each eye sees an object from a different angle. The brain coordinates the image picked up by each eye so a solid, three dimensional object is seen. The eye is held in place by six muscles, which allow it to swivel in many directions.

Cross section of the eye

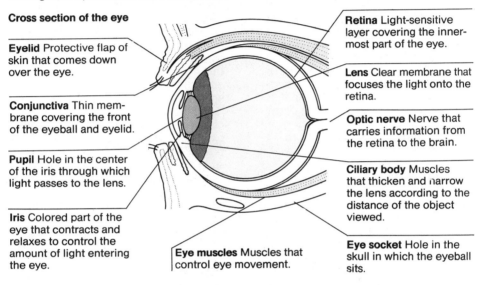

Eyelid Protective flap of skin that comes down over the eye.

Conjunctiva Thin membrane covering the front of the eyeball and eyelid.

Pupil Hole in the center of the iris through which light passes to the lens.

Iris Colored part of the eye that contracts and relaxes to control the amount of light entering the eye.

Eye muscles Muscles that control eye movement.

Retina Light-sensitive layer covering the inner-most part of the eye.

Lens Clear membrane that focuses the light onto the retina.

Optic nerve Nerve that carries information from the retina to the brain.

Ciliary body Muscles that thicken and narrow the lens according to the distance of the object viewed.

Eye socket Hole in the skull in which the eyeball sits.

The ear

The ear is an important organ for hearing and for balance. The ear consists of three parts—the outer, middle and inner ear. The part of the ear you see is the outer ear. All three sections of the ear are involved with hearing. Balance is controlled in the inner ear alone.

Cross section of the ear

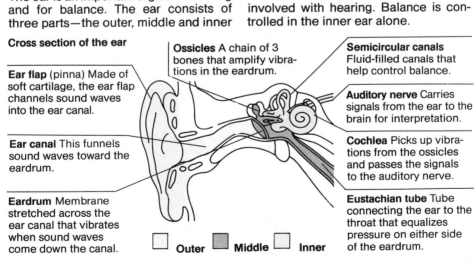

Ear flap (pinna) Made of soft cartilage, the ear flap channels sound waves into the ear canal.

Ear canal This funnels sound waves toward the eardrum.

Eardrum Membrane stretched across the ear canal that vibrates when sound waves come down the canal.

Ossicles A chain of 3 bones that amplify vibrations in the eardrum.

Semicircular canals Fluid-filled canals that help control balance.

Auditory nerve Carries signals from the ear to the brain for interpretation.

Cochlea Picks up vibrations from the ossicles and passes the signals to the auditory nerve.

Eustachian tube Tube connecting the ear to the throat that equalizes pressure on either side of the eardrum.

☐ **Outer** ◼ **Middle** ☐ **Inner**

19

Organs and glands

Housed in the center of the body cavity are the organs that deal with digestion, breathing and blood circulation. The glands produce hormones, which control the functioning of the organs and growth and development.

Glands that swell

The glands that swell during an illness are not glands in the true sense because they do not secrete hormones. They are *lymph nodes*, part of the lymphatic system that is responsible for helping the body to fight infection. When infection occurs, more white cells are produced throughout the body and sent to the lymph nodes nearest the area of infection so germs can be destroyed. This causes the lymph nodes to swell, and they may be slightly tender. Lymph nodes are situated all over the body. Those in the neck are most commonly activated by infection, but the other main sites are the armpit and groin.

Glands behind the ear These glands swell if your child has an ear infection.

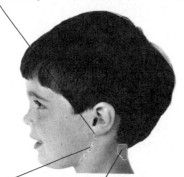

Glands below the ear and the jaw These are the glands most commonly affected by tonsillitis.

Glands in the back of the neck These swell if, for example, your child has German measles.

Circulatory system

The blood is the body's main transportation system. It carries oxygen from the lungs and nourishment from digested food around the body. It carries waste matter, such as carbon dioxide, away from the body cells. Blood loaded with oxygen comes from the lungs into the left side of the heart. The heart pumps this blood into the main artery, the *aorta*. This subdivides into smaller arteries, ending in thin-walled capillaries in the body cells. It is in the capillaries that the nourishment and oxygen carried by the blood are passed into the cells. Waste matter, such as carbon dioxide, is picked up. The capillaries then join to form veins. The veins join to form larger veins, finally forming two veins, the *superior vena cava* and *inferior vena cava*, which carry blood back into the right side of the heart. From here, the blood is pumped up into the lungs, where the carbon dioxide is exchanged for oxygen, then carried back into the left side of the heart.

Organs and glands

Thyroid gland Regulates the general rate of growth and development of the body.

Esophagus (gullet) Passage that carries food and drink from the mouth to the stomach.

Heart Muscular organ that pumps blood around the body at regular intervals.

Stomach Muscular organ where food is broken down by digestive juices.

Pancreas Produces digestive juices for use in the breakdown of food in the intestine. It also produces the hormone insulin, which regulates the amount of sugar in the blood.

Liver Gland that secretes bile and regulates blood chemistry.

Small intestine Long, narrow tube, up to 22 feet long in an adult, in which digestion of food is completed. Nearly all the nutrients are absorbed there.

Appendix Narrow, wormlike protrusion near the junction of the small and large intestine. Its purpose is unknown.

Rectum Organ where feces are stored before being expelled from the body.

Pituitary gland This controls the body's growth and development and ensures all the hormone-producing glands (the endocrine system) function properly.

Windpipe (trachea) Passage that carries air from the nose and mouth to the lungs.

Lungs Two organs (one slightly larger than the other) that expand to take air into the body and relax to push used air out.

Diaphragm A large dome-shaped sheet of muscle that separates the organs of the chest and the abdomen. It moves up and down to help breathing in conjunction with the intercostal muscles.

Spleen Destroys worn-out red blood cells and recycles iron from them.

Adrenal gland

Kidney

Large intestine Wider and much shorter than the small intestine, water and undigested food pass into it from the small intestine. The water is reabsorbed, but the undigested waste products pass on to the rectum as feces.

21

Organs and glands

Organs of the lower abdomen

These include the two kidneys, the bladder (with the ureters and urethra they comprise the urinary system) and the reproductive organs.

Male reproductive system

The male sex glands, the *testes* (testicles), are situated on the outside of the body in the scrotal sac. They produce sperm and testosterone, the hormone that controls the development of the sex organs and the secondary sexual characteristics, such as broad shoulders and muscular arms and legs.

From puberty on, all the organs of the reproductive system enlarge. The testes then begin to manufacture sperm, first in small quantities, then in increasingly larger amounts.

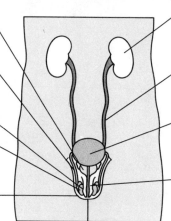

Prostate Small gland at the base of the bladder.

Vas deferens Tube connecting the penis and the testis along which sperm pass.

Penis Male sex organ.

Testes Glands where sperm are manufactured; they also produce the male sex hormones.

Scrotal sac Pouch that surrounds the testes.

Kidneys Two organs that filter the blood, removing any waste products from it. They also make urine.

Ureters Tubes connecting the kidneys and the bladder. There is one for each kidney.

Bladder Expandable bag in which liquid waste (urine) is stored before being excreted.

Urethra Passage that carries urine and fluid containing sperm (seminal fluid) out of the body.

Female reproductive system

At birth, the uterus is extremely small, and it does not begin to grow until puberty. However, ovaries already contain all the eggs that will ever be produced and released during a girl's fertile life. Female sex hormones, estrogen and progesterone, are manufactured by the ovaries. At puberty, their production begins to follow a monthly pattern, which stimulates the beginning of the menstrual cycle.

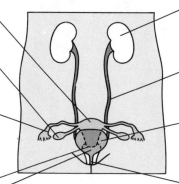

Uterus (womb) Organ in which a developing fetus is carried.

Ovaries The organs where the female sex hormones are produced and the eggs are stored.

Fallopian tubes Tubes linking the uterus and ovaries. These are the tubes into which the egg is released during the menstrual cycle.

Cervix Entrance to uterus.

Kidneys Two organs that filter the blood, removing any waste products from it. They also make urine.

Ureters Tubes connecting the kidneys and the bladder. There is one for each kidney.

Bladder Expandable bag in which liquid waste (urine) is stored before being excreted.

Vagina Female genital passage leading to the cervix.

Urethra Tube that carries urine out of the body.

Caring for
a sick child

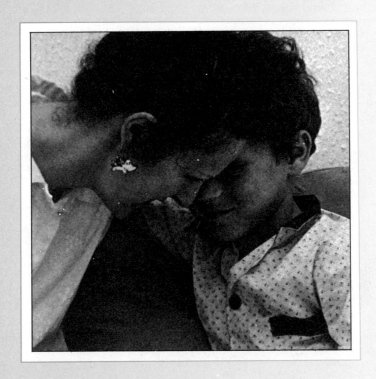

Calling the doctor

Most parents know instinctively when their child is getting sick; the child may not be as active as usual; he may refuse his food; he may become clingy. However, you are not always able to diagnose exactly what is wrong nor are you necessarily able to tell whether the child's symptoms are serious or potentially serious. An ill child is always distressing, and the situation can be made even more tense if you cannot decide whether or not to call the doctor.

There are some circumstances, after a serious injury, for example, when medical help *must* be sought immediately. For most parents, these situations are obvious. But there are many more situations where the seriousness isn't as clear cut. This is where the worry comes in. "Are my child's symptoms normal, or are they potentially serious?" Most doctors do not mind if you seek their advice, even if it's just for reassurance. Always follow your instincts and, if you are ever in doubt, call your doctor.

If your child is already undergoing treatment from your doctor and you are worried about his progress, call your doctor again. Don't take your child to an emergency room unless it is a true emergency. The doctor in the emergency room will not be able to change your child's treatment without consulting your own doctor first.

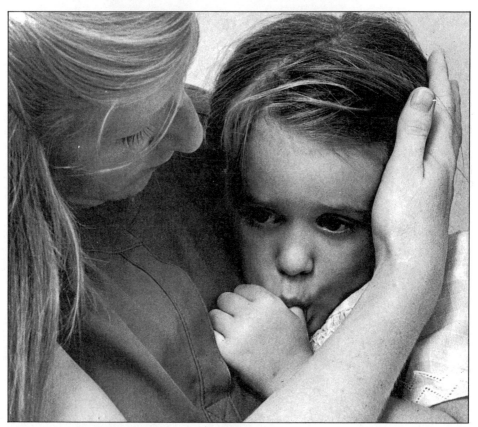

You will almost certainly know when your child is getting ill.

Calling the doctor

When to call your doctor

Listed below are the circumstances under which you should *always* call your doctor. For further information *see pages 52 to 262.* The following are important signs, so never ignore them.

Temperature
● A raised temperature of over 102F (38.6C).
● A raised temperature of over 100F (37.5C), plus any other obvious signs of illness.
● A raised temperature accompanied by a convulsion or a raised temperature if your child has had convulsions in the past.
● A raised temperature accompanied by a stiff neck and headache.
● A temperature below 95F (35C).
● A temperature that drops, then rises again suddenly.
● A temperature of more than 100F (37.5C), for more than 3 days.

Diarrhea
● If your baby is under 6 months old.
● If diarrhea is accompanied by pain in the abdomen, a temperature or any other obvious signs of illness.

Vomiting
● If your baby is under 6 months old.
● Prolonged, violent vomiting.
● Dizzy spells, nausea and headaches.
● If your child vomits or feels sick and has a pain in the right side of his abdomen.

Loss of appetite
● If your baby stops eating suddenly or is less than 6 months old and doesn't seem to be thriving.
● If your child usually has a good appetite, but refuses food for a day and seems listless.

Pain and discomfort
● If your child feels sick and dizzy and has headaches.
● If your child complains of blurred vision, especially if he's recently had a bump on the head.
● If your child has severe pains that occur at regular intervals.
● If your child has a pain in the right side of his abdomen and feels sick.

Breathing
● If your child's breathing is labored, and his ribs are being sharply drawn in with each breath.
● If the breathing is noisy.

Emergencies

Call the paramedics or take your child to the nearest emergency room if you notice *any* of the following:
● Your child has stopped breathing (*see page 283*).
● Your child is breathing with difficulty, and his lips are turning blue.
● Your child is unconscious (*see page 291*).
● Your child has a deep wound that has resulted in a serious loss of blood (*see page 292*)
● Your child has a serious burn (*see page 296*).
● Your child has a suspected broken bone (*see page 73*).
● Your child has chemicals in his eyes (*see page 133*).
● Your child's ear or eye has been pierced (*see pages 123 and 135*).
● Your child has been bitten by an animal or snake (*see pages 65 and 221*).
● Your child has eaten a poisonous substance (*see page 299*).

Calling the doctor

What to tell your doctor

Your doctor will need to know the answers to specific questions to help him make a diagnosis and to gauge the severity of the illness or injury. The doctor needs as much information as possible. If necessary, write down everything that you think might be helpful on a piece of paper, and have it with you when you are speaking to the doctor so you do not forget anything. He will probably need to know the following from you:

● Your child's age.
● Whether your child has a temperature. If so, what it is; how long he has had it; have there been any fluctuations and, if so, what they were.
● If your child has a fever, did it come on quickly?

● Are your child's neck glands swollen?
● Has your child vomited?
● Has your child had diarrhea?
● Has your child complained of any kind of pain and, if so, where is the pain?
● Has your child suffered from dizziness or blurred vision (particularly if he's recently had a bump on the head)?
● Has your child had a convulsion? If so, how long did it last?
● Has your child lost consciousness?
● Did your child eat the last meal offered and has he eaten within the past 3 hours?

What to expect from your doctor

There are certain things you should expect your doctor to do. Make sure he answers all your questions fully.

Your doctor should give your child a

Taking your child's pulse

The pulse is the wave of pressure that passes along each artery every time the heart beats. You can feel the pulse wherever an artery lies close to the skin. The most common site for taking the pulse is at the wrist (radial pulse). The pulse can also be taken in the neck (carotid pulse), although this is normally done if you suspect that the heart has stopped beating altogether (*see page 288*).

The pulse rate varies with age. It is normally faster after exercise and slower after resting. A young baby's heart will beat about 160 times a minute; by the time he is age 1, it will beat about 100 to 120 times a minute. By the time he is 7 or 8 years, it will have slowed down to the adult rate of 80 to 90 beats a minute. A normal pulse is regular and strong; any abnormality, such as a fast, weak pulse or a slow pulse, may indicate your child is ill.

If your child is under 1, it is generally easier to place your hand on his chest and count the actual heartbeats rather

than trying to find one of his arteries because babies are generally quite chubby.

Taking the radial pulse

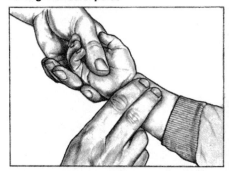

1 Support your child's wrist with your thumb, and place 3 fingers in the hollow below the palm of his hand on the thumb side just below the wrist creases.

2 Count the number of beats you can feel in 15 seconds and multiply this figure by 4 to get the number of beats in a minute.

Calling the doctor

thorough examination. If your child has an earache, the doctor should examine his ears. If he has abdominal pain, your doctor should examine his abdomen without his clothes on. If he has a sore throat and a cough, your doctor should listen to his chest, check his ears and examine his throat and feel his neck glands. You should not accept a prescription for your child without an examination first.

Below is a list of things you should expect your doctor to do or tell you or that you should remember to ask him.

Expect your doctor to
● Examine your child thoroughly.
● Give you an honest opinion of what is wrong. If your doctor does not know what is wrong, you should expect him to tell you what further investigations are necessary to obtain a clear diagnosis.
● Tell you the implications of the illness or condition. If, for example, your child has an acute attack of sinusitis or a middle-ear infection, your doctor should tell you your child may need antibiotics to eradicate it completely.
● Not give you medicine if he is sure there is nothing wrong. He would be wrong to give you something simply because you have gone into the office expecting to be treated. Respect him for not being pressured into giving you a prescription.
● Answer all your questions—be persistent until you are completely satisfied.
● Give you as much information as possible about the medicines prescribed for your child—whether to give them before or after a meal, whether there are any side effects and whether there are any special precautions to take.
● Warn you about possible complications and danger signs to look out for.

Things to ask your doctor
● If your child has a recurrent condition, such as cold sores or boils, ask your

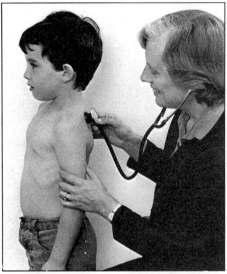

Your doctor will give your child a thorough examination.

doctor what you can do if you notice the symptoms recurring.
● Ask your doctor for home-nursing tips.
● If your child has a chronic condition, ask your doctor if there is anything you can do yourself at home to help the condition. For example, if your child has infantile eczema, there's quite a lot you can do, such as add oil to the bath water, use special soap, gently rub in moisturizing ointments and creams, even when the skin is clear.
● If your child has an infectious disease, ask your doctor about the incubation period (for the benefit of your friends whose children have come in contact with your child), the length of time your child will be infectious and how long he will have to stay out of school.

27

Temperature

In children, normal body temperature ranges from 96.8F (36C) to 100.4F (38C). Any temperature over 100F (37.5C), taken orally or 100.4F (38C), taken rectally, is classed as a fever. Hypothermia develops if the temperature falls below 95F (35C). Body temperature varies according to how active your child has been and the time of day. It is lowest in the morning because there is little muscle activity during sleep and highest in the late afternoon after a day's activity. It will also be high after your child has been running around.

An abnormally hot forehead may be the first indication your child has a temperature. To be accurate, you must take your child's temperature with a thermometer (*see opposite* and *page 30*). The temperature control center in the brain is primitive in young children, and a temperature can shoot up more rapidly than in adults. When a fever is present, take your child's temperature again after 20 minutes, just in case it was only a transitory rise. Never regard a high temperature as an accurate reflection of your child's health; it is only one sign of illness. A child can be very ill without a temperature or quite healthy with one.

Thermometers

There are two main types of thermometer: mercury thermometers and liquid-crystal (forehead) thermometers. Mercury thermometers are the most accurate means of assessing a temperature. Made of glass, with a hollow tube running up the center, they register temperature when the mercury expands and moves up the tube to a point on the scale. Try to buy one with a short reading time so your child does not have a chance to get fidgety. It is also useful to have a low-reading thermometer because babies and young children lose heat quickly, and this can be dangerous (*see page 300*). With babies up to 1½ years, use a rectal thermometer. After that age, he'll tolerate his temperature being taken under his armpit. By the time your child

---

Types of thermometers

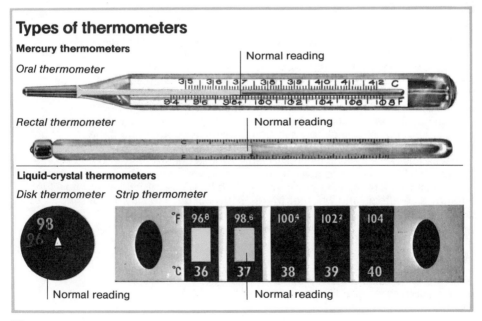

Mercury thermometers

Oral thermometer

Normal reading

Rectal thermometer

Normal reading

Liquid-crystal thermometers

Disk thermometer   *Strip thermometer*

Normal reading

Normal reading

Temperature

is 6 or 7, you can probably take his temperature orally, as long as you are sure you can trust him not to bite the thermometer.

Liquid-crystal thermometers are plastic thermometers with a heat sensitive panel on one side and numbers or panels on the other side. When the sensitive side is placed on the forehead, the numbers or panels light up. They are not as accurate as mercury thermometers, but they are quick, safe and easy to use.

Reading thermometers

The temperature registered on a liquid-crystal thermometer is the number or panel that remains lit up. Mercury thermometers are more difficult to read. Hold the thermometer between your finger and thumb, and turn it until you can see a thick silver line. The actual body temperature is the point on the scale reached by the mercury.

Tips for taking your child's temperature

- Never take your child's temperature if he has been running around.
- Never leave your child alone with a thermometer in his mouth.
- If there is an accident and the thermometer breaks in your child's mouth, remove the pieces of glass quickly and carefully. The mercury is unlikely to spill from its tube. If it does, tell your child to spit out as much as he can, then mop up the rest with a dry tissue.
- Make sure there is no break in the mercury inside the thermometer— if there is, the reading will not be accurate.
- If your thermometer is cracked, throw it away immediately.
- Wash the thermometer after use with soap and cold water or alcohol.
- Always store the thermometer in its own case.

Using forehead thermometers

There are several different types of forehead thermometer, but they all work on the same principle. The two main types are shown below. Always read the manufacturer's instructions carefully before you begin.

Using the disk

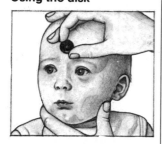

Place the disk in the center of your child's forehead. Leave it for 15 seconds. Numbers will light up in sequence before coming to rest at the reading for your child's temperature.

Using the strip

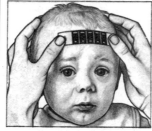

1 Hold the strip against your child's forehead with both hands, keeping your fingers clear of the numbered panels. Make sure the strip is flat against your child's forehead.

2 Leave it for about 15 seconds. Numbers and colored panels will light up in sequence, as at left, before coming to rest at the reading for your child's temperature.

Temperature

Using a mercury thermometer

Whether you are using a rectal or an oral thermometer, hold it by the top end, and shake it down sharply until the mercury falls below the 95F (35C) mark. Always wash the thermometer in cold water or alcohol after use. Never wash it with hot water because it can crack the glass.

Using a rectal thermometer

1 Lubricate the bulb of the thermometer with baby cream or oil.

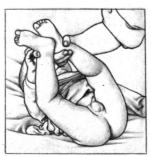

2 Lay your baby on his back, and remove his diaper. Grasp his heels, keeping your fingers between his ankles so they do not rub together. Lift up his legs or lay him face down across your lap, and place one hand over his back to keep him from wiggling.

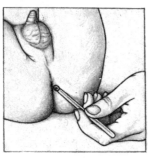

3 Gently insert the thermometer into his rectum about 1 inch, and hold it in place.

4 Leave the thermometer in place for 2 minutes (or according to manufacturer's instructions), then remove and read.

Using an oral thermometer

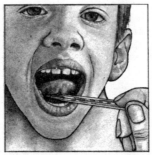

1 Ask your child to open his mouth and raise his tongue. Place the thermometer under his tongue.

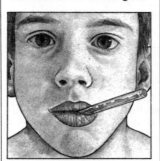

2 Ask your child to place the tip of his tongue firmly behind his lower front teeth—this will hold the thermometer in place. Then ask him to close his lips—but not his teeth—over the thermometer so the seal is airtight. Make sure he is not gripping the thermometer with his teeth.

3 Leave the thermometer in your child's mouth for 2 minutes (or according to the manufacturer's instructions), then remove and read.

Armpit method

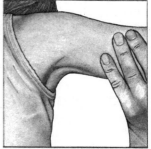

1 Sit with your child on your lap, facing away from you. With the thermometer in your right hand, raise your child's arm to expose the armpit.

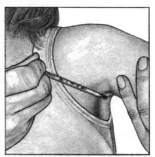

2 Place the thermometer into the armpit, and lower your child's arm over it. Hold the arm down for 2 minutes (or according to manufacturer's instructions), then remove and read.
Note: The temperature reading when taken in the child's armpit will be about 1F (0.6C) lower than the child's actual body temperature.

Temperature

Treating a raised temperature

The raised temperature that accompanies an illness is the body's way of responding to infection. It is a sign the body is marshalling its defenses (*see page 139*). This is a good sign. If your child has a high temperature, he will be uncomfortable and irritable. A temperature, particularly in young children, can lead to convulsions (*see page 96*).

Removing bedclothes

Remove your child's clothes and any blankets so that his body cools down by radiation. Leave him covered with only a sheet. If his temperature rises over 102F (38.6C), he may be more comfortable left uncovered but wearing a short-sleeved cotton T-shirt and underpants or a diaper.

Medicines

The most efficient way of reducing your child's fever is to give him medicine. The most effective medicines for reducing a fever are acetaminophen or aspirin, but some children suffer from side-effects from aspirin. It is a stomach irritant and can cause vomiting. In addition, aspirin should never be given to children with influenza or chickenpox because of the danger of Reye's syndrome (*see page 208*).

Acetaminophen is as good as aspirin and has fewer side effects, so it's probably the best choice with children. It also has the advantage that it is available in liquid or chewable tablets, so it is much easier to give to young children.

Whether you are using acetaminophen or aspirin, it is very important not to give your child more than the recommended dose—but don't give him less either. Do not give medication to your child for longer than 2 days without consulting your doctor.

Tepid sponging

If your child's temperature is over 104F (40C) for longer than ½ hour, and removing his bedclothes hasn't helped, try tepid sponging. Always use tepid water, never cold. Tepid water causes the blood vessels in the skin to dilate, aiding heat loss. Cold water causes the blood vessels to contract and retain heat. *Never* use alcohol.

1 Half fill a bucket with water that is comfortable to your elbow or the inside of your wrist. Put several clean face cloths or sponges in it. Place dry towels around your child so the bed doesn't get wet.

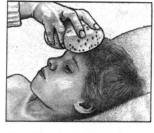

2 Wring one of the cloths or sponges out slightly so it is still dripping. Starting from the head, and using brisk gentle strokes, sponge the entire body. Change the sponge when it feels warm.

3 Take your child's temperature after awhile. If it has dropped to 100F (37.5C), stop sponging. If his temperature has not dropped, keep sponging. Stop when the temperature has dropped.

4 Cover him with a cotton sheet, and watch him carefully. Be careful not to let him get too cold. Repeat tepid sponging if his temperature rises again.

Medicines

When you take your child to the doctor, he may prescribe some form of medicine for your child. Ask your doctor to give you as much information as possible about the medicine. Ask if there are likely to be any side effects or whether there are foods that should be avoided or special precautions to take while your child is taking the medication (*see page 27*).

Most medicines for young children are in a sweetened syrup form to make them more palatable. They can be given with a spoon tube or dropper. Droppers and tubes are often more suitable for babies who haven't learned to swallow from a spoon. Some medicines for older children come in tablet or capsule forms.

On most occasions, your child will be cooperative, but nearly everyone has been faced with the situation of trying to give medicine to a child who refuses to take it. It is very important that your child takes any medicine prescribed when he is ill. This is one occasion when blackmail is justified. Be firm but never harsh, cruel or threatening, and never punish your child for being difficult about taking medicine. Very occasionally, a child will resist physically; in this case, there is no alternative but to be forceful and to hold your child down.

Giving medicine to a baby or young child

It can be difficult to administer medicine to babies because they wiggle. You will need to enlist the help of another adult or older brother or sister. Position your baby so that he is slightly raised—never have your baby lying flat while giving him medicine because he may inhale the medicine into his lungs.

Using a spoon

1 Hold your baby in the crook of your arm. Gently open his mouth by pulling down his chin. If necessary, get someone to do this while you hold him.

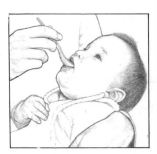

2 Place the tip of the spoon on his lower lip. Raise the angle of the spoon, and let the medicine run into his mouth.

Using a dropper

1 Hold your baby as described at left, and put the specified amount of medicine into the glass tube.

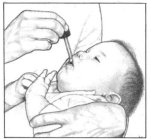

2 Place the dropper in the corner of your baby's mouth, and release the medicine gently.

Using a spoon tube
Pour the required dose into the tube. Hold your baby as described at left. Place the mouthpiece on his lower lip, and let the medicine run into his mouth.

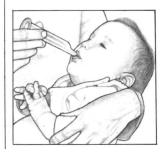

Using your finger
If your baby will not take his medicine from a spoon or a dropper, measure the required dose into a container. Dip your little finger into it, then let your baby suck it off your finger.

Medicines

Giving medicine and tablets to older children

Children do not usually mind medicine too much and often want to pour medicine out for themselves rather than let you give it to them. Below are a few tips that may help if your child is difficult. For example, tablets can be crushed and mixed with jam. Medicines can sometimes be mixed with a favorite drink. Capsules, however, should not be broken unless your pharmacist says it's all right.

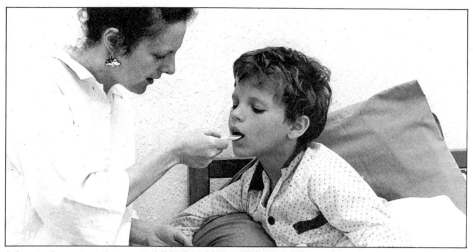

It is very important that your child takes his medicine exactly as prescribed.

Tips for giving medicine

Giving medicine to babies

● Get someone else to help.
● If you are on your own, wrap a blanket around your baby's arms so you can stop him struggling and hold him steady.
● Only put a little of the medicine in his mouth at a time.
● If your baby spits the medicine out, get the other person to hold his mouth open while you pour the medicine into the back of his mouth. Gently, but firmly, close his mouth.

Giving medicine to older children

● Suggest your child holds his nose while taking the medicine, so he doesn't taste it.
● Don't forcibly hold your child's nose because he may inhale some of the medicine.
● Mix liquid medicine with another syrup.
● Don't add liquid medicine to a drink because it will sink to the bottom of the glass. You won't be sure your child has had the whole dose.
● Show your child you have his favorite drink ready to wash the taste of the medicine away. Do this even if you would not normally allow your child to have it very often.
● Help your child brush his teeth after taking any liquid medicine to prevent syrup sticking to his teeth.
● Crush tablets between two spoons, and mix the powder with jam or ice cream.

Medicines

Giving drops

Ear, nose or eye infections are generally treated with external drops. It is always easier to administer drops to a baby or young child if you lay him on a flat surface before you begin. Enlist the help of another adult or an older child to keep him still and hold his head steady. An older child will probably be more co-operative; you only need to ask him to tilt his head.

Ear drops	Nose drops	Eye drops

Ear drops

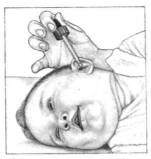

1 Lay your baby on his side with the affected ear up. Let the drops fall into the center of his ear.

2 Hold your baby steady until the drops have run into the canal.

Nose drops

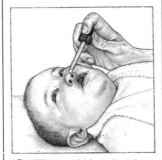

1 Tilt your baby's head back slightly. Gently drop liquid into each nostril.

2 Count the number of drops as you put them in. Two or 3 drops at a time are normally sufficient. Any more will run down his throat and cause him to cough and splutter.

Eye drops

1 Get someone to hold your baby still and tilt his head slightly so his affected eye is lowest. This way, no drops can run from the affected eye to the other eye.

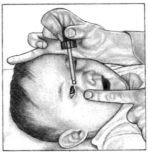

2 Very gently pull his lower eyelid down, and let the drops fall between his eye and his lower lid.

Tips for giving drops

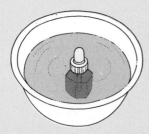

● Warm nose drops and ear drops slightly by standing them in warm, *not hot,* water for a few minutes. Your child won't be shocked when they drop into his nose or ear.

● Do not let the dropper touch your child's nose, ear or eye, or you will transfer the germs back to the bottle. If the dropper does touch your child, wash it thoroughly before putting it back in the bottle.

● Over-the-counter drops should *not* be used for longer than 3 days without consulting a doctor. They can cause worse irritation and inflammation than the condition you were treating in the first place.

Medicines

Medicine chest

Always keep some medicines in the house in case of emergency in the middle of the night when you may not be able to get to a drugstore easily. Keep them somewhere obvious so you can find them quickly when you need them. Never mix pills in the same containers, and never keep unused prescription medicines. Keep all medicine out of reach of children.

You should also have a first-aid kit. Keep all the equipment in a clean, dry, airtight box. Put it somewhere it can be found in an emergency.

Medicines to avoid

The following items, commonly given as useful, should be avoided:
● Any over-the-counter product containing local anesthetic because they can cause allergies. They are generally found in creams for insect stings.
● Any skin creams containing antihistamines—unless prescribed by your doctor. They can cause skin allergies.
● Over-the-counter products containing aspirin.
● Mouth washes, gargles, eye, nose and ear drops unless your doctor has specifically recommended them.

Medicine chest
1 Mercury thermometer—keep 2 in case one breaks.
2 Forehead thermometer.
3 Baby aspirin.
4 Acetaminophen.
5 Calamine lotion for soothing skin irritations, sunburn and stings.
6 Syrup of ipecac to make your child vomit in case of non-corrosive poisoning (*see page 299*).

First-aid kit
7 Box of Band-aids.
8 Wound dressings—large dressings that consist of a gauze pad attached to a bandage.
9 Packet of skin closures.
10 Cotton.
11 Mild antiseptic cream.
12 Gauze dressings.

13 Surgical tape.
14 Elastic bandages for supporting sprains and strains.
15 Open-weave bandages.
16 Triangular bandage.
17 Blunt-ended tweezers, safety pins and scissors.

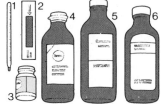
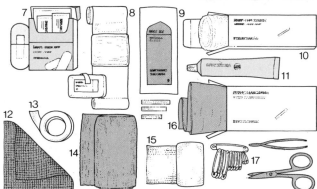

Useful household items

● Packages of frozen peas or ice cubes in plastic bags for cold compresses.
● Newspaper—when folded this makes an excellent splint.
● Elastic belt for supporting a strain or sprain.

● Baking soda—this can be added to your child's bath to relieve itching.
● Salt—this can be added to your child's bath to cleanse wounds.
● Vinegar—mixed with water, it can be used to soothe jellyfish stings.

Nursing a sick child

Few parents escape being called upon to look after a sick child—all children fall ill at some time. Babies often become very clingy when they are ill and may cry more than normal because they do not understand what is happening to them. If a baby is breast-fed, he will probably want to be fed more often, as much for the comfort of being near you as anything else. Bottle-fed babies will also want to be cuddled and will want smaller feedings more often. If your baby has recently given up his bottle, you may find he wants it back again.

Older children also become insecure when they are ill and want to be around people. Nursing a child does not require any special skills, just love. Few things can go wrong. If a child's condition takes a turn for the worse, most parents will spot it immediately. Use your common sense. If you're worried, take your child to your doctor. If any medicines are prescribed, make sure you give them *exactly* as directed (*see page 32*), and follow any nursing tips your doctor gives you. Try

Tips for nursing your child

- Use cotton sheets—they are more comfortable for a child with a temperature.
- Change sheets regularly, particularly if he has a fever—clean sheets feel better.
- Put a bathrobe and socks or slippers on over his pajamas if he does not want to stay in bed all the time.
- Leave a box of tissues near his bed.
- Leave a bowl or bucket beside your child's bed if he feels sick so he doesn't have to run to the bathroom.
- If your child vomits, hold his head and comfort him while he is being sick. Give him a mint or strongly flavored sweet, or help him brush his teeth to take away the aftertaste.

to be cheerful and optimistic because children are often frightened by being ill and will be quick to pick up any tension from you.

Should my child stay in bed?

Take your lead from your child. There's no need to keep a child with a fever in bed, though he should stay in a draftfree room where the temperature is fairly constant. The room does not have to be particularly hot—if it is comfortable for you, it should be warm enough for your child. If your child is really ill, he will probably want to stay still and will sleep a lot, but when he is awake he will want to be around other people.

If your child wants to be out of bed and playing, let him do so around the house.

Should I isolate my child?

There is no point in keeping your child isolated if he has an infectious illness, such as chickenpox or measles. However, he is still contagious as long as he has the rash, so he should stay home. The practice of sterilizing everything used by the child during his illness is out-of-date. This is because it has been shown that most infections are caught and passed on within 48 hours, although the symptoms may not appear in that time. Obviously, if your child has a more serious infection that does need isolation, such as hepatitis (*see page 158*) or meningitis (*see page 177*), your doctor will arrange for your child to be admitted to the hospital or advise you on the necessary precautions. Also, if your child has German measles (*see page 146*), warn any women you think may be pregnant.

Feeding a sick child

Most children with a fever don't want to eat, so never force your child to eat. As long as he is getting plenty of liquid, your

Nursing a sick child

child can survive perfectly well for 2 or 3 days on very little food. When the illness is over, your child's appetite will return. As soon as it does, take advantage of it, and let your child eat as heartily as he wants to.

If he does want to eat, there is no particular food that is especially necessary when your child is ill, so forget the rules and spoil him a little by giving him his favorite foods until he is well again.

Getting a sick child to drink

Your child can survive without much food when he is ill, but it is very important for him to drink as much as possible to replace any fluid lost in sweating, vomiting or diarrhea. A child with a fever needs to drink at least 1½ fluid ounces (45ml) of liquid per pound of body weight a day. This should be increased to 3 fluid ounces (90ml) per pound if he is vomiting

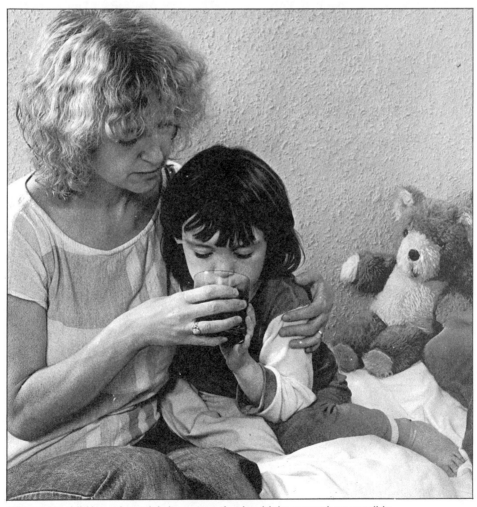

When your child has a fever, it is important that he drinks as much as possible.

Nursing a sick child

or has diarrhea (*see page 115*). Get your child to drink as often as you can, even a little every ½ hour while he's awake. Help an older child by leaving his favorite drink by the bed. Remind him every so often to take a sip. Soda is often tolerated better than fruit juice in an upset stomach.

Occupying a sick child

When your child is ill, spoil him a little. Let him play with games that have not been allowed in bed. Even messy activities like painting will not cause too much mess if you put a large sheet of plastic over the bed.

Be easy on yourself, and relax the rules on tidiness—you can always clean up later. Whatever you do, don't make a fuss, and don't nag your child to be tidy. Sit down and spend time with him. Read him stories, play games or sing him songs, help him with his coloring, painting or building.

Let your child watch television or listen to the radio while he is ill—have the television in his room or in the room where you are both sitting. Buy him some new toys, and give them to him one at a time. If he isn't feeling too ill, try wrapping them up and play a game with the package. Ask him to guess what's in the packages, and let him tear off the wrapping. Ask his friends to come and see him, and let them play for a short time.

If your child is not in bed all the time, there's no reason to keep him indoors on a warm day, even if he has a mild fever. But don't let him exercise too strenuously. If he wants to stay outside

---

Feeding and drinking tips

Feeding your child
● Give your child small meals more often than you would normally.
● Don't scold your child for not eating. He will eat again as soon as he gets better.
● Give your child his favorite foods.

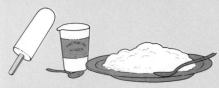

● If your child has a sore throat, give ice cream, frozen fruit juice or yogurt to soothe his throat.
● If your child is feeling slightly sick, give him mashed potatoes.
● As soon as your child's appetite returns, let him eat as much as he wants.

Making drinks more interesting
● Give your child a glass to drink out of that is normally reserved for adults.

● With a young child or baby, get him to sip drinks from a teaspoon. Make it seem like a game by using a long-handled spoon.

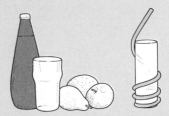

● Give your child diluted, defizzed soda or fresh fruit juices, such as pear, apple, orange or watermelon. Dilute them with soda water to make them more interesting.
● Use an interesting straw, such as a curly or bendy one.
● If your child does not like milk, make it more attractive by adding milkshake mixes or ice cream.
● Vary the drinks as much as possible.

Nursing a sick child

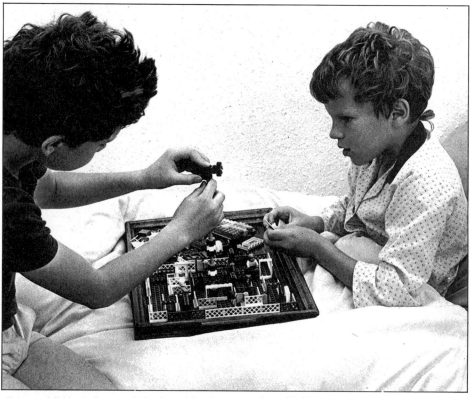

If your child is well enough, invite a friend over to play with him.

for longer than a few minutes, he is probably getting better anyway.

Getting better

As your child gets better, his appetite will return, and he will probably be more active. As soon as his temperature is back to normal in the morning and evening, he is probably ready to go back to school.

But if he has been suffering from an infectious illness, check with your doctor first.

A young child may have regressed slightly while he was ill. For example, if he was just out of diapers you may have to start toilet training again. Try not to worry about this too much, and don't scold him.

39

Your child in hospital

You'll be doing your child a big favor if you always encourage him to think about hospitals as friendly places. Try to take him with you if you are visiting a family friend or relative.

Preparing your child

If your child has to go into the hospital, for an operation, for example, and you are given sufficient warning, prepare him by discussing as many aspects of his stay as possible. Talk about it with the rest of the family, and get him used to the idea.

Answer all his questions honestly. Don't make promises you can't keep, and don't tell lies. If he is having an operation, he will probably ask you if there will be any pain or discomfort after the operation. If you say that nothing is going to hurt and it does, he won't trust you again. Explain there will be some discomfort, but it won't last long.

Another good way to prepare him for a hospital stay is to read him a book about someone who goes to the hospital. You could also buy him a toy stethoscope, and play doctors and nurses with him. Encourage him to be the doctor or nurse, and suggest he make up a hospital bed for his favorite teddy bear or toy.

When he is in the hospital

Few children's wards are frightening places. However, it is very important for parents to be with their children as much as possible while they are in the hospital. Because of this, almost all hospitals now allow parents to stay in the hospital with their child, particularly if he is very young. Many hospitals have sleeping facilities for parents with children up to age 6.

When you are there, ask the nurses how you can help with the daily routine. You will probably be encouraged to bathe and change your child and help with his feeding. You can read books

What to take to the hospital

If you can, you and your child should pack his suitcase together a few days before he has to go in.
☐ Three pairs of pajamas.
☐ Bathrobe and slippers.
☐ Three pairs of ankle socks.
☐ Hair brush and comb.
☐ Bag with soap, toothbrush and toothpaste.
☐ Bedside clock.
☐ Portable radio or cassette player with headphones.
☐ Favorite books and portable games.
☐ Favorite picture or photograph to place by his bedside.

and play games with him and any other children who want to join in. If your child is well enough and will be in the hospital for a while, ask his school teacher to give you the work he would normally be doing at school.

If you cannot be with your child all day, try to arrange so someone he knows well is with him at other times.

Back home from the hospital

It's quite normal for a child to behave a little oddly when he comes out of the hospital. Your child's sleeping and eating patterns may have changed. Hospital meals, and certainly bedtimes, tend to be earlier than you'd have them at home. Secondly, because your child has been away from his domestic discipline, you may find he will make a fuss about small points like brushing his teeth. Don't be too hard on him at first. Give him time to readjust to being home before you insist that he fits in with the old routine.

Visual
diagnosis
guides

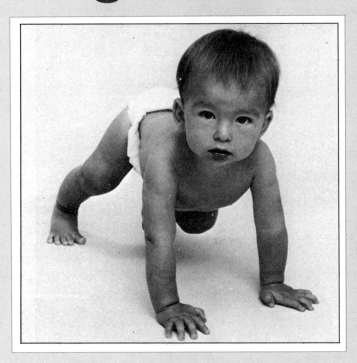

How to use this section

This section is designed to help if you don't know what has caused your child's symptoms, and are therefore unsure which A-Z entry to look up. Because it is impossible to give a definitive medical diagnosis from only one or two symptoms, this section instead helps you make an educated guess as to the possible cause. For ease of reference, the body is illustrated in six sections (see below), and the symptoms relating to those parts are dealt with accordingly. To use the guide, turn to the page dealing with the affected part of the body and look for the symptom most similar to the one your child is suffering from (if your child has more than one symptom, look up the major one first). Then turn to the A-Z entry suggested as a possible cause for more detailed information. If you cannot find the symptom you are looking for, turn to the major index on page 315 and either look up the symptom itself (for example, headache) or the part of the body affected (head).

Listed below are the parts of the body that may be affected, and the page on which you will find them. Problems affecting the skin in general, such as rashes, are also listed.

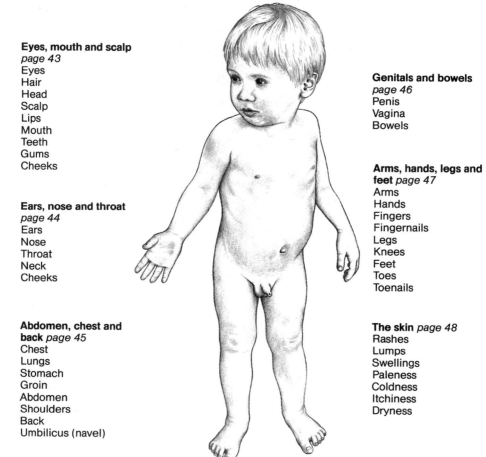

Eyes, mouth and scalp
page 43
Eyes
Hair
Head
Scalp
Lips
Mouth
Teeth
Gums
Cheeks

Ears, nose and throat
page 44
Ears
Nose
Throat
Neck
Cheeks

Abdomen, chest and back *page 45*
Chest
Lungs
Stomach
Groin
Abdomen
Shoulders
Back
Umbilicus (navel)

Genitals and bowels
page 46
Penis
Vagina
Bowels

Arms, hands, legs and feet *page 47*
Arms
Hands
Fingers
Fingernails
Legs
Knees
Feet
Toes
Toenails

The skin *page 48*
Rashes
Lumps
Swellings
Paleness
Coldness
Itchiness
Dryness

Eyes, mouth and scalp

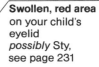

Thick, yellow scales over part or all of your baby's scalp *possibly* Cradle cap, see page 100

White flakes on your child's scalp *possibly* Dandruff, see page 107

Bald patches of red or gray scaly rings *possibly* Ringworm, see page 210

Itchy head with tiny pearl-white eggs clinging to the hair roots *possibly* Lice, see page 174

Severe headache and pain when neck is stretched *possibly* Meningitis, see page 177

Swollen, red area on your child's eyelid *possibly* Sty, see page 231

Red, scaly eyelids, with dandrufflike scales clinging to your child's eyelashes *possibly* Blepharitis, see page 69

Sore, watery eye *possibly* a Foreign body in the eye, see page 133

Weepy, sore, red eyes that may be gummed together in the morning *possibly* Conjunctivitis, see page 93

Weepy, red-rimmed, itchy eyes accompanied by sneezing *possibly* Hay fever, see page 149

One or both of your baby's eyes wander *possibly* Strabismus, see page 230

Pus oozing from the inner corner of your baby's eye *possibly* Sticky eye, see page 227

Small, white raised ulcerated area inside the mouth *possibly* Aphthous mouth sore, see page 182

Large, red area with a yellow center, usually on the inside of the cheek *possibly* Mouth sore, see page 182

Creamy-yellow or white frothy patches inside your baby's mouth, that become raw or bleed when wiped off *possibly* Oral thrush, see page 239

Tiny, itchy blisters around the nostrils and lips *possibly* Cold sore, see page 88

Tiny blisters that ooze and crust over *possibly* Impetigo, see page 164

Small cracks on the lips *possibly* Chapping, see page 82

Swollen red area on your baby's gum, accompanied by dribbling *possibly* Teething, see page 235

Painful, throbbing sensation in the tooth *possibly* Toothache, see page 245

Ear, nose and throat

Blotchy red rash that starts behind the ears then spreads to the rest of the body, accompanied by swollen neck glands *possibly* German measles, see page 146

Brown-red rash of small spots that starts behind the ears then spreads to the rest of the body, usually preceded by a runny nose and red, sore eyes *possibly* Measles, see page 176

Tiny white or yellow spots on and around a newborn baby's nose *possibly* Milia, see page 178 *Or* Infantile acne, see page 52

Nasal speech and mouth breathing *possibly* Adenoids, see page 243

Pain in and around the ear *possibly* Otitis media, see page 195 *Or* Toothache see page 245 *see also* Earache, page 124

Pussy discharge from the ear *possibly* Otitis media, see page 195

Pain inside the ear canal, made worse when the earlobe is pulled *possibly* Otitis externa, see page 193

Impaired hearing, accompanied by a sensation of fullness in the ear *possibly* Wax in ears, see page 258 *Or* Serous otitis, see page 216 *Or* Foreign body in the ear, see page 123

Sneezing, with a runny nose and itchy eyes *possibly* Hay fever, see page 149

Runny nose, often with a sore throat and fever *possibly* a Common cold, see page 91 *Or* Influenza, see page 165

Bleeding nose *possibly* Nosebleed, see page 189 *Or* Foreign body in the nose, see page 188

Swelling on either or both sides of the face *possibly* Mumps, see page 184

Hoarse cough or loss of voice *possibly* Croup, see page 101 *Or* Laryngitis, see page 172

Swollen neck glands with a sore throat that may be accompanied by a fever *possibly* Tonsillitis, see page 243 *Or* Mononucleosis see page 179 *Or* Scarlet fever, see page 213

Abdomen, chest and back

Rapid, difficult breathing in a baby under 1, following a common cold *possibly* Bronchiolitis, see page 75

Whooping sound during a coughing fit as air is breathed in *possibly* Whooping cough, see page 259

Dry cough, with a fever and rapid, labored breathing *possibly* Bronchitis, see page 76

Flat, red or pink rash starting on the trunk and spreading to the neck and limbs, usually after a high fever *possibly* Roseola infantum, see page 211

Intensely itchy, small blisters that appear in clusters on the trunk then spread to the rest of the body *possibly* Chickenpox, see page 83

Nausea and vomiting while traveling *possibly* Motion sickness, see page 181

Legs drawn up as if in pain to your baby's stomach with fits of crying *possibly* Colic see page 89

Painless bulge in the groin that increases in size when your child coughs or strains *possibly* Inguinal hernia, see page 160

Weeping, umbilical cord stump that crusts over *possibly* Umbilical-cord infection see page 249

Projectile vomiting in a newborn baby where milk shoots out forcefully from the mouth after feeding *possibly* Pyloric stenosis, see page 205

Severe spasmodic cramps in a baby under 12 months, with vomiting and red, jelly-like stools containing blood and mucus *possibly* Intussusception, see page 168

Pain starting around the navel then moving to the lower right area of the groin *possibly* Appendicitis, see page 56

Painless bulge near the navel that increases in size when your child strains or coughs *possibly* Umbilical hernia, see page 160

Genitals and bowels

Hard, pebblelike stools and pain in the lower abdomen
possibly Constipation,
see page 94

Loose, frequent bowel movements
possibly Diarrhea,
see page 114

Red, jellylike bowel movements containing blood and mucus, in a baby under 1, accompanied by severe abdominal pain
possibly Intussusception,
see page 168

Loose, frequent bowel movements accompanied by vomiting shortly after eating
possibly Food poisoning,
see page 141

Pimply red rash on area normally covered by your baby's diaper
possibly Diaper rash,
see page 112
Or Thrush,
see page 239

Small, threadlike worms around the anus, with intense itchiness
possibly Worms,
see page 261

Red, swollen tip of penis
possibly Balanitis,
see page 65

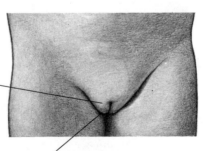

Smoky, dark-colored or red-brown urine
possibly Hepatitis,
see page 158

Irritation of the vulva
possibly Foreign body in the vagina,
see page 251
Or Worms,
see page 261
Or Vulvovaginitis,
see page 256

Frequent, painful passing of urine, accompanied by fever
possibly Urinary-tract infection,
see page 250

Arms, hands, legs and feet

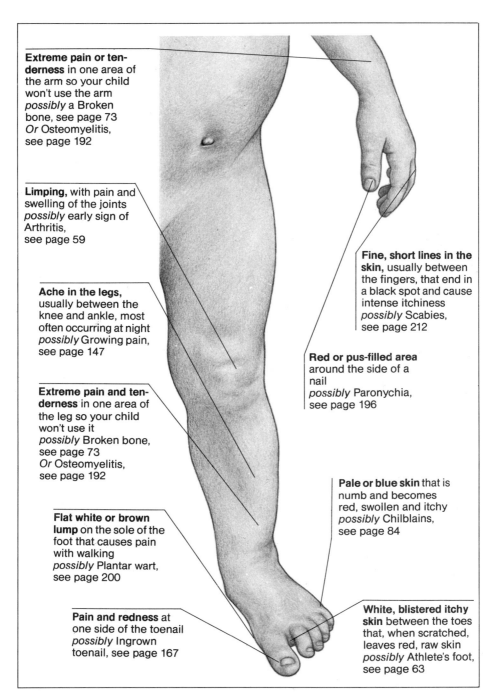

Extreme pain or tenderness in one area of the arm so your child won't use the arm *possibly* a Broken bone, see page 73 *Or* Osteomyelitis, see page 192

Limping, with pain and swelling of the joints *possibly* early sign of Arthritis, see page 59

Ache in the legs, usually between the knee and ankle, most often occurring at night *possibly* Growing pain, see page 147

Extreme pain and tenderness in one area of the leg so your child won't use it *possibly* Broken bone, see page 73 *Or* Osteomyelitis, see page 192

Flat white or brown lump on the sole of the foot that causes pain with walking *possibly* Plantar wart, see page 200

Pain and redness at one side of the toenail *possibly* Ingrown toenail, see page 167

Fine, short lines in the skin, usually between the fingers, that end in a black spot and cause intense itchiness *possibly* Scabies, see page 212

Red or pus-filled area around the side of a nail *possibly* Paronychia, see page 196

Pale or blue skin that is numb and becomes red, swollen and itchy *possibly* Chilblains, see page 84

White, blistered itchy skin between the toes that, when scratched, leaves red, raw skin *possibly* Athlete's foot, see page 63

The skin

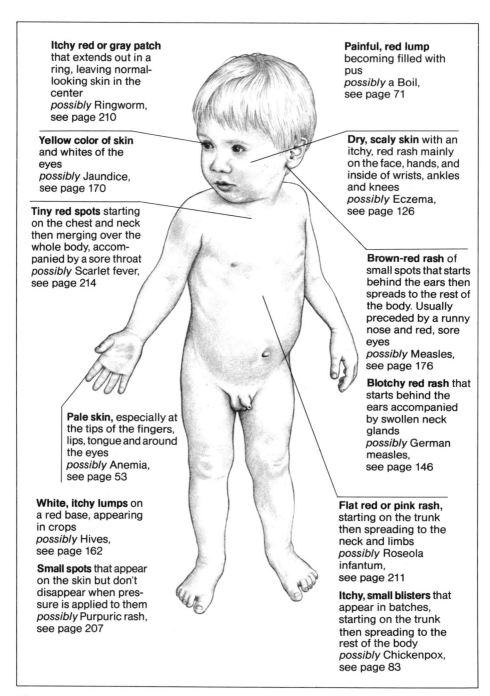

Itchy red or gray patch that extends out in a ring, leaving normal-looking skin in the center
possibly Ringworm, see page 210

Yellow color of skin and whites of the eyes
possibly Jaundice, see page 170

Tiny red spots starting on the chest and neck then merging over the whole body, accompanied by a sore throat
possibly Scarlet fever, see page 214

Pale skin, especially at the tips of the fingers, lips, tongue and around the eyes
possibly Anemia, see page 53

White, itchy lumps on a red base, appearing in crops
possibly Hives, see page 162

Small spots that appear on the skin but don't disappear when pressure is applied to them
possibly Purpuric rash, see page 207

Painful, red lump becoming filled with pus
possibly a Boil, see page 71

Dry, scaly skin with an itchy, red rash mainly on the face, hands, and inside of wrists, ankles and knees
possibly Eczema, see page 126

Brown-red rash of small spots that starts behind the ears then spreads to the rest of the body. Usually preceded by a runny nose and red, sore eyes
possibly Measles, see page 176

Blotchy red rash that starts behind the ears accompanied by swollen neck glands
possibly German measles, see page 146

Flat red or pink rash, starting on the trunk then spreading to the neck and limbs
possibly Roseola infantum, see page 211

Itchy, small blisters that appear in batches, starting on the trunk then spreading to the rest of the body
possibly Chickenpox, see page 83

A~Z
of common
complaints

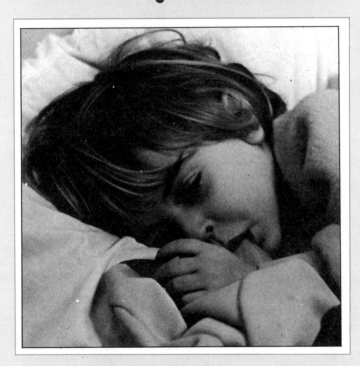

How to use this section

The A-Z of Common Complaints is the focus of the book, covering all the most common childhood complaints. The entries take two basic forms. In the majority, a detailed description of the illness is given, with a possible-symptoms box for easy reference, a list of what to check for first and treatments that might be given. In some cases, no symptoms box is given because the symptom is the complaint's name.

Long-term complaints, such as cerebral palsy and spina bifida, are dealt with in a discussion. There is no checklist for *What should I do first?* nor do the headings *Is it serious?* or *Should I call the doctor?* appear. Instead, the treatments and procedures following diagnosis of a long-term ailment are given under the heading *What can be done?*

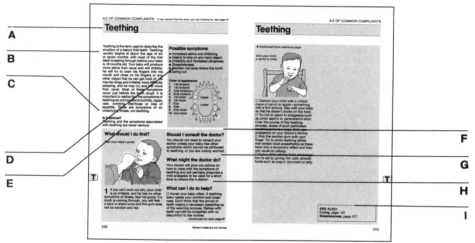

A Heading
Name by which the complaint is commonly known.

B Introduction
Gives a description of the complaint, explaining why it arises and how it is likely to develop.

C Is it serious?
States whether or not the complaint is serious and the conditions under which it would become serious.

D Possible symptoms
Lists the symptoms that are likely to occur with the given complaint. Your child may have some or all of them. He may or may not develop them in the order given, although it is the most likely sequence of appearance.

E What should I do first?
Details what you should do if you suspect your child has a certain complaint. This may involve action to determine whether your child definitely has the complaint (taking his temperature, checking for a rash); may suggest home treatments that will provide immediate relief for your child while you contact the doctor (tepid sponging for fever or calamine lotion for itchiness). If your child's case is an emergency, the section will say so and will suggest you call an ambulance or go to an emergency room.

F Should I consult the doctor?
This will tell you the circumstances under which you should seek medical assistance. There are four levels of immediacy.
1 Emergency
In a life-threatening situation, you will be told to call an ambulance or go to the emergency room.
2 Consult your doctor immediately
This means call your doctor at once—even in the middle

How to use this section

of the night—because your child needs medical attention now. If the complaint is life-threatening and there is any risk of a delay in seeing the doctor, the entry will tell you to call an ambulance or go to the emergency room.

3 Consult your doctor
This means call your doctor to make an appointment as soon as possible. If your child's symptoms develop when the office isn't open, don't worry, but do call as soon as the office opens.

4 Consult your doctor for advice
Your child has no serious problem, but it may be one that worries him or you. Make an appointment to talk to your doctor about it whenever it is convenient.

G What might the doctor do?
The treatment most likely to be given to your child is outlined.

H What can I do to help?
Makes suggestions as to what you can do to assist the doctor in the treatment of your child, as well as home treatment and nursing tips for the complaint itself.

I See-also box
A cross-referencing system to other articles within the A-Z. You may be referred to another complaint because it could be the possible cause of your child's symptoms, or it may be of background interest to the complaint in question.

A-Z Index

Acne, infantile

Acne is usually a problem of adolescence, triggered by the rise in hormonal levels at puberty. The sebaceous glands in the skin, which produce sebum to keep the skin soft and lubricated, become blocked by tiny keratin plugs so the sebum cannot escape. This results in inflammation and infection and the typical spots or pimples. Quite commonly, mild acne can occur in the first months after birth, when a baby's hormonal levels are in a similar state of flux. This form of acne is called infantile acne.

Is it serious?
Infantile acne is not serious and doesn't distress the baby though you may be upset by your baby's appearance.

Possible symptoms
● Red spots, sometimes with yellow pustules, usually across the cheeks, forehead and chin where the sebaceous glands are most numerous.

What should I do first?

1 Leave the pimples alone, and don't use any adult soaps or cosmetics.

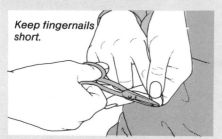

Keep fingernails short.

2 Keep your baby's fingernails short, and put mittens on him to keep him from scratching the pimples and breaking the skin.

Should I consult the doctor?
Consult your doctor for advice if the spots get worse or if you are concerned about them.

What might the doctor do?
☐ Your doctor will reassure you that the condition will clear up in 4 to 6 weeks.

What can I do to help?
☐ Try to ignore your baby's spots; they will go away eventually.

Words in **bold** are A-Z entries

Anemia

Anemia is due to a reduction in the number of normal red cells in the blood or a reduction in the amount of hemoglobin, the oxygen-carrying pigment derived from iron that gives red cells their color. This reduction can be caused by inadequate production of red cells in the bone marrow, by lack of iron and other blood-forming substances, by diseases such as **leukemia, sickle cell anemia** and thalassemia (an inherited blood disorder), by excess blood loss or by infection.

Is it serious?
Anemia may be a symptom of a serious disease.

Possible symptoms

- Pale skin, especially at the tips of the fingers, the lips, around the eyes and on the tongue.
- Fatigue, lethargy and weakness.
- Shortness of breath on exertion.
- Dizziness.
- Raised pulse rate.

What should I do first?

1 If your child seems listless and pale, and he is not eating well, call your doctor.

Should I consult the doctor?

Consult your doctor if you think your child is anemic. Anemia should always be investigated promptly and thoroughly by a doctor. Don't rely on home remedies.

What might the doctor do?

☐ Your doctor will take blood samples and send them for analysis.
☐ If anemia is due to iron deficiency, your doctor will probably prescribe supplements of iron and may advise you to include more iron-rich foods in your child's diet.
☐ If your child is suffering from an inherited defect in the hemoglobin in his blood (as occurs with thalassemia), he will need treatment with drugs for life and perhaps blood transfusions to relieve the chronic symptoms.

What can I do to help?

☐ Make sure your child is eating a well-balanced diet as prescribed by your doctor or a dietician. Iron-rich foods include liver, egg yolk, dark green leafy vegetables and nuts. Vitamin C helps in the absorption of iron, so give your child a glass of orange juice with his egg, for example.

SEE ALSO:
Dizziness, *page 118*
Leukemia, *page 173*
Sickle cell anemia, *page 218*

Apnea

An apnea is literally a period during which breathing stops. Short periods of apnea are normal during sleep, especially dreaming. A normal, healthy baby may hold his breath for up to 10 seconds. During what is medically termed an "apnea," breathing stops for more than 20 seconds. Apnea is more likely to occur in very premature babies, less than 32 weeks gestation, or when a baby has a blocked nose, as occurs with a **common cold.**

Is it serious?

Apnea is serious because it can be a sign of a major underlying condition, such as a heart defect. Prolonged apnea may cause such a lack of oxygen to the brain that brain damage and even death result. Apnea is believed to be one of the mechanisms that causes Sudden Infant Death Syndrome (SIDS).

Possible symptoms

- Lack of breathing (the chest does not rise and fall) for periods exceeding 20 seconds.
- Total lack of movement.
- Pallor.
- Blue skin color around the lips and tongue.

What should I do first?

1 If you notice your baby has periods when he stops breathing, time the events, even if he does not actually turn blue or very pale. If the periods last about 10 seconds, this may be normal, especially if they occur when he is asleep. If they last longer than 20 seconds, shake his arm or leg to stimulate him.

2 During one of these periods, if he can't be roused, make sure there is nothing obstructing his breathing by pressing down on his chin to open his mouth and look inside.

3 If there is no visible obstruction, loosen any clothing around your baby's neck.

4 Make a loud noise to startle your baby, such as clapping your hands or shouting.

5 If there is still no response, put your baby over your knee, face down, so his tongue cannot fall back and obstruct the airway. With both

hands around his body, squeeze gently a couple of times.

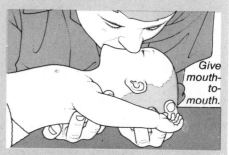

Give mouth-to-mouth.

6 If this fails, start mouth-to-mouth resuscitation immediately (*see page 287*). Ask someone to call an ambulance. If you are alone, go to the phone and dial 911 or call an ambulance. Take your baby with you and continue the mouth-to-mouth resuscitation.

Continued on next page ▶

Words in **bold** are A-Z entries

Apnea

◀ *Continued from previous page*

Should I consult the doctor?

Consult your doctor immediately if your baby has a period of apnea. Call an ambulance immediately or take your baby to the nearest emergency room if you cannot rouse your child during an attack.

What might the doctor do?

☐ If your baby has not started breathing, the doctor or paramedic will administer oxygen by face mask, mouth-to-mouth resuscitation or intubation (a tube is inserted directly into your baby's airway under anesthetic to aid breathing). Your baby will be admitted to the intensive-care unit, where his breathing will be maintained with a mechanical ventilator until he can breath on his own again.
☐ Your baby will be treated for any side effects of the period during which he was without oxygen, such as convulsions.
☐ Your doctor will test for a possible cause of the apnea, such as an infection or heart defect.
☐ If your baby has 1 episode of apnea, your doctor may provide you with an apnea monitor. This small device, similar to a radio, is attached to a sensor on the baby's stomach or to the crib mattress. The monitor gives off an alarm if the baby does not breathe for a preset time.

What can I do to help?

☐ Learn to manage the monitor. Even if it gives off the occasional false alarm, it should be reassuring to know you will be alerted if your baby's breathing stops for any period of time.
☐ Learn CPR (cardiopulmonary resuscitation, *see page 286*).
☐ Find a local support group.

SEE ALSO:
Common cold, *page 91*

Appendicitis

Appendicitis occurs when infection causes the appendix to become inflamed and swollen. The appendix is a small tube—about 3 inches (8cm) long—that lies on the right side of the abdomen at the junction of the large and small intestines. The tube has one blind end and a small opening at the other. The opening may become partly or completely blocked, leading to a buildup of bacteria. This can result in infection, which may necessitate surgical removal of the appendix (appendectomy). Appendicitis is rare in babies under 1 year, but appendectomy is the most common emergency operation among children.

Is it serious?

Appendicitis is not a serious condition if it is diagnosed early. However, if the symptoms are mistaken for something else, such as **constipation**, and there is any delay in treatment, the buildup of pus in the blocked appendix can cause the appendix to burst. This is called *peritonitis.*

Possible symptoms

● Abdominal pain, starting around the navel, then moving down to the lower right abdomen.
● Slight temperature, rarely above 100F (37.5C).
● Loss of appetite.
● Vomiting.
● Diarrhea or constipation.

Site of appendix

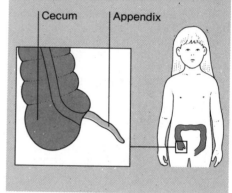

Cecum | Appendix

What should I do first?

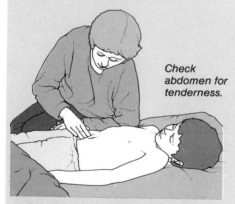

Check abdomen for tenderness.

1 If your child complains of an abdominal pain for more than a couple of hours, lay him flat on his back and examine his stomach. Press gently about an inch to the right of, and just below, the navel. Pain on gentle pressure and sharp pain when you suddenly remove your hands are characteristic signs of appendicitis. Consult your doctor immediately.

2 If your child is constipated and you suspect appendicitis, don't give him laxatives. They can cause the appendix to burst if it is already inflamed.

3 Don't give your child anything to eat or drink. If an appendectomy is necessary, it will be performed under general anesthesia and may be delayed if your child doesn't have an empty stomach.

Continued on next page ▶

Words in **bold** are A-Z entries

Appendicitis

◀ Continued from previous page

Should I consult the doctor?

Consult your doctor immediately if you suspect appendicitis. Any delay could spread the infection to the intestines.

What might the doctor do?

☐ Your doctor will examine your child's abdomen and ask you when the pain started and what other symptoms there were. Diagnosis of this condition is difficult, and your doctor will probably arrange for the transfer of your child to the hospital for confirmation of the diagnosis and for surgical removal of the appendix.

What can I do to help?

☐ Ask the hospital if you can stay with your child after the operation. Many hospitals now allow a parent to do so. Your presence will reassure your child and should speed his recovery.

☐ Encourage your child to rest and eat normally when he comes home from the hospital, usually about 5 days after the operation. You will be advised by your doctor how to care for your child at home. Your child should be fit and well again in about 2 to 3 weeks.

SEE ALSO:
Constipation, *page 94*

Appetite, loss of

A sick child nearly always loses his appetite. Loss of appetite can be a general sign of ill health and can be accompanied by a fever. It is also a symptom of a problem in the stomach and intestines, such as **gastroenteritis**, or it may be from a **sore throat**, if swallowing is painful. Minor disorders, such as **motion sickness**, usually cause your child to lose his appetite, but this will be only temporary. Don't worry about loss of appetite being a symptom of an underlying problem if your child misses one meal because of fatigue or because you've had a battle of wills at mealtime. This is perfectly normal, and your child will make up for it in the following meals.

Is it serious?

If your child refuses to eat for 24 hours and you can find no reason for the loss of appetite, it is a cause for concern.

What should I do first?

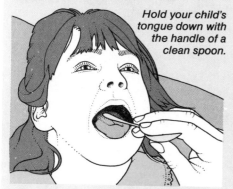

Hold your child's tongue down with the handle of a clean spoon.

1 If your child refuses food for a day but is taking plenty of fluid, check his temperature, and examine his throat for possible inflammation of the tonsils. With the handle of a spoon, depress his tongue gently and ask him to say a long "aaah."

2 Check to see if your child is suffering from **earache.** An ear infection, such as **otitis media,** could be painful enough to cause him to lose his appetite.

3 Check for abdominal pain (*see page 56*). Pain in the lower right of the abdomen may mean **appendicitis**.

4 Check to see if there is any pain when your child passes urine. This could be a sign of a **urinary-tract infection**.

5 If your child's temperature is normal, and you can find no evidence of illness, and he still refuses food, get him to drink plenty of fluid.

Should I consult the doctor?

Consult your doctor if appetite loss persists, even without other symptoms, for more than 24 hours.

What might the doctor do?

☐ Your doctor will examine your child to see if there is any physical reason why he is not eating. If none can be found, your doctor will probably keep a check on your child's condition.

What can I do to help?

☐ Make sure your child gets plenty of nutrients by disguising them in drinks. Enrich a milkshake with an egg and 1 teaspoon of wheat germ.

SEE ALSO:
Appendicitis, *page 56*
Earache, *page 124*
Gastroenteritis, *page 144*
Motion sickness, *page 181*
Otitis media, *page 195*
Sore throat, *page 220*
Tonsillitis, *page 243*
Urinary-tract infection, *page 250*

Words in **bold** are A-Z entries

Arthritis

Arthritis is the inflammation of a joint. This is usually accompanied by swelling, pain, stiffness and tenderness. Arthritis may be caused by an injury to a joint, or by an infection in the joint, when it is called *septic arthritis*. In rare cases, it may be caused by **rheumatic fever**, or by a malfunctioning of the body's defense mechanism which leads the antibodies to attack the body's own tissues, causing inflammation and a fluctuating temperature. This is called *Still's disease* or *juvenile rheumatoid arthritis*. Still's disease starts between age 2 and 5 and affects mainly girls.

If your child is ill with an infectious disease such as **influenza** or **measles**, he may have arthritic pains in his joints. These will, however, disappear once the infection has passed.

Is it serious?
Arthritis is a serious disorder that can lead to permanent deformity.

Possible symptoms

- Pain and swelling in a joint or several joints.
- Limping if hip or knee joints are affected.
- General aches and pains all around the body.
- A temperature of 104F (40C) or higher, or a temperature that fluctuates from normal to 102F (38.9C).
- Loss of appetite.

What should I do first?

1 Check to see if your child has a temperature. If it is as high as 104F (40C), and there is pain in the joints, treat this as an emergency. This could be septic arthritis. If his temperature fluctuates from normal to as high as 102F (38.9C), and he seems unwell, consult your doctor immediately. This could be Still's disease.

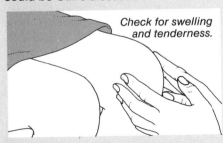
Check for swelling and tenderness.

2 If you notice that your child is limping, check his joints for swelling and tenderness by pressing on and around them.

3 If your child has had an injury to a joint and he complains of aches and pains, check the joint for tenderness and swelling.

4 If pain is felt by your child between the joints and not on the joint itself, this could be a **growing pain**. Check calf and thigh muscles for tenderness.

5 Don't give your child any pain-killing drugs until you have seen your doctor.

Should I consult the doctor?

Consult your doctor immediately if your child has a high, fluctuating temperature and a painful, swollen joint. Consult your doctor if you notice your child limping.

Continued on next page ▶

Arthritis

◀ Continued from previous page

What might the doctor do?

☐ Your doctor will examine your child and ask about any other symptoms or illnesses your child may have had over previous months.

☐ If your doctor suspects arthritis, your child will probably be referred to a specialist for examination and blood tests to find a definite cause. Your child may have to stay in the hospital to complete any necessary tests.

☐ If your child has septic arthritis, he will be given antibiotics intravenously to eradicate the infection in the joint.

☐ If your child has Still's disease, he may be prescribed aspirin and anti-inflammatory drugs. He will be taught a set of exercises to increase mobility in the affected joints.

What can I do to help?

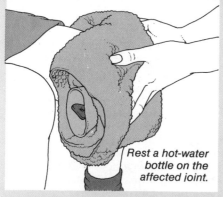

Rest a hot-water bottle on the affected joint.

☐ Wrap a hot-water bottle in a towel or turn the heating pad on low, and rest it on the affected joint. Heat is sometimes soothing and can help get the joint moving.

☐ Apply a cold compress to a joint if it is hot and swollen. Wrap a plastic bag filled with ice cubes in a piece of cloth, and apply it directly to the joint.

☐ Make sure your child has plenty of rest and a protein-rich diet.

☐ Gently massage the joints. Sometimes this can relieve aches and pains.

☐ Take your child for regular 30-minute swimming sessions. Swimming in warm water is excellent exercise for arthritis sufferers. Check with your doctor before doing this.

☐ Practice the special exercises at home with your child if the physio-therapist agrees.

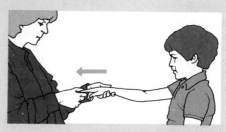

Pull gently on each finger to keep the finger joints from stiffening.

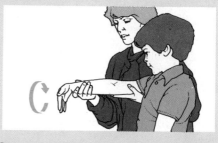

Support your child's arm, and ask him to do circles in the air with his hands. Hold his forearm steady so only the wrist joint moves.

SEE ALSO:
Growing pain, *page 147*
Influenza, *page 165*
Limp, *page 175*
Measles, *page 176*
Rheumatic fever, *page 209*

Words in **bold** are A-Z entries

Asthma

Asthma is an allergic disease which affects the air passages (*bronchi*). It is a "twitchiness" in response to environmental factors, viruses or allergies. When it occurs, the bronchi constrict and become clogged with mucus, making breathing difficult. An asthma attack can be frightening because the feeling of suffocation can cause panic, making breathing more difficult. The initial cause of the wheezing may be allergies and is usually airborne. Once asthma is established, emotional stress and exercise can also bring on an attack.

Children often wheeze before age 2 but usually are not diagnosed as asthmatic until 2. The condition may run in families and may be accompanied by other allergic diseases, such as **eczema** or **hay fever**. Most children get better as they get older.

Many babies under 1 wheeze if they suffer from **bronchiolitis**, when their small air passages become inflamed. They are not necessarily suffering from asthma. As they grow and their air passages widen, the wheezing stops. Infection, not an allergic reaction, is the usual cause of this wheezing.

Is it serious?

Asthma attacks can be frightening, but with medication and advice from your doctor, your child should suffer no serious complications.

Possible symptoms

- Persistent cough.
- Labored breathing; breathing out becomes difficult and the abdomen may be drawn inward with the effort of breathing in.
- Sensation of suffocation.
- High-pitched whistling sound.
- Blueness around the lips (cyanosis) only if wheezing is severe.

Area affected

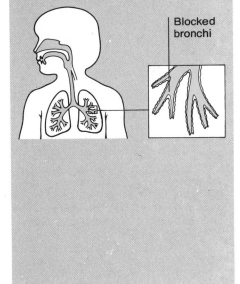

Blocked bronchi

What should I do first?

1 Consult your doctor immediately if your child is having an asthma attack.

2 If the attack occurs when your child is in bed, prop him in a sitting position with pillows. Or sit him in a chair with his arms braced against the back to take the weight off his chest. This allows the chest muscles to force air out more efficiently.

3 Stay calm. A show of anxiety may make your child more fearful.

4 Try to take your child's mind off the asthma attack. Sing to him or read to him to try to help him forget about the wheezing.

Continued on next page ▶

Asthma

◀ *Continued from previous page*

Should I consult the doctor?

Consult your doctor immediately if your child has an asthma attack.

What might the doctor do?

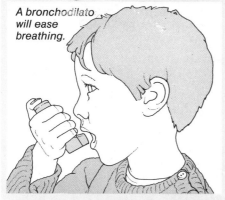

A bronchodilator will ease breathing.

☐ Your doctor will probably treat the attack with a shot of adrenalin or a bronchodilator drug, which opens up the bronchi by relaxing the muscles in the linings. A severe attack may require treatment in the hospital, where bigger doses of drugs may be given by inhalant or by intravenous drip.

☐ If there is some evidence of a chest infection, antibiotics will be prescribed.

☐ Your doctor will discuss prevention of further attacks. If he feels the wheezing is due to allergies, he may perform skin tests to determine the cause. Your doctor will arrange for you to have a supply of a bronchodilator drug, either in liquid, capsule or aerosol form or as capsules for insertion in an inhaler. This should be taken as soon as an attack begins. Your doctor will ask you to inform him if your child has a severe attack or if an attack does not respond to 2 doses of the bronchodilator.

☐ Your doctor may prescribe a steroid drug if other simpler measures don't prevent further attacks. A small dose of steroid may be inhaled 3 or 4 times a day, or a dose may be given in tablet form.

What can I do to help?

☐ If your doctor failed to pinpoint the allergen, try to track it down yourself. Notice when the attacks occur and at what time of the day or year. Avoid obvious allergens, such as feather pillows, and keep the dust down in your house by vacuuming floors rather than sweeping them.

☐ Many asthmatics are allergic to animals. If you have a pet, ask a friend to look after it for a couple of weeks, and see if your child's asthma attacks are reduced.

☐ Make sure your child has the prescribed drugs nearby at all times. Inform his school about the possibility of attacks occurring.

☐ Encourage your child to stand and sit up straight so his lungs have more space. Don't let him get overweight because this puts an extra burden on his lungs.

☐ Moderate exercise can help his breathing, but too much can bring on an asthma attack. Swimming, however, can be especially helpful.

☐ If the wheezing is precipitated by a cold virus, start the bronchodilator at the first sign of a cough.

☐ Don't smoke around your child.

SEE ALSO:
Bronchiolitis, *page 75*
Eczema, *page 126*
Hay fever, *page 149*

Words in **bold** are A-Z entries

Athlete's foot

This is a fungal infection that affects the soft area between and underneath the toes. In an advanced stage, it also affects the nails. It is contagious and is usually picked up by walking barefoot in communal areas, such as shower rooms, gyms and swimming pools, where infected feet have been. The infection is aggravated by sweaty feet because the fungus, *tinea,* which also causes **ringworm** elsewhere on the body, thrives in warm, moist conditions.

Is it serious?

Athlete's foot is a common condition, requiring simple treatment and good hygiene to cure it. It is contagious, so act quickly to keep the infection from spreading.

Possible symptoms

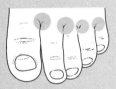

Possible sites of blistered skin

● White, blistered skin between and underneath the toes. The area is itchy and, when scratched, splits and leaves raw, red skin underneath.
● Dry, peeling skin.
● Thick, yellow toenails.

What should I do first?

1 If your child has itchy feet, check the area between and underneath the toes for white blisters and redness.

2 Check underneath the foot for blisters and cracking.

3 Check the condition of the toenails.

4 Buy an anti-fungal foot powder or cream at the drugstore. After washing and drying the feet thoroughly, apply the treatment, following the manufacturer's instructions.

5 Emphasize to your child that he must not go barefoot until the condition has cleared up.

6 Keep your child's towel and bathmat separate from the rest of the family's, and wash them every day.

Should I consult the doctor?

Consult your doctor if the underside of the foot is already affected or if the nails are distorted or yellowing. Consult your doctor if the self-help measures fail to improve the condition within 3 or 4 weeks.

What might the doctor do?

□ If the fungus has affected the toenails, your doctor will prescribe an anti-fungal medication that may need to be taken for as long as 9 months.
□ If you consulted your doctor because self-help measures failed, your doctor will prescribe another antifungal cream and will advise you on the correct procedure for good foot hygiene.

What can I do to help?

□ Make sure your child has clean socks every day, preferably made from natural fibers, such as cotton or wool.
□ Rotate your child's shoes, especially his running shoes, so they have a chance to dry out between wearings.

SEE ALSO:
Ringworm, *page 210*

Autism

The word autism is used to define a behavior pattern in which a child suffers from a profound inability to relate to other people, including his parents. The autistic child lives in curious isolation. For example, even though not deaf, he may not appear to hear what is being said to him and may never speak or may speak in an unusual way. With hindsight, parents may remember their autistic child was not a cuddly baby, he seldom if ever smiled and he never indicated a desire to be picked up by stretching out his arms.

There have been many theories about the cause of this rare disorder since it was first described in 1943. But it is now clear that it is not induced by parental behavior and is not a reaction to environ-mental factors. Autism cannot usually be diagnosed until it is realized that speech has not developed by the normal time, if at all. By this time you will probably have noticed your child is withdrawn and spends hours in solitary play. Quite often your child will adopt behavior rituals, such as touching certain objects in a set sequence or rocking backward and forward. Disruption of these routines can bring on severe temper tantrums. This behavior reflects the child's need to surround himself with an environment that never varies. Some autistic children have a heightened sensitivity to certain objects, and they may constantly look carefully at their own hand and finger movements or rub surfaces as if to appreciate the textures.

Possible symptoms

- Social withdrawal.
- Hearing abnormalities.
- Avoidance of eye contact.
- Speech disorders.
- Repetitive behavior patterns.
- Indifference to pain.

What can be done?

Autistic children usually attend special schools from an early age. If parents cannot manage at home, treatment in a therapeutic residential setting may be advised. Many different therapies for autism have been tried, but success in all of them has been limited. Intensive psychotherapy has been disappointing, and medication with tranquilizers is useful only in controlling aggressive behavior. Behavior therapy and holding therapy (in which the parent is encouraged to hold the child close for as long as possible to build up physical and emotional contact) have been useful. All therapy needs to be prescribed and supervised by experts in this field.

Words in **bold** are A-Z entries

Balanitis

Balanitis is the inflammation of the tip (*glans*) of the penis in uncircumcised boys. It may be caused by **diaper rash**, an allergic reaction to the detergent in which your child's clothing is washed or by a tight foreskin in boys over the age of 5. Up until this age, the foreskin is normally tight.

Is it serious?
The condition is not serious, though it is important for your child's comfort to treat it promptly. If balanitis is recurrent, your son may need to be circumcised.

Possible symptoms

● Red, swollen tip to the penis.
● Pussy discharge from the tip.
● A foreskin that cannot be drawn back.
● If your child is still in diapers, a general inflammation around the buttocks and in the genital region.

What should I do first?

1 As soon as you notice any redness around the tip of the penis, carefully and gently try to draw back the foreskin. Don't force it. Leave it alone if your son is under 5 years old. If the foreskin won't retract, leave it alone and consult your doctor.

2 If the foreskin will retract, wash and dry the penis thoroughly. Apply an antiseptic ointment.

3 If the condition is part of diaper rash, change your child's diapers frequently. Wash and dry the area thoroughly at every diaper change, and liberally apply a barrier cream over the area covered by the diaper, including the penis.

Should I consult the doctor?

Consult your doctor if your child complains of pain, if you cannot retract the foreskin or if home treatment fails to relieve the swelling within 48 hours.

What might the doctor do?

☐ Your doctor may prescribe an antibiotic cream to relieve the inflammation.
☐ If the foreskin is tight, your doctor

will regularly check it. If the foreskin has failed to stretch by the time the boy is 6 the condition may need to be corrected surgically with **circumcision.** Your doctor will refer you to a surgeon who will assess your child to see if he really needs to be circumcised.

What can I do to help?

☐ Always change your child's diapers frequently to prevent the recurrence of diaper rash.
☐ Teach your child good personal hygiene from an early age. Until the age of 5, regular bathing will keep the penis adequately cleaned. After this age, encourage your child to draw back the foreskin and wash the area daily.
☐ If an allergic reaction has caused balanitis, try changing your laundry detergent. Make sure your child's clothing is thoroughly rinsed.

SEE ALSO:
Diaper rash, *page 112*
Circumcision, *page 86*

Bedwetting

Children master bladder control at different ages. Just as they develop skills at different rates, their ability to hold urine for long periods varies. Although 1 in 10 normal boys still wets the bed at age 5, most children become dry at night between the ages of 3 and 4. A child should not be classified as a bedwetter while he is still training his bladder to last the 10 to 12 hours of nighttime sleep.

A return to bedwetting once a child has gained bladder control may be a sign of increased tension and anxiety. This often happens as a result of an important occasion, such as the arrival of a new baby in the house or starting school. A few children, especially girls, may have a physical reason for their incontinence, such as a **urinary-tract infection** or some abnormality of the urinary system. If bedwetting is accompanied by increased thirst and frequent urination during the day, this could be a symptom of **diabetes**.

Is it serious?

Although irritating for parents, bedwetting is not a serious problem.

What should I do first?

1 Put a rubber sheet on the bed, and cover it with a top sheet.

2 Examine your own behavior. You may be the source of the problem. You may be pushing your child too hard or creating a tense atmosphere.

3 Make sure your child empties his bladder before going to bed. If he wishes, leave a potty chair in his room so he doesn't have to go any distance to the bathroom.

4 Limit fluid intake after dinner.

Should I consult the doctor?

Consult your doctor if you and your child are becoming discouraged or if you suspect there may be some physical cause of the problem, such as a urinary tract infection, which causes the urine to have an unpleasantly fishy odor.

What might the doctor do?

☐ Your doctor will examine your child and take a urine sample to exclude the possibility of a urinary tract infection or a malformation of the urinary tract.
☐ Your doctor may recommend a special pad for your child's bed that sets off an alarm when moistened with urine. Your child can learn to react to this alarm and get up and go to the bathroom. This system is useful only if your child is over 6 and doesn't object to it.

What can I do to help?

☐ Don't scold your child, no matter how tiresome it becomes.
☐ Make a chart, and give your child a star for every dry night.
☐ Limit the amount of liquid you give your child before bedtime.
☐ Don't try anything, such as the alarm pad, that your child objects to. It will only increase the tension.
☐ Try bladder stretching. Encourage your child to drink lots of fluids, then try to hold off urinating for as long as possible.

SEE ALSO:
Diabetes mellitus, *page 111*
Urinary-tract infection, *page 250*

Words in **bold** are A-Z entries

Birthmark

A birthmark is a skin discoloration caused by a collection of small blood vessels or pigment just below the surface. The birthmark, which can be flat or raised, may be present at birth or may appear in the first months of life.

Dark-brown birthmarks are circular and may have hair growing out of them. These are called moles, and they are usually permanent.

Storkbites are small, pink and spidery and appear on the back of the neck, the upper eyelids or the nose. They usually disappear within a few years.

A *Mongolian spot* looks like a blue bruise in the skin and is usually found on dark-skinned people. It occurs most often on the lower back or buttocks.

A *strawberry nevus* is a raised red mark with a bumpy surface that is sometimes shaped like a strawberry. It usually disappears by the time your child is 5, but before it does, it enlarges alarmingly, growing darker or lighter, before gradually disappearing. It is most common in girls and can bleed spontaneously.

A *port wine stain* looks exactly like its name—a red-purple patch on the skin. When it appears on the face, it is called the Sturge-Weber syndrome. It can appear over much of the face and forehead or the limbs. It is usually large. This is the most distressing birthmark because it doesn't disappear, though it can fade to a paler pink. It is more common among blond children.

Is it serious?

A birthmark is almost always harmless and many will disappear by the age of 5.

What should I do first?

1 Don't rush into treatment because many birthmarks disappear spontaneously.

2 If a strawberry nevus bleeds, place a clean gauze pad or handkerchief over the mark. It should stop bleeding after a minute or so.

Should I consult the doctor?

Consult your doctor for advice if you feel the birthmark is disfiguring and your child may suffer in the future.

What might the doctor do?

☐ If the birthmark is unsightly, your doctor may refer you to a plastic surgeon. Birthmarks can be treated with many different techniques, including tattooing and laser therapy. If you decide against cosmetic surgery, your doctor may prescribe special camouflage makeup for your child.

What can I do to help?

☐ If the mark is unsightly and disturbs you and your child, use the camouflage makeup.

☐ Try not to show your child you are anxious about the birthmark.

Bites

B

Most children love animals, but because they are not always as gentle with them as they should be, bites do occur. The most common animal bites—from dogs and cats—leave puncture marks; humans leave teeth marks. Insect bites leave a welt resembling **hives**—a white center on a red base. They are extremely itchy, but the pain and localized reaction usually fade in 3 to 4 hours. Flea bites, normally from a pet, leave itchy welts.

Are they serious?
Animal, human and insect bites are rarely serious. However, they could become infected.

What should I do first?

1 For animal bites, capture the dog or cat, if possible, so authorities can evaluate the animal for rabies.

2 Reassure your child, and try to calm him down.

3 For animal and human bites, wash the wound with soap and water to

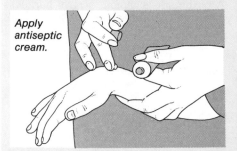

Apply antiseptic cream.

remove blood, saliva or dirt. Apply an antiseptic cream, and put a clean dressing over the wound.

4 For insect bites, apply calamine lotion, ice, baking soda or meat tenderizer to relieve the irritation.

Should I consult the doctor?

Consult your doctor immediately if the bite is from a bat, wild animal or stray animal that is acting strangely. Consult your doctor if the wound is bleeding heavily or if, after 12 hours, the area looks red and swollen.

What might the doctor do?

□ Your doctor will ask you when your child had his last **tetanus** shot. If it is needed, he will give him a tetanus booster.
□ If the wound is infected, your doctor will probably prescribe antibiotics.
□ Your doctor will determine if your child needs to start rabies shots.

What can I do to help?

□ Call animal-control authorities for quarantine of the animal, especially if its rabies-shot status is in question.
□ Emphasize to your child the need to treat animals carefully and not tease them. In most cases, if a pet caused the injury, it will be an isolated incident, and you should not need to get rid of the animal.
□ Clean the carpet, curtains and furniture if you suspect your child has been bitten by fleas. A special flea powder to dust furniture is available from veterinarians. Take your pet to the vet for treatment.
□ If your child is being bitten by mosquitoes, apply an insect repellent to his skin or clothes. At night, spray his room with an insect repellent.

> **SEE ALSO:**
> **Hives,** *page 162*
> **Tetanus,** *page 238*

Blepharitis

Blepharitis is an inflammation of the skin around the edges of the eyelids and usually affects both eyes. Inflammation can become worse if the area is infected; **sties** may occur. Blepharitis is often accompanied by **dandruff** and may be part of a condition known as seborrheic **eczema**.

Is it serious?
Even though the condition may initially be a minor irritant, it should be treated because it can recur.

Possible symptoms

- Red, scaly eyelids.
- Discharge of pus from the eyelids, which dries to look like dandruff clinging to eyelashes.

B

What should I do first?

1 If you notice your child rubbing his eyelids, check to see if the area seems red and scaly or if eyelashes are matted together with pus.

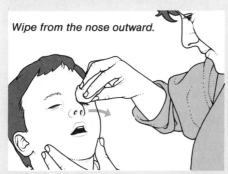
Wipe from the nose outward.

2 Don't use any over-the-counter creams or eye lotions. Wash away the discharge morning and night with warm water and a little baby shampoo. Use a clean cotton swab for each eye. Wipe from the nose outward.

3 Check for **cradle cap** or dandruff on the scalp.

Should I consult the doctor?

Consult your doctor if the washing treatment doesn't clear the scaliness and redness in a week.

What might the doctor do?

☐ Your doctor may prescribe a soothing, anti-inflammatory skin cream to help the inflammation.
☐ If your child has seborrheic eczema, your doctor may prescribe special shampoo and scalp lotion.
☐ If there is an infection, such as a sty, your doctor may prescribe antibiotic ointment or eye drops to remove discharge.

What can I do to help?

☐ Pay particular attention to hygiene. If your child's eyelids are infected, the infection can be easily spread to other members of the family. Wash your hands thoroughly before and after you administer the treatment.
☐ Discourage your child from touching his eyes.
☐ Apply a thin layer of petroleum jelly to your child's eyelids at night. Scales will wash away easily in the morning.

> SEE ALSO:
> **Cradle cap,** *page 100*
> **Dandruff,** *page 107*
> **Eczema,** *page 126*
> **Sty,** *page 231*

Blister

B

A blister is a fluid-filled bubble of skin that forms as a result of **burns** or friction or as a result of exposure to extremes of temperature. Blisters vary in size, depending on the cause. Their purpose is to form a cushion to protect the new layer of skin growing underneath. The fluid is eventually reabsorbed by the body. The outer surface dries out and peels away, leaving the healed skin behind. If the blister is broken before healing takes place, there is risk of infection.

Is it serious?
A blister is not usually serious.

Possible symptoms

● Raised surface of the skin, filled with fluid, which may be 1 or 2 inches across.

What should I do first?

1 Don't prick a blister that has formed as a result of friction, burning or extremes of temperature. Leave intact.

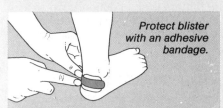

Protect blister with an adhesive bandage.

2 Protect blisters where friction may cause them to burst. For example, if the blister is a result of poorly fitting shoes or wearing shoes without socks, change your child's shoes. Put two pairs of socks on your child, or use special sponge pads or corn plasters to protect the blister.

3 If the blister bursts, keep it clean and dry. Cover it with an adhesive bandage.

Should I consult the doctor?

Consult your doctor if the blister is the result of a scald or **sunburn.** Consult your doctor if the blister becomes pussy, if red streaks extend outward from it, if the skin surrounding it becomes red, tender or swollen or if your child complains of pain.

What might the doctor do?

☐ If the blister is large, it may require bursting. Your doctor will do this.
☐ If the blister is infected, your doctor will prescribe antibiotics.

What can I do to help?

☐ Limit the time your child wears new shoes to help his feet toughen up.

SEE ALSO:
Burn, *page 79*
Frostbite, *page 143*
Sunburn, *page 232*

Words in **bold** are A-Z entries

Boil

A boil is a large, tender, red lump that results when a hair follicle becomes infected with bacteria (*staphylococci*). (If the infection occurs farther up the hair follicle, near the skin's surface, it is called a *pimple*.) The pus-filled lump gradually comes to a white or yellow head and bursts after about 2 or 3 days. It may heal on its own, without bursting, and slowly disappear. Because the hair follicles are so close together, the bacteria can infect a wide area, causing more boils to occur. This is most likely to occur on the face. The boils usually appear on areas where there are pressure points, such as where a collar rubs or on the buttocks.

Is it serious?

Although unsightly, a boil is not serious. However, it can be extremely painful, especially if it develops over a bony area, such as the jaw or forehead, where the skin is stretched tight.

Possible symptoms

- Large, painful, red lump.
- Increasing tenderness and throbbing as pus builds up inside the lump. After a day or 2 the red lump forms a white or yellow pus-filled center, which may or may not burst.

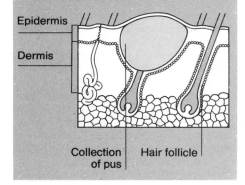

Cross section of skin

What should I do first?

1 If your child complains of throbbing pain, stop him from scratching or touching the area.

Wash boil with warm, soapy water.

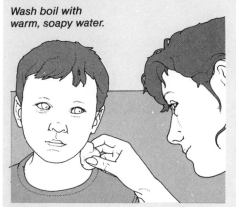

2 Wash the skin with warm, soapy water.

3 Do not squeeze the boil, even when it comes to a head. Squeezing may spread the infection to the surrounding area and make the outbreak much worse.

Should I consult the doctor?

Consult your doctor if the boil does not come to a head in 5 days or if the boil is causing your child a lot of pain because it is situated over a bony area or in an awkward place, such as the armpit. Consult your doctor as soon as possible if you notice red streaks spreading out from the center of the boil. This may mean the infection is spreading.

Boil

◀ Continued from previous page

What might the doctor do?

□ Your doctor will examine the boil and the surrounding area. If he can feel pus under the skin, he will probably lance the boil with a small scalpel and drain the pus, thus reducing pain immediately.

□ If there is an infection and it has spread to the surrounding area, or if your child has had a number of boils over the previous months, your doctor may prescribe an anti-infective cream to treat the skin's surface or an oral antibiotic to prevent the internal spread of the infection.

□ If there are crops of boils, your doctor may prescribe a special antiseptic to put in the bath water.

□ If the boils are recurrent, your child will be referred to a dermatologist to find out the underlying cause.

What can I do to help?

Put a pad over boil to prevent friction.

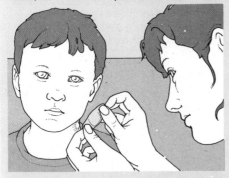

□ If the boil is in a place where clothing might rub it, put a thick pad over the dressing to prevent any friction.

□ Once the boil has burst, keep the area clean.

□ Keep your child's towel and face cloth separate from the family's.

□ If your child has a boil on the buttocks and is still in diapers, try to leave diapers off as much as possible. Change them frequently, and use an antiseptic cream around the site of the boil.

Broken bone

Children's bones are like young, flexible twigs on a tree. They do not snap as easily as the harder bones of an adult. A *greenstick fracture* is most common in children; the bone bends rather than breaks. In this type of fracture, minimal damage occurs in the surrounding tissue. A *simple fracture* is one where the bone breaks in one place. In a *compound fracture,* the bone sticks through the skin and may damage the blood vessels and muscles. If the bone breaks through the skin or is exposed by a deep wound, this is also known as an *open fracture.*

Is it serious?

A broken bone should always be treated promptly by a doctor for a number of reasons. The bone has to be set correctly, and any damage to surrounding organs or tissues has to be repaired. There is also a risk of infection if the break is an open fracture and the bone is exposed to the air.

Possible symptoms

- Pain.
- Swelling around the site of the injury.
- Bruising around the site of the injury.
- Possible deformation of the affected area.
- Inability to move the affected area normally or without pain.

Types of fracture

Greenstick   Simple   Compound

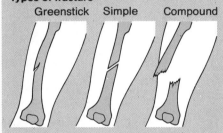

What should I do first?

1 Call an ambulance if the bone is sticking through the skin. Otherwise, take your child to the emergency room.

2 If the broken limb appears bent or curved, don't try to straighten it. If a bone has broken through the skin or if there is a wound leading down to the fracture, drape a sterile dressing or gauze over the wound. Don't attempt any cleaning, and *don't* touch the wound!

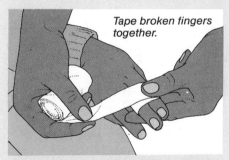

Tape broken fingers together.

3 If there is no bone sticking through the skin, but your child cannot move the affected area without pain, immobilize the joints above and below the break to prevent worsening of the injury. For an arm, put it in a sling. For a leg, tie the knees and ankles together. Take your child to the nearest emergency room if you can, but call an ambulance if the legs are affected, because you may need help.

Continued on next page ▶

Broken bone

B

◀ Continued from previous page

4 Don't give your child anything to eat or drink. He may need a general anesthetic, and this will be delayed if his stomach is not empty.

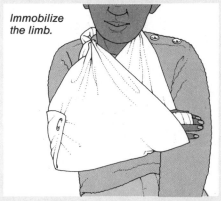

Immobilize the limb.

5 Keep your child warm and as calm as possible while you get medical help. If possible, raise the affected part after immobilizing it.

Should I consult the doctor?

Call an ambulance if the bone is sticking through the skin or if a leg is broken. Take your child to the emergency room if you suspect your child has a broken bone.

What might the doctor do?

☐ The hospital doctor will X-ray your child to determine the extent of the damage. With a straightforward break, the bone will be immobilized by strapping with a tight bandage or by setting it in a cast.

☐ If the break is a compound fracture, the bones will be manipulated into position, under general anesthetic, before being immobilized in a cast.

☐ If there is an open wound with the broken bone, antibiotics will be given to prevent infection.

☐ If your child has a bad break in his leg, he may have to remain in the hospital in traction. The damaged bone is pulled apart and held in the correct position for healing with a system of pulleys and weights.

What can I do to help?

☐ If your child has a cast, make sure it stays dry. Help your child lead as normal a life as possible while the bone heals. Most broken bones in children heal in 6 to 10 weeks, depending on the severity of the fracture.

☐ If your child has to remain in the hospital in traction, make his stay as entertaining as possible by bringing in his favorite games and toys, as well as new books and perhaps a personal cassette machine. Try to stay with him if you can.

Words in **bold** are A-Z entries

Bronchiolitis

Bronchiolitis is inflammation of the smallest airways in the lungs (*bronchioles*). It is usually caused by a virus and occurs in babies under 1 year old. The condition may start as a **cough** or **common cold**. The virus causes the lining of the small airways to swell and fill with mucus. This results in a cough with sputum and often wheezing. A few babies will have breathing difficulties.

Is it serious?
Bronchiolitis can be serious because it may cause breathing difficulties.

Possible symptoms

● Rapid breathing—over 60 breaths per minute.
● Drowsiness.
● Breathing difficulties.
● Raised temperature sometimes.
● Blueness of the lips and tongue.

Area affected

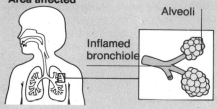

Alveoli

Inflamed bronchiole

What should I do first?

1 If your baby is distressed because of difficulty with breathing, and he starts to turn blue around the lips, treat this as an emergency. Call your doctor immediately, or take your child to the nearest emergency room.

2 Try to soothe your baby. Crying makes the breathing problem worse.

3 If you are breast-feeding, offer the breast frequently. This helps keep your baby's fluid levels up. Offer your bottle-fed baby frequent fluids.

4 Take your baby's temperature every 6 hours and more often if he appears hot. If the temperature is over 100F (37.5C), give your baby acetaminophen to bring his temperature down.

5 Do not smoke anywhere near your baby, and don't allow others to do so.

Should I consult the doctor?

Consult your doctor immediately or take your baby to the nearest emergency room if he has obvious breathing problems or if there is any sign of blueness around his lips and on his tongue. Consult your doctor immediately if you notice any deterioration in your baby's condition after he has had a cold or cough.

What might the doctor do?

☐ Some babies with extreme bronchiolitis are admitted to the hospital overnight for observation.

What can I do to help?

☐ If your baby is admitted to the hospital, stay with him if the hospital allows it.
☐ Try to keep your baby away from other children and adults who have coughs and colds.
☐ Don't smoke around your baby.

SEE ALSO:
Common cold, *page 91*
Cough, *page 98*

Bronchitis

Bronchitis is inflammation of the membranes that line the larger airways leading to the lungs. The condition may arise because a minor upper-respiratory tract infection, such as a **common cold** or **sore throat**, reduces your child's resistance to infection. The infection, which may be viral or bacterial, causes the lining of the air passages to swell and mucus to build up, making breathing difficult. There is also a dry hacking **cough,** which, after 1 or 2 days, produces phlegm. If this is swallowed, the child may vomit.

Is it serious?
In children over 1 year old, bronchitis is not usually serious. In rare cases wheezing and **vomiting** may be troublesome enough to require hospitalization.

Possible symptoms
- Raised temperature.
- Dry hacking cough, changing to a cough that produces green or yellow phlegm.
- Rapid breathing, over 40 breaths per minute, with wheezing.
- Breathing difficulties.
- Loss of appetite.
- Vomiting with the cough.
- Blueness of the lips and tongue.

What should I do first?

1 If your child has recently had a cold, sore throat or ear infection and his condition worsens, take his temperature. If your child has a fever, take his temperature every 4 hours. If it is as high as 103F (39.5C), lower it with tepid sponging, (*see page 31*), or acetaminophen.

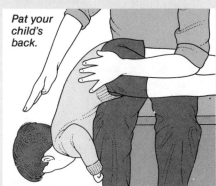

Pat your child's back.

2 If your child is coughing persistently, check if there is any phlegm. If there is, encourage your child to

cough it up. Hold him over your lap if he doesn't understand how to do this. Pat him on the back.

3 Keep offering your child liquids; even if he won't eat, encourage him to take plenty of fluids to prevent the risk of **dehydration** and to keep mucus loose.

4 Don't give him cough suppressants if there is phlegm because he needs to cough it up.

5 Keep your child calm, quiet and warm.

Should I consult the doctor?
Consult your doctor immediately or take your child to the nearest emergency room if your child is breathing with difficulty, drawing in his chest with every breath or if there is any sign of blueness around his lips and on his tongue. This should be treated as an emergency. Consult your doctor if your child's upper-respiratory tract infection gets worse.

Continued on next page ▶

Words in **bold** are A-Z entries

Bronchitis

◄ *Continued from previous page*

What might the doctor do?

☐ If your child is in great distress because of breathing difficulties or vomiting, your doctor may admit him to the hospital so he can be given oxygen to help with breathing or given intravenous fluids to combat dehydration if your child has been vomiting.

☐ Your doctor will prescribe antibiotics if a bacterial infection is present. If your child's bronchitis is caused by a virus, your doctor will advise you on the nursing procedures for bronchitis because there will be no specific medication. Ask your doctor to show you how to help your child cough up the phlegm.

What can I do to help?

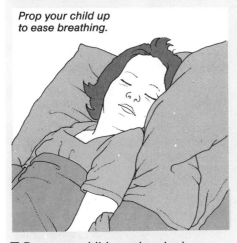

Prop your child up to ease breathing.

☐ Prop your child up when he is sleeping so he can breathe more easily.
☐ Keep your child quiet.
☐ Don't smoke around your child.

SEE ALSO:
Common cold, *page 91*
Cough, *page 98*
Dehydration, *page 109*
Sore throat, *page 222*
Vomiting, *page 255*

B

Bruise

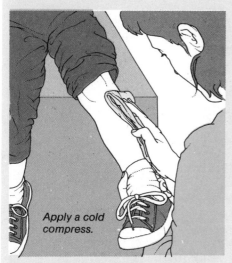

A bruise is a purple-red stain in the skin. It is usually the result of a blow or bump that ruptures the small blood vessels near the skin's surface. Children with fair skin bruise more easily than children with olive skin. It usually takes 10 to 14 days for a bruise to disappear completely. As it fades, it changes to maroon, then green or yellow as the blood pigments break down and are reabsorbed by the body.

Is it serious?
A bruise is rarely serious. If one appears without reason, it may relate to uncommon, but serious, conditions such as **leukemia** and **hemophilia**.

Possible symptoms
- Purple-red mark on the skin that fades to maroon, then green or yellow.
- Tenderness for a day or 2.
- Swelling, if the bruise is over a bone.

What should I do first?

1 A minor bruise needs no treatment, just a hug and reassurance if your child is upset.

Apply a cold compress.

2 If the bruise is large, apply a cold compress, for half an hour or so. This will contain the bruising.

Should I consult the doctor?

Consult your doctor immediately if pain on the site of the bruise gets worse after 24 hours. An underlying bone could be broken. Consult your doctor immediately if a bruise appears spontaneously, with no apparent cause.

What might the doctor do?

□ Your doctor will examine your child to determine if there is a **broken bone** and prescribe accordingly.
□ Your doctor will refer you to a specialist if your child suffers from recurrent bruising or bruises that appear spontaneously. This could indicate hemophilia or leukemia.

What can I do to help?

□ Encourage your child to wear protective gear when he rides his bike.

SEE ALSO:
Broken bone, *page 73*
Hemophilia, *page 157*
Leukemia, *page 173*

Words in **bold** are A-Z entries

Burn

A burn is an injury to the skin following exposure to heat from fire, hot liquids, chemicals, sun or electric current. The severity of a burn depends on the situation and the cause. In a *superficial burn*, there may be just a reddened patch of skin or a fluid-filled **blister**. In a *deep burn*, layers of skin may actually be removed. Only small, superficial burns should be treated at home. No matter how minor a burn may seem to be or how painless, there will always be some damage to the underlying tissue. In deep burns there may not always be pain because nerve endings have been damaged.

Are they serious?

Apart from the most superficial burns, all burns should be treated seriously because of possible scarring, risk of infection and shock. Electrical burns are serious because they may be deep but appear minor.

Possible symptoms

● Raw, red areas.
● Fluid-filled blisters.
● Small blackened area after an electric current has touched the skin.

What should I do first?

For small, superficial burns

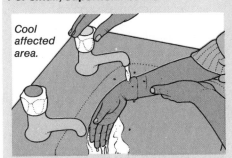

Cool affected area.

1 Cool the affected area by placing it under cold running water for 10 to 15 minutes or as long as your child can tolerate it. Or apply ice cubes if only a small area is affected.

2 Cover the burn with a dressing or a clean handkerchief. The dressing should extend beyond the injured area. Don't apply any cream or lotion, especially butter or fat.

3 Give your child acetaminophen to relieve pain.

4 Raise the affected part slightly so blood flow to the area is slowed. It won't be so painful.

Continued on next page ▶

Burn

B

◄ *Continued from previous page*
For major, deep burns or any electrical burn

1 If the burns were caused by chemicals, put on rubber gloves or use a cloth or towel to keep chemicals from getting on your skin. Remove your child's clothing. Clothes will continue to burn him until they are removed. Do not remove any clothing that is sticking to the skin.

2 If your child has suffered an electric shock, first break his contact with the electricity by turning off the current or knocking him away with a non-conducting material, such as wood (*see page 298*).

3 Cool the affected area by running cold water over the skin.

4 Cover the affected area with a sterile dressing or any clean, non-fluffy material, such as a handkerchief or pillowcase. Don't apply any cream or lotion, especially butter or fat.

5 Lay your child down with his legs raised and supported and his head turned to one side. This prevents

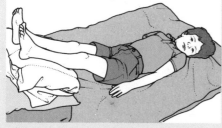

Raise your child's legs.

shock by keeping the essential blood supply in the vital organs. Wrap him in a clean sheet to reduce the risk of infection.

6 Take your child to the nearest emergency room by ambulance or by car if someone else can drive.

Should I consult the doctor?

Only small, superficial burns should be treated at home. Consult your doctor immediately or take your child to the nearest emergency room for all deep burns, burns on your child's face or any electric burn. Consult your doctor as soon as possible if a superficial burn does not heal in a week or if the area becomes red and swollen and pus forms, indicating infection.

What might the doctor do?

☐ The doctor will evaluate the burn and treat your child accordingly.
☐ If the burn has become infected, the doctor will cover the area with an antibiotic dressing. Your child may also be prescribed antibiotics to clear up the infection.

What can I do to help?

☐ Try to safeguard your child against hazards in the home by putting safety guards around the stove and fireplace and childproof plugs in unused electric sockets.
☐ Teach your child about the dangers of fire and burning as soon as he is old enough to understand.
☐ Check labels when you buy clothing for your child to ensure fabric is non-flammable.
☐ Turn pot handles away from the stove edge when you are cooking.
☐ Install a smoke alarm as a warning device.
☐ Install fire extinguishers in your home.
☐ Keep emergency numbers by the phone.

SEE ALSO:
Blister, *page 70*
First aid, *page 297*

Words in **bold** are A-Z entries

Cerebral palsy

Cerebral palsy is the name given to disorders of the brain that occur early in life and result in a lack of full control of physical movement. In some children, the damage occurs in pregnancy. In others, it occurs during a difficult labor, when the baby may suffer from lack of oxygen. Cerebral palsy may also result if a premature baby has severe breathing problems, with bleeding in the brain and lack of oxygen contributing to the condition. Other, less common problems that may damage the parts of the brain controlling movement, thus giving rise to cerebral palsy, are serious head injury and meningitis.

Because the more sophisticated voluntary control centers of the brain do not function in the first months of life, cerebral palsy may not be apparent at birth. After 9 months, it may show itself if the child is slow to sit up, is generally unsteady or cannot grasp and hold an object. Cerebral palsy may affect one side (the right arm and leg), both legs with the arms hardly affected at all or all four limbs and the trunk. Walking is delayed but usually possible. If the limbs tend to be stiff and fixed in certain postures, the child is technically termed "spastic." If he is prone to frequent, purposeless, writhing movements, he is said to be "athetoid."

Cerebral palsy is not a progressive disease which steadily gets worse. It is not uncommon for children with cerebral palsy to have normal intelligence and normal social capabilities.

Possible symptoms

- Delayed sitting.
- Delayed walking.
- Stiffness in arms and legs.
- Persistent abnormal postures.

What can be done?

The treatment for cerebral palsy consists of trying to develop the child's physical, mental and social capabilities to the fullest. It is important for the child to be fully assessed by a specialist and a physiotherapist so he can be given treatment at an early age. Stretching exercises will prevent fixed deformity of the limbs. Orthopedic appliances, such as braces, and in some cases surgery, can improve mobility. Education, such as speech therapy, can compensate for the physical disability.

Where there is no mental handicap, the outlook for the child is extremely good. Children can adjust to severe lack of motor function as long as their intellectual capacity is good and they can make themselves understood. The reaction of the family is of great importance. Parents must guard against feeling sorry for the child. If there are other children in the family, the child must be treated, as nearly as possible, in the same way as they are, though this may be hard for parents. As with all disabled children, the emphasis should be on what the child *can* do rather than on what he cannot.

Chapping

C

Chapped areas are small cracks in the skin that can be painful if they are deep. In nearly all cases, chapping is preceded by drying out of the skin due to its exposure to cold air or to hot, dry air. Chapping is most common in exposed parts of the body such as on the lips, fingers, hands and ears.

Is it serious?
Chapping is not serious.

Possible symptoms

- Small cracks in the skin, most commonly on the lips, fingers, hands and ears.
- Bleeding if cracks are deep.

What should I do first?

1 Keep your child's skin moisturized with cream.

2 Keep your child warm in cold weather, particularly his hands and ears.

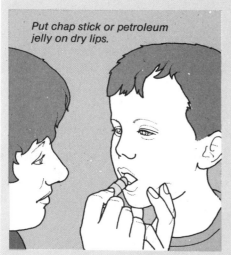

Put chap stick or petroleum jelly on dry lips.

3 In hot, dry air, be sure skin, especially lips, is covered with moisturizer, such as chap stick or petroleum jelly. Try to use a chap stick with sunscreen.

Should I consult the doctor?

Consult your doctor if the chapped areas fail to heal or become red, tender and filled with pus.

What might the doctor do?

☐ Your doctor will give you advice on how to stop your child's skin from drying to the point of cracking. He may prescribe a cream or ointment to keep skin moist.
☐ If there is an infection, your doctor will prescribe antibiotics.

What can I do to help?

☐ Don't wash your child with soap too often during cold weather. Soap dries the skin and makes it rough. Cream or baby lotion can be used instead of soap to cleanse the skin.
☐ Be sure skin is protected in hot, dry air.

SEE ALSO:
Chilblains, *page 84*

Words in **bold** are A-Z entries

Chickenpox

Chickenpox is a common, infectious, childhood disease. It has an incubation period of 7 to 21 days and causes only mild symptoms. Some sufferers may have a headache and fever, though the majority give no indication of illness except for the characteristic itchy chickenpox spots. Spots cover most of the body and can even appear in the mouth, anus, vagina or ears. They appear in crops every 3 to 4 days and quickly develop tiny **blisters** that leave a scab. Your child is infectious until all the lesions are scabbed and there are no new lesions for 24 hours. Spots may leave shallow scars if the child scratches too vigorously.

Is it serious?

Chickenpox is not serious. However, in rare cases, the chickenpox virus may cause **encephalitis** or be complicated by a condition called **Reye's syndrome**.

Possible symptoms

Sites of rash

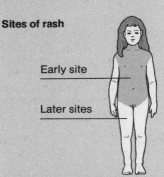

Early site

Later sites

- Small blisters appearing in new batches every 3 or 4 days, usually starting on the trunk, then spreading to the face, arms and legs, and eventually scabbing over.
- Intense itchiness.
- Headache and fever.

What should I do first?

1 Help stop itchiness by applying calamine lotion to the rash or giving your child warm baths in which you have dissolved a handful of baking soda.

2 Keep your child away from other children. Don't send him to school or the nursery until the lesions have scabbed over.

3 If your child has a fever, give appropriate doses of acetaminophen. Aspirin should *not* be used.

4 Cut your child's fingernails short and discourage scratching.

Should I consult the doctor?

Call your doctor to confirm that your child has chickenpox. Consult your doctor as soon as possible if any spots develop a redness with swelling, which indicates infection, or if the child is unable to stop scratching. Consult your doctor immediately if your child is feverish, complains of neckache, or seems confused and lethargic when he should be feeling better.

What might the doctor do?

☐ Your doctor will prescribe an antibiotic cream if the spots are infected.

What can I do to help?

☐ If your child is still in diapers, change them frequently, and leave them off when possible to allow the spots to scab over.

SEE ALSO:
Blister, *page 70*
Encephalitis, *page 128*
Itching, *page 169*
Reye's syndrome, *page 208*

Chilblains

Chilblains are areas of red, itchy skin that result from hypersensitivity to cold. When the skin of a cold-sensitive child is exposed to cold and damp, blood vessels beneath the skin close up to conserve heat. This causes the skin to become numb and pale. When the blood vessels dilate with warmth, the skin becomes red and itchy. Chilblains usually appear on the ankles, hands and feet and on the back of the legs.

Are they serious?
Chilblains are not serious, but they are irritating.

Possible symptoms

● Pale, numb skin, particularly on the hands and feet.

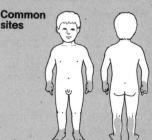
Common sites

● Red, swollen, itchy skin when the area warms up.

What should I do first?

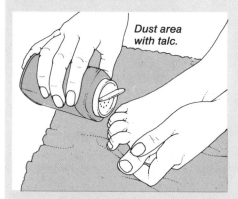
Dust area with talc.

1 If your child has been out in the cold without sufficient warm clothing, then complains of itchiness, dust the skin with talcum powder to ease the irritation.

2 Keep your child from breaking the skin of the affected areas by covering with clothing or putting mittens or gloves on your child.

Should I consult the doctor?

Consult your doctor if chilblains give your child a great deal of discomfort.

What might the doctor do?

☐ Your doctor may prescribe a vaso-dilator cream to improve circulation.

What can I do to help?

☐ Keep all susceptible parts on your child's body covered and warm in damp, cold weather.
☐ Put thermal insoles in your child's shoes to keep his feet warm.

SEE ALSO:
Frostbite, *page 143*

Words in **bold** are A-Z entries

Choking

Choking is the body's way of dislodging a foreign body—usually food or a toy—that has entered the airway instead of the passage to the stomach. If there is enough air getting through to the lungs, your child should be able to cough to bring the object back up into his mouth.

Is it serious?
If your child is coughing very feebly or if he is gasping for breath or turning blue in the face, this is serious. It should be treated as an emergency (*see page 294*). If the airway is totally blocked, your child will become unconscious.

Possible symptoms
- Spluttering or coughing.
- Gasping for breath.
- Blueness around the lips (cyanosis).
- Unconsciousness.

C

What should I do first?

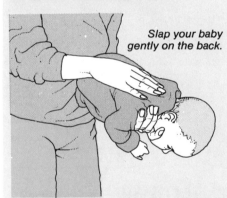

Slap your baby gently on the back.

1 With a baby, lay him along your forearm, with his head held firmly in your hand. His head should be below his chest. Give him 4 light slaps on his back with your other hand. With an older child, lay him across your knee with his head tipped forward, holding him firmly by the waist. Hit him sharply between the shoulder blades.

2 If the foreign body is coughed into the throat and you can see it, try to hook it out with a finger. Hold the child steady with your other hand to prevent him from reinhaling the object. Be very careful not to push the object farther into his throat.

Should I consult the doctor?

Call for an ambulance immediately. While waiting for medical assistance, keep slapping your child on his back to try to dislodge the foreign body. If your child loses consciousness, lay him in the recovery position (*see page 285*) until help arrives. Stay with him, and if he stops breathing, start giving mouth-to-mouth resuscitation (*see page 286*).

What might the doctor do?

The paramedic will try to revive your child if necessary and remove the foreign body if it is still lodged in the throat.

What can I do to help?

☐ Keep small toys out of your child's mouth because of the risk of choking. Toys small enough to be swallowed should not be given to children under 3.
☐ Never leave a small child unattended when he is eating.
☐ Never give peanuts, hot dogs, grapes or popcorn to a child under 3.
☐ Never prop up your baby's bottle.

Circumcision

Circumcision is the surgical removal of the skin at the tip of the penis—the foreskin. It is still the most common surgical procedure carried out on boys, and it is usually done for religious and social reasons. It is required in Jewish and Muslim communities and is the social norm in most Western countries.

A medical reason for circumcision is *phimosis*, but this condition is uncommon. Phimosis is the name given to an abnormal tightness of the foreskin, which keeps the skin from being drawn back over the tip (*glans*) of the penis. A tight foreskin can result in infections, such as **balanitis**, because the penis cannot be properly cleaned. It may also cause problems with urination and pain with erections during adolescence. The foreskin is normally tight until the age of 4 or 5. After this time if the foreskin fails to loosen naturally, circumcision may be recommended.

Is it serious?
Circumcision is not a serious operation. But with any surgery there can be complications. These include infection, bleeding and, very rarely, scarring of the penis.

Possible symptoms
● Foreskin cannot be drawn back over the tip of the penis after age 5.
● Urine does not come out in a steady stream. It either dribbles out slowly, or the foreskin balloons with the pressure of the urine, which sprays out in all directions.

What should I do first?

1 Decide if it is necessary to have your baby boy circumcised. If you are not Jewish or Muslim, and there is no medical reason for it, you may decide not to have the procedure done.

2 If your child is under 4 years old, don't try to pull the foreskin back to check if it's too tight. It will be tight naturally.

3 If your child is over 4, check whether the foreskin is still tight.

4 Note whether your child's urine dribbles out or whether the foreskin balloons with the pressure of urine.

Should I consult the doctor?

Consult your doctor after your baby's birth if you want him circumcised. Arrangements are often made with your pediatrician before the baby is born, so the procedure can be done in the hospital. Consult your doctor if the foreskin has not loosened naturally by the time your child is age 5 or 6. Consult your doctor if you or your child have forced the foreskin back and it will not slide forward again.

Continued on next page ▶

Words in **bold** are A-Z entries

Circumcision

◀ Continued from previous page

What might the doctor do?

☐ Before agreeing to circumcision, your doctor will ask if there is any family history of bleeding, such as **hemophilia.** If there is, a full investigation must be carried out first. Babies who are premature or who weigh less than 5½ pounds should not be circumcised until the pediatrician is satisfied with his condition. If there is any abnormality of the opening of the urethra, circumcision will be postponed.

☐ If your baby is circumcised within the first few days of birth, this is usually done without a general anesthetic. In some hospitals, a plastic bell-shaped device is used with a small ring of plastic that is left on the penis. The ring and extra skin drop off after a few days.

☐ If your older child has a tight foreskin, your doctor will refer him to the hospital for circumcision. The foreskin will be removed under general anesthesia and your child will usually be discharged the same day.

☐ If the foreskin has been pulled back and won't return to its normal position, your doctor will return it. He will probably regularly check your child, in case circumcision is necessary.

What can I do to help?

☐ If necessary, gently wipe the penis with a face cloth and warm water, or just pour warm water over the penis.

☐ Change your baby's diapers regularly. Never leave your baby in a dirty or wet diaper.

☐ Check the penis for bleeding or pus. Consult your doctor immediately if there is any discharge.

☐ If your child is older, let him go without pants. Anything that rubs on a recently circumcised penis will make it sore.

☐ Often a healing circumcision looks infected, but it is just the normal granulation of tissue.

☐ Give your newly circumcised older child a bowl of warm water to pour over his penis when he urinates. There will be some pain urinating for about 48 hours after the operation.

C

SEE ALSO:
Balanitis, page 65
Hemophilia, page 157

Cold sores

C

Cold sores are tiny **blisters** that form around the nostrils, mouth area and, occasionally, genitals. Blisters break open and weep before they crust over and disappear. Cold sores are caused by a virus (*Herpes simplex*) that lives permanently in the nerve endings of some adults and children. Tiredness, stress and a rise in skin temperature—perhaps caused by a cold or by going out in the sun—activate the virus. The first attack takes the form of **mouth sores**. Subsequent attacks, which tend to occur when children are run down, take the form of blisters.

Are they serious?
Cold sores are not serious unless they occur near the eye, where they may cause an ulcer to form on the front of the eyeball.

Possible symptoms

Common sites

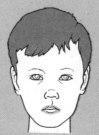

● Raised red area, usually around the nostrils and lips, which tingles and feels itchy. Tiny blisters then form on the spot.
● Weeping blisters that crust over.

What should I do first?

1 After blisters form, stop your child from touching the area. Keep his hands clean.
2 Apply hydrogen peroxide to cold sores to dry them up, or smear a soothing cream, such as petroleum jelly, on them to keep them moist while the virus runs its course. One or the other treatment may give your child some relief.

Should I consult the doctor?

Consult your doctor if a cold sore is near your child's eye. Consult your doctor if cold sores become redder and develop pussy centers, which indicates they have become infected with bacteria. Ask your doctor's advice if your child suffers from recurrent cold sores.

What might the doctor do?

□ If cold sores become infected, your doctor will prescribe an antibiotic ointment that lubricates the area and treats the infection.
□ Your doctor may prescribe an antiviral cream to spread over the affected area regularly to help contain an attack.

What can I do to help?

□ Make sure your child uses his own towel and face cloth.
□ Don't let your child kiss other children. The virus can be transmitted this way.
□ If your child tends to develop cold sores after exposure to sunlight, use sunblock on his lips or nose when he plays in the sun.

SEE ALSO:
Blister, *page 70*
Mouth sores, *page 182*
Sunburn, *page 232*

Words in **bold** are A-Z entries

Colic

Colic, as applied to a baby under 4 months old, describes a crying spell during which the baby's face becomes red and both legs are drawn up to his stomach as if he is in great pain. This crying spell may come in the early evening but can be any part of the day. During the other part of the day the baby is generally contented. Crying can reach screaming pitch and last 1 to 3 hours. It doesn't usually stop as a result of the proven methods of soothing. Colic is so common it is regarded by pediatricians as normal, but for parents it can be difficult to endure. The cause of the apparent spasmodic pain is unknown.

Is it serious?
The fact your baby is contented during the rest of the day means this crying bout is not related to a serious physical problem. Colicky babies are usually healthy and thriving.

Possible symptoms

● Your baby can't settle at a particular time of day and cries no matter what you do to calm him.

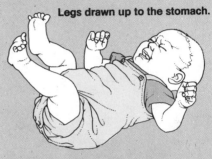

Legs drawn up to the stomach.

● He becomes red-faced and draws his legs up into his stomach as if in pain.
● He may wake from a short sleep with a startled cry.

What should I do first?

1 Try all the methods of soothing your baby that work at other times of the day. This may mean you are constantly offering the breast or bottle, changing diapers, burping, nursing rocking, walking with him held over your shoulder, putting the baby in a sling against your body, playing music for constant background noise or walking him in his stroller or carriage.

Continued on next page ▶

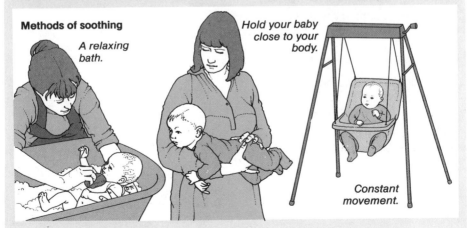

Methods of soothing

A relaxing bath.

Hold your baby close to your body.

Constant movement.

Colic

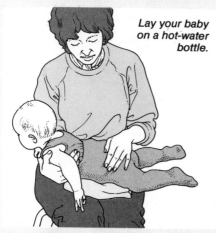

◄ Continued from previous page

Lay your baby on a hot-water bottle.

2 Lay him on his tummy over a hot-water bottle wrapped in a towel.

3 Try using a pacifier. Your baby may need to suck a lot.

4 Don't use any over-the-counter medicines without your doctor's advice.

5 Bathe your baby at the difficult time of the day. A warm bath may relax him and this will pass the time when the crying seems worst.

Should I consult the doctor?

Consult your doctor if you find you can't cope with the nightly crying sessions.

What might the doctor do?

☐ Your doctor will reassure you that your baby is healthy. Your doctor may discuss the use of medication to calm your baby down.

☐ If you are being driven to the breaking point, call your doctor immediately.

What can I do to help?

☐ Make sure you look after yourself. Sleep during the day, if you can, when the baby sleeps. You'll be better able to cope with the bad times.

☐ Invite friends in to share the time of day when your baby cries. A relaxed atmosphere may calm you and your baby.

☐ Talk to other parents who have had colicky babies. When you realize you are not alone and that colic does pass, you may find it easier to bear.

SEE ALSO:
Crying, *page 102*

Words in **bold** are A-Z entries

Common cold

The common cold is caused by a virus. We cannot kill viral infections, so there is no specific cure for a cold. The virus enters the body through the nasal passages and throat, causing inflammation of the mucous membranes lining these passages. This gives rise to the symptoms of a runny nose and **sore throat.** It takes the body's defenses up to 10 days to overcome the virus.

Is it serious?
The common cold is not a serious illness, but because it lowers the body's resistance, complications such as **bronchitis** or **pneumonia** can arise. Regard a cold more seriously in a baby because even minor cold symptoms, like a blocked nose, can cause feeding problems. There is also a greater chance of complications.

Possible symptoms
- Sneezing.
- Runny or blocked nose.
- Raised temperature.
- Coughing.
- Sore throat.
- Aching muscles.
- Irritability.
- Swollen nasal passages.

C

What should I do first?

1 If your child has any cold symptoms, take his temperature to see if he has a fever. If he doesn't have a temperature, keep him warm and comfortable. He doesn't need to go to bed unless he wants to. If he has a temperature around 100F (37.5C). that does not subside within 4 to 5 hours, put him to bed and try to bring his temperature down (*page 31*).

2 Don't give your child any cough medicines without your doctor's advice.

Should I consult the doctor?

Consult your doctor if you think your child has developed another infection. Consult your doctor if your baby isn't eating well because of the cold, seems distressed or if he has a hacking cough that causes sleepless nights.

What might the doctor do?

☐ If there is another infection present, your doctor will treat it accordingly.

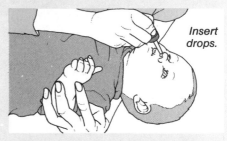

Insert drops.

☐ Your doctor may prescribe nose drops to be given before a feeding. Don't use nose drops more frequently than your doctor suggests or for a long period because they can damage the lining of the nose.
☐ Your doctor may prescribe a cough suppressant or an expectorant for a bad cough.

Continued on next page ▶

Common cold

◀ *Continued from previous page*

What can I do to help?

☐ With a baby, help him breathe more easily by raising his head by elevating one end of the crib.

☐ Give your child plenty to drink. Even if he isn't hungry, make sure he keeps up his fluid intake.

☐ Help your child blow his nose properly by having him blow one nostril at a time.

☐ If possible, keep the air in your child's room humid so the lining of his nose is not further irritated by a dry atmosphere. Do this by using a cool-mist vaporizer.

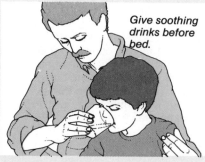

Give soothing drinks before bed.

☐ To ease your child's sore throat and clear nasal passages, give him a warm drink of freshly squeezed lemon juice and water before putting him to bed.

☐ Use saline nose drops to help clear nasal passages. Buy them at the drugstore or make your own. Add ¼ teaspoon of table salt to ½ cup water. Use with a bulb-type syringe that has been washed with soap and water.

Smear on petroleum jelly to prevent chaffing.

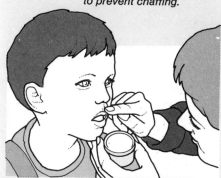

☐ If constant blowing makes your child's nose and upper lip sore, smear on a little petroleum jelly to prevent chaffing.

SEE ALSO:
Bronchitis, *page 76*
Cough, *page 98*
Croup, *page 101*
Fever, *page 139*
Pneumonia, *page 201*
Sore throat, *page 222*

Words in **bold** are A-Z entries

Conjunctivitis

Conjunctivitis is an inflammation of the *conjunctiva,* which is the membrane covering the eyeball and the inside of the eyelid. Inflammation may be caused by a viral or bacterial infection or by injury from a **foreign body** or chemicals. It may be the result of an allergic reaction. The eyes become red and weepy, and they can be painful or extremely itchy. They may be irritated by bright light. The condition, which may affect one or both eyes, can be contagious.

Is it serious?
Although conjunctivitis is not a serious eye infection, it should always be treated by a doctor.

Possible symptoms

● Weepy, red eye that feels sore or itchy.
● Intolerance to bright light.
● Discharge of pus causing eyelashes to stick together after a night's sleep.

Cross section of the eye

Eyelid | Conjunctiva | Eyeball

What should I do first?

1 Check to see if there is a foreign body in the eye. If possible remove it (*see page 133*).

2 Before consulting your doctor, bathe each eye with a solution of 1 teaspoonful of salt in a glass of warm water. Using a new ball of cotton for each eye, begin at the inner corner of the eye and wipe outward.

3 If only one eye is affected, reduce friction between the conjunctiva and other parts of the eye by keeping your child's eye closed. Tape a gauze pad over the area. Hold it in place with a lightly tied bandage.

4 To prevent the spread of infection, encourage your child to keep his hands clean and not to rub his eyes. Be sure you wash your hands after treatment.

Should I consult the doctor?

Consult your doctor if you suspect conjunctivitis, especially if there is sign of injury or reduced vision.

What might the doctor do?

□ If the condition is caused by an infection, your doctor will prescribe antibiotic eye drops or ointment. If the infection does not respond to treatment within a few days, your doctor may refer you to an eye specialist.
□ If the irritation is caused by an allergy, such as **hay fever**, your doctor will prescribe anti-inflammatory eye drops and antihistamine medication.
□ If there is a foreign body in your child's eye, your doctor will remove it.

What can I do to help?

□ Emphasize to your child that the infection can be spread by his hands. He should keep them clean and use a separate face cloth and towel.
□ If your child suffers from hay fever, keep him away from freshly mown lawns during the worst hay fever months.

SEE ALSO:
Eye, foreign body in, *page 133*
Hay fever, *page 149*

Constipation

A child who is constipated passes hard, pebblelike stools; this may cause discomfort or actual pain when the stools are passed. Constipation describes the consistency of stools, not the regularity or frequency of bowel movements. During babyhood, constipation is unlikely for breast-fed or bottle-fed babies. When a child starts on solid food, he can suffer from constipation if his diet doesn't contain enough fresh fruit and vegetables and liquids. By the age of 2 or 3, constipation may become a problem for a different reason. Some parents are so obsessed with the importance of "regularity" during the period when their child is learning bowel control that the child reacts by holding back the stools as a weapon in a battle of wills.

As a guiding rule, if your child is happy and healthy and shows no signs of discomfort when going to the bathroom, and if his stools are not as hard as pebbles, he is not constipated.

If your child's stools are hard and dry during a period when, because of illness he is feverish or has been vomiting, this is not true constipation. The body compensates for loss of fluid from vomiting or fever by absorbing water from the stools.

Possible symptoms
- Hard pebblelike stools.
- Pain in the lower abdomen.
- Blood on diaper or underpants.

Bowel activity should return to normal when the illness has passed.

If your child involuntarily soils his underpants when he was previously toilet trained, you might think he has diarrhea. It could be a condition called **encopresis**. Chronic constipation leads to hard stools becoming impacted in the intestine, and loose, watery stools leak out past the blockage.

Is it serious?
Occasional constipation is not serious and can be avoided by means of a diet high in fiber. Chronic constipation can be a serious matter because it can cause problems in later life. Blood in the stools may indicate an underlying disorder and should always be cause for concern.

What should I do first?

1 If your child strains when passing stools and complains of pain, check the consistency of what he has passed.

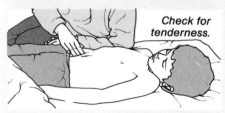

Check for tenderness.

2 If he complains of stomach pain, check the right side of his abdomen below his navel (*see page 56*) for possible **appendicitis**.

Should I consult the doctor?

Consult your doctor immediately if you suspect appendicitis. Consult your doctor if your child complains of pain when moving his bowels. Consult your doctor immediately if you notice red blood on his diaper or underpants. The passing of a large, dry stool may have injured his anal passage. This is called an *anal fissure*, and your child may be reluctant to pass any more stools for fear of the pain caused by this tiny crack.

Continued on next page ▶

Words in **bold** are A-Z entries

Constipation

◀ *Continued from previous page*

What might the doctor do?

☐ Your doctor will prescribe a very mild laxative, specially formulated for babies and children, which is safe to give your child for short periods. He may also give you advice about your child's diet.

☐ If your doctor suspects an anal fissure, he will examine your child's rectum. If there is a tiny crack, he will gently lubricate the anal passage to help the skin to heal.

What can I do to help?

☐ Never use laxatives unless your doctor advises it. They encourage a lazy bowel.

☐ If your child has been prescribed a laxative, follow the manufacturer's instructions precisely.

☐ Make sure your child is getting plenty to drink.

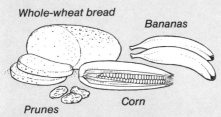

Whole-wheat bread

Bananas

Prunes

Corn

☐ Include as many natural, unprocessed foods in your child's diet as possible, with some fiber in the form of whole grains—such as brown rice and whole-wheat bread—and fresh fruit and vegetables. It is not a good idea to scatter bran over your child's meal. This can deplete certain minerals in the diet. A few stewed prunes or dried figs can produce a soft stool within 24 hours.

☐ Don't leave your child sitting on the toilet for long periods of time. He may get the impression he must perform or lose your approval.

☐ Don't rush your school-age child when he is in the bathroom. if the pace is hectic in the morning, make sure he has time to go to the bathroom without the anxiety of having to rush off to school. Many children prefer to go to the bathroom at home because they find the school facilities lack privacy.

C

> **SEE ALSO:**
> **Appendicitis,** *page 56*
> **Encopresis,** *page 129*

Convulsion

A convulsion is a fit or seizure that occurs when the brain reacts abnormally. During the convulsion, your child loses consciousness, becomes rigid for some seconds while holding his breath, then rhythmically bends and straightens his arms and legs for some minutes. Your child may cry out at the beginning of the seizure. He may urinate, and he may defecate. When the convulsion is over, your child will be in a confused state, and he may want to sleep.

The most common cause of convulsions is a raised temperature that accompanies a viral infection, such as **influenza**. This type of convulsion is called a *febrile convulsion* and generally occurs between the ages of 6 months and 6 years. The tendency to suffer from febrile convulsions often runs in families. Convulsions may also be caused by **meningitis**, **encephalitis** and, rarely, chemical abnormalities of the blood, such as a low level of glucose in diabetics. **Epilepsy** is another cause of convulsions. Sometimes no specific cause is found.

Is it serious?
Though dramatic and frightening, a convulsion is not life-threatening. But it should be treated seriously.

Possible symptoms
- Sudden rise in temperature.
- Crying out and loss of consciousness.
- Rigid phase with the breath held.
- Rhythmic jerking of the limbs.
- Urination and/or defecation.
- Confusion and drowsiness.

What should I do first?

1 As soon as your child loses consciousness, place him in the middle of the floor. With a baby or young child, roll him on his side. This ensures that his tongue does not fall backward and obstruct the airway.

2 Don't leave your child alone for a moment.

3 Don't try to stop him from jerking his limbs. You may injure him.

4 Don't try to force anything into his mouth, and never try to force the teeth apart if they are clenched.

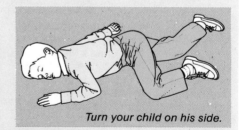
Turn your child on his side.

5 As soon as the violent movements have ceased, turn your child on to his side so he won't inhale his tongue or saliva.

Continued on next page ▶

Words in **bold** are A-Z entries

Convulsion

◀ *Continued from previous page*

Should I consult the doctor?

Consult your doctor immediately as soon as the convulsion has passed. If there is someone with you, ask him to call the doctor while you stay with your child. If the seizure hasn't stopped in 15 minutes, take your child to the nearest emergency room or call an ambulance if you are alone. Any fit that continues for 20 minutes should be stopped with an anti-convulsant drug.

What might the doctor do?

☐ If the convulsion is continuing, your doctor will give your child an injection of an anti-convulsant drug.
☐ If your child is under 2 when he has his first convulsion, your doctor may perform tests to exclude any serious cause of convulsions, such as meningitis.
☐ With an older child, your doctor will admit him to the hospital if the cause of the convulsion is not clear. Tests will be carried out, and the doctor will advise whether or not anti-convulsant drug treatment is needed.
☐ Your doctor will give you advice on

how to avoid a rapid rise in temperature in the future. Children usually outgrow febrile seizures by age 6.

C

What can I do to help?

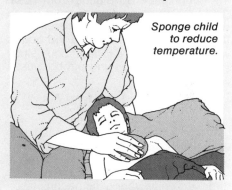

Sponge child to reduce temperature.

☐ Once the convulsion is over, if your child is feverish and has a high temperature, remove his clothing and cool his skin with tepid sponging (*see page 31*). Cover him with a light sheet when he sleeps.
☐ Don't give him any over-the-counter medicines without your doctor's advice.
☐ Stay calm.

SEE ALSO:
Encephalitis, *page 128*
Epilepsy, *page 131*
Fever, *page 139*
Influenza, *page 165*
Meningitis, *page 177*

Cough

A cough is a symptom of an illness or the body's way of reacting to an irritant in the throat or air passages. A cough may bring up phlegm from the chest and clear mucus from the air passages, such as during an attack of **asthma**. The cause of a dry cough is usually an irritation and not an infection. The irritation provoking the cough may be mucus from nasal discharge from a **common cold** which dribbles down and tickles the back of the throat. A dry cough may be the body's way of bringing up a foreign body stuck in the windpipe. Coughing may be caused by "passive smoking." If adults around your child smoke a lot, the smoke may irritate your child's throat and cause a cough. Children may also adopt a cough or clearing of the throat as an attention-seeking device, when it becomes a **tic** or mannerism.

Is it serious?
A cough is not usually serious, although it can be irritating. However, a cough that causes breathing difficulties is serious and should be treated as an emergency.

What should I do first?

1 If your child is coughing up phlegm, lay him over your lap as if you were going to spank him. Pat him gently on the back to help him bring up the phlegm.

2 Don't give your child cough-suppressant medicines for a cough that produces phlegm unless your doctor tells you to.

3 If you think that your child has a foreign body in his throat, call your doctor.

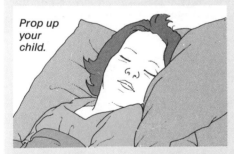
Prop up your child.

4 If your child is coughing at night, prop him up with pillows. This will keep mucus or nasal discharge from dribbling down the throat.

5 Use a cool-mist vaporizer in your child's room.

6 Give your child lots of fluid.

Should I consult the doctor?

Consult your doctor if your child's cough doesn't get better in 3 or 4 days or if your child is not getting any sleep at night. Consult your doctor immediately if your baby develops a hacking cough or if your child's coughing is accompanied by rapid, labored or wheezy breathing. This could be **croup** or asthma.

What might the doctor do?

☐ If your child's cough is part of an infection, such as **pneumonia**, **bronchitis** or croup, your doctor will prescribe antibiotics to clear up the infection.

☐ If your child is suffering from a viral infection, your doctor will tell you how to relieve the symptoms and help your child cough up phlegm.

Continued on next page ▶

Words in **bold** are A-Z entries

Cough

◄ *Continued from previous page*
☐ If the cough is part of an asthmatic condition, your doctor may prescribe bronchodilator drugs that help to widen the air passages.

☐ Your doctor may prescribe nose drops to administer sparingly to your child before he goes to bed. These drops ease congestion and prevent mucus from dripping down the back of the throat.

☐ Your doctor may prescribe a cough medicine—either a cough suppressant (to soothe the throat and reduce irritation) or an expectorant (to encourage coughing up of phlegm).

What can I do to help?

☐ Keep your child quiet and warm so that any minor infection does not spread into the lungs and cause a more serious condition, such as bronchitis.

☐ Don't let your child run around too much during the day. Breathlessness can bring on a coughing attack.

Lying on the stomach cuts down mucus irritation.

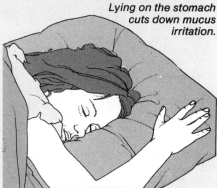

☐ Encourage your child to lie on his stomach or his side at night so mucus will not drip into his throat.

☐ Keep the air in your child's room moist by using a cool-mist vaporizer.

☐ Don't smoke at home, and don't take your child into smoky atmospheres.

SEE ALSO:
Asthma, *page 61*
Bronchitis, *page 75*
Common cold, *page 91*
Croup, *page 101*
Otitis media, *page 195*
Pneumonia, *page 201*
Tic, *page 242*

Cradle cap

Cradle cap is a thick, yellow encrustation on the scalp. It occurs mainly in babies, although children up to 3 can have cradle cap. Yellow scales appear in small patches, or they can cover the entire scalp. Cradle cap is not due to poor hygiene. Babies who suffer from it probably just have oily scalps.

Is it serious?
Cradle cap may appear unsightly, but it is harmless unless it is accompanied by red, scaly areas elsewhere on your baby's body, in which case he may have seborrheic **eczema**.

Possible symptoms
● Thick, yellow scales over part or all of the scalp.

What should I do first?

1 Don't try to remove the scales with your fingers. If they don't brush out, they must be loosened first.

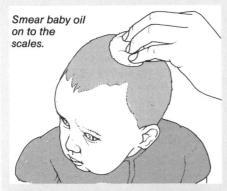

Smear baby oil on to the scales.

2 Smear a little baby oil or petroleum jelly on your baby's scalp, and leave it on overnight. This makes the scales soft and loose, and they will wash away easily when you shampoo.

3 Don't use anti-dandruff shampoos without consulting your doctor.

Should I consult the doctor?

Consult your doctor if the cradle cap is accompanied by red, scaly areas elsewhere.

What might the doctor do?

□ Your doctor may prescribe a special shampoo to prevent scales from forming. He can tell you how to prevent cradle cap with brushing and other home treatments.

What can I do to help?

□ You can keep scales from building up by brushing your baby's hair daily, even if there is little of it, with a soft-bristled brush.

□ Never rub the scalp hard when washing your child's hair. Shampoo removes dirt in seconds, so you only need to bring the shampoo to a lather, then rinse it thoroughly. Use a soft hairbrush to clean scales from hair and head.

□ If the cradle cap becomes hard and thick, you may have to continue the baby oil or petroleum jelly treatment over a 10-day period to loosen all the encrustations.

SEE ALSO:
Dandruff, *page 107*
Eczema, *page 126*

Words in **bold** are A-Z entries

Croup

Croup is the name given to the sound made when air is breathed in through a constricted windpipe, past inflamed vocal cords. It usually occurs only in young children who are susceptible because their air passages (*bronchi*) are narrow and become blocked with mucus when inflamed. This is most common with a virus, such as a **common cold**, or an infection, such as **bronchitis**. In rare cases, croup can be caused by an inhaled foreign body. In older children, the condition is less serious and is called **laryngitis**.

The first attack of croup can come on quickly, usually at night, and it may last a couple of hours. Your child will have a croaking cough and labored breathing.

Is it serious?
If your child has a severe attack of croup, he could develop breathing difficulties— a serious condition called **epiglottitis**.

Possible symptoms
● Croaking cough.
● Labored breathing when the lower chest caves in at every inhalation.
● Wheezing.
● Face turning gray or blue.

C

What should I do first?

1 Stay calm, and try to calm your child so he won't panic.

2 Your child's air passages will be soothed by moist air. If the air outside is cool and damp, take him to the window or go outside. Get him to take a deep breath of air. Or take him into the bathroom, and turn on the hot water to make it steamy.

3 Prop your child up in bed with pillows, or hold him on your lap. It will be easier for him to breathe if he is sitting up.

4 Use a cool-air vaporizer in the bedroom when he sleeps.

Should I consult the doctor?

Consult your doctor immediately if your child's skin turns gray or blue and he has to fight for breath. Consult your doctor to tell him that your child has croup.

What might the doctor do?

□ In a serious attack your doctor will give your child oxygen.
□ You will be given advice on what to do should there be another attack.
□ If the attack is caused by a foreign body, your doctor will remove it.

What can I do to help?

□ In future attacks, stay with your child and follow your doctor's instructions.

SEE ALSO:
Bronchitis, *page 76*
Common cold, *page 91*
Epiglottitis, *page 130*
Laryngitis, *page 172*
Nose, foreign body in, *page 188*

Crying

All babies cry, but some cry much more often than others. Crying is a baby's means of communicating, and you will soon be able to recognize whether the crying is a symptom of an illness or not. By the age of about 6 weeks, your baby will be spending part of his waking hours by taking in his surroundings and making gurgling noises instead of just crying, feeding and sleeping. By 6 months, babies spend most of their waking time playing and communicating in many ways. A baby who cries rather than plays by the age of 6 months may be an anxious child or cutting teeth or one who is easily bored, or, in a minority of cases, one who has some physical illness.

Most healthy babies stop crying as soon as they are fed, cuddled and made comfortable. If there are certain times of the day (especially in the evening) when nothing stops the crying, your baby could be suffering from **colic**, which is a common cause of crying in babies. A toddler will usually cry only for obvious reasons of illness or injury or as a show of temper.

Is it serious?
Crying is not normally serious. Persistent crying can, however, cause problems if you become angry, resentful and over-tired. A crying baby is a common cause of child abuse.

What should I do first?

1 Pick your baby up, and cuddle him or give him a pacifier if he finds sucking calming.

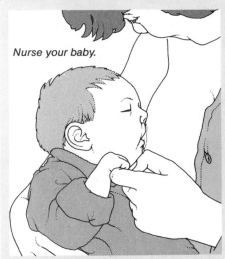

Nurse your baby.

2 Feed him, or give him a few sips of cool water.

3 Change your baby's diaper, and make sure he isn't too hot or too cold in what he's wearing.

Should I consult the doctor?

Consult your doctor if the crying seems to be following a different pattern from usual and there are symptoms of illness, such as **diarrhea**, **fever** or **vomiting**. Consult your doctor as soon as possible if you are exhausted by your active baby and you think you might lash out in anger.

What might the doctor do?

☐ Your doctor will question you about the extent of your baby's crying. He will examine your baby for any symptoms of illness. If your baby is healthy, your doctor will probably reassure you there is nothing to be worried about.

Continued on next page ▶

Words in **bold** are A-Z entries

Crying

◀ Continued from previous page

What can I do to help?

□ Try to think of ways to help yourself if you have a particularly demanding baby. Rest whenever you can, and take turns with your partner if your baby is difficult at night and seems to need little sleep.

□ Stay calm yourself. Try not to resent your baby's need to be close to you.

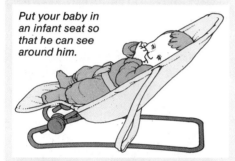

Put your baby in an infant seat so that he can see around him.

□ Keep your baby near to you when he is awake. Put him in an infant seat or stroller so he can watch you work. Carrying him round in a sling may also give him comfort and reassurance.

□ Always go to your crying baby. Parental apathy and lack of response may result in a failure to thrive, and it can inhibit a child's attachment to others in later life. There is no such thing as spoiling a baby.

SEE ALSO:
Colic, *page 89*
Common cold, *page 91*
Diarrhea, *page 114*
Failure to thrive, *page137*
Fever, *page 139*
Sleeplessness, *page 219*
Teething, *page 235*
Vomiting, *page 254*

Cuts and scrapes

A *cut* is an injury that breaks the skin and underlying tissue, causing bleeding. A *scrape* is an injury in which the skin's surface is not actually broken, but rubbed so blood vessels under the skin's surface ooze slightly. Small cuts and scrapes can be treated at home and should be cleaned up and dressed to keep germs from entering and causing infection. The best dressing for a cut or scrape is a Band-aid or a piece of sterile gauze held in place with adhesive tape so air can get to the wound. Skin-closure tapes can be used to hold edges of a cut together and prevent it from healing in a gaping shape.

Are they serious?
Few cuts and scrapes are serious enough to need medical attention. However, if a cut is deep (from a nail or an animal bite) there is a risk of **tetanus** or another infection developing. If it is very bloody, there is the risk of shock (*see page 293*).

What should I do first?
If the wound is large and bleeding

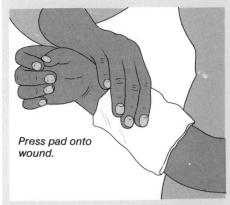

Press pad onto wound.

1 Get medical help immediately. Take your child to the emergency room. Before you go, press directly on the wound with a clean pad, a handkerchief or your hand if you have nothing else.

2 Elevate the affected part to slow the blood flow. Lay your child down.

3 Place a sterile dressing over the cut, and tie it in place with a knot directly over the wound to keep pressure on it until you get medical help.

If the wound is a scrape or small

1 Hold the affected area under cold running water or wash with soap and water or antiseptic lotion.

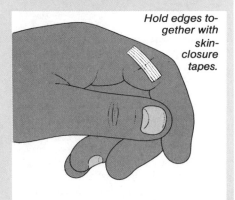

Hold edges together with skin-closure tapes.

2 Pat the skin dry. Hold the edges of a straight cut together with special tape to help the cut heal neatly. Apply a sterile dressing, held in place with adhesive tape, if the cut or scrape needs it.

3 If the scrape is on the face or is very large, such as the result of a bike accident, take your child to the doctor.

Continued on next page ▶

Words in **bold** are A-Z entries

Cuts and scrapes

◀ Continued from previous page

Should I consult the doctor?

Consult your doctor immediately or take your child to the emergency room if the wound is large, if bleeding persists after 10 minutes of pressure, if the wound is very deep and bloody, if the wound is on the face, if the wound is gaping, if there is dirt or a foreign body in the wound that you can't get out, if the wound is deep but only has a small puncture hole in the skin or if your child was playing in an area where horses are kept and the wound has been contaminated by dirt or gravel. Consult your doctor if, after a day or 2, you notice red streaks extending from the wound. This could be a sign of infection.

What might the doctor do?

☐ The doctor will clean the wound and stitch it, if necessary, under local anesthetic. Any wound on the face will be stitched to minimize scarring.
☐ If the bleeding doesn't stop, a blood vessel may have been lacerated. This will be tied off under anesthesia.

☐ If there is a deep wound or a wound contaminated with dirt, the doctor will ask you when your child last had a tetanus booster. If there is any doubt, your child will be given a tetanus shot.
☐ If there is any sign of infection, the doctor will cover the area with an antibiotic dressing. He may also prescribe antibiotics to be taken by mouth to eradicate the infection.

What can I do to help?

☐ Change the dressing daily.
☐ When you change the dressing, check for any redness extending from the wound. If you notice any, contact your doctor immediately.
☐ A scrape covers a larger area, and it may need to be protected against rubbing. Use a dry gauze strip, and hold it in place with surgical tape. Don't apply any adhesive dressing directly on the wound because it will be painful to remove.
☐ Put a handful of salt in your child's bath water to clean the skin and help stop infection.

C

> **SEE ALSO:**
> **Tetanus,** *page 238*

Cystic fibrosis

Cystic fibrosis is a rare, congenital disease. It is present at birth and inherited from both parents. If the mother and father are healthy but each carries one defective gene for cystic fibrosis, each child conceived has a 25% chance of inheriting two defective genes and being born with cystic fibrosis. The disease causes several glands in the body to be defective, particularly the glands in the lining of the bronchial tubes. Instead of producing the normal thin mucus, the bronchial glands produce a thick, sticky phlegm, which results in blockages of the air passages. This leads to lung infections. When small parts of the lungs collapse, pneumonia results. This is a common and recurrent infection in those who suffer from cystic fibrosis.

In the intestines of a child with cystic fibrosis, the pancreas fails to produce certain vital enzymes. These enzymes aid digestion, breaking down food so it can be absorbed by the body more easily. Lack of these digestive enzymes means food is poorly absorbed, which leads to diarrhea and foul-smelling stools. Food goes undigested, so the body does not absorb many of the nutrients essential to good health. The child will be small, underweight and fail to thrive. Bouts of diarrhea may alternate with constipation, which can actually block the intestine.

Possible symptoms

- Recurrent chest infections with a cough and some breathing difficulty.
- Diarrhea, alternating with constipation.
- Greasy, foul-smelling stools.
- Failure to thrive.
- Swollen abdomen and wasted limbs.

What can be done?

There is no cure for cystic fibrosis, but early detection of the condition lessens the chance of permanent damage to the lungs. The definitive test for cystic fibrosis is a sweat test because there is an increased salt level in the sweat of sufferers. This test will be done on brothers and sisters of a child with cystic fibrosis or if a baby has recurrent bouts of pneumonia or fails to thrive. It will be carried out when the baby is old enough to perspire (around 3 months).

A child with cystic fibrosis has to have a special diet, vitamin supplements and enzyme replacements, which can be taken by mouth. Fat in the diet is reduced. Physiotherapy and breathing exercises must be done daily to loosen and drain mucus from the lungs. Respiratory infections are treated with antibiotics or bronchodilator drugs.

Words in **bold** are A-Z entries

Dandruff

Dead cells are shed constantly from the surface of the skin. On the scalp they tend to become trapped and build up because of the hair. This buildup of cells is called dandruff. It is not a disease, nor is it infectious or contagious. It is simply a variation of normal. The amount of dandruff seen on the scalp varies from person to person according to how rapidly skin cells are shed and how oily the scalp is. If the scalp is irritated, such as by vigorous rubbing or a medicated shampoo, more dead cells will be shed. If dandrufflike flakes appear on your child's eyelashes, this may be part of seborrheic **eczema** called **blepharitis**.

Is it serious?

Dandruff is never serious, but it can be embarrassing, particularly as your child gets older. Although dandruff cannot be prevented if your child's scalp is oily, it can be controlled.

Possible symptoms

● Flakes of white skin that are present on the scalp and can be easily wiped away with a finger.
● White flakes that appear on your child's shoulders after hair brushing.

What should I do first?

1 If you notice white flakes on your child's scalp, try to wipe them off with your fingers. If they move easily, this is dandruff. If not, don't pick at them. It could be an infestation of **lice**.

2 Wash your child's hair every other day using baby shampoo.

3 Don't rub the scalp hard to get rid of the dandruff. It will make it worse by stimulating the scalp.

Should I consult the doctor?

Consult your doctor if home treatment fails to get rid of the white flakes.

What might the doctor do?

☐ Your doctor will reassure you and advise you how to cope with dandruff.

What can I do to help?

☐ Don't use anti-dandruff shampoos more than once every 2 weeks. Avoid those containing selenium; it can irritate a child's scalp. Wash your child's hair with baby shampoo at other times.

SEE ALSO:
Blepharitis, *page 69*
Eczema, *page 126*
Lice, *page 174*

Deafness

D

Deafness, either partial or total, is usually the result of a congenital defect—that is, present at birth—or caused by an illness during a baby's first 6 weeks of life. There may be some residual hearing, so with early diagnosis, hearing aids will help develop speech. A child may also suffer a non-permanent hearing loss as the result of an ear infection, such as **serous otitis** or **otitis media,** or a buildup of wax in the external ear canal. The problem for parents is how to recognize whether their child is deaf or not. It isn't easy to spot deafness in a newborn baby. But sometimes deaf newborns won't have a "startle-reflex" to loud noises. All babies make gurgling noises up to the age of 6 months, and loud noises don't seem to disturb very young babies. However, after about 4 to 6 months, a deaf baby may become quiet because he hasn't been stimulated by his own or other people's voices.

Is it serious?

If a baby can't hear properly, learning to talk can be a difficult task. Much of a child's language is learned before he starts to talk. Therefore, the longer a child is unable to hear, the greater will be the delay in communicating. Even partial deafness will interfere with speech development.

What should I do first?

Test your child's hearing by making a fairly loud noise when his head is turned away from you. See if he turns around. Make sure he doesn't see you. If he responds, make the sounds gradually fainter and note the level at which he ceases to hear.

Should I consult the doctor?

Consult your doctor if you suspect a hearing problem. Consult your doctor immediately if your child has had an ear infection and you detect some hearing loss.

What might the doctor do?

☐ Your doctor will perform routine hearing tests on your child and examine his ears. If a hearing difficulty is diagnosed, your doctor will refer your child to an ear, nose and throat specialist for audiometric tests to determine the extent of deafness. In most cases, a hearing aid will be fitted. A baby can wear a hearing aid from 6 months. Your child will probably have aids fitted to both ears even if the hearing difficulty is only in 1 ear. You will be given advice on how to talk to your child.
☐ If the deafness is the result of repeated attacks of otitis media, surgery may be necessary to insert tubes and drain the fluid causing the deafness.

What can I do to help?

☐ Don't be concerned if your child remains silent for several months after hearing aids are fitted. It may take time for him to start to use what he's hearing by way of speaking the words.
☐ Communicate with your child as clearly as you can. Make sure everyone else talks to him clearly but never shouts.
☐ If your child goes to school, ask if he can sit near the front of the class so his school work won't suffer as a result of the disability.

SEE ALSO:
Otitis media, *page 195*
Serous otitis, *page 216*
Wax in the ear, *page 258*

Words in **bold** are A-Z entries

Dehydration

The body needs adequate supplies of water to carry essential minerals through the system, both to maintain body chemistry and to get rid of waste. If your child loses water by **vomiting**, **diarrhea** or **fever** and doesn't take in enough to replace the lost fluid, dehydration will result. Diarrhea in babies can cause dehydration to develop fairly quickly because the intestines don't have enough time to absorb water.

Dehydration will be compounded if your baby or child has a fever and is losing fluid through perspiration. The body chemistry will be upset, essential nutrients will be lost and the volume of blood circulating through the body will be dangerously lowered.

Is it serious?

Dehydration can be extremely serious and should be treated as an emergency. If dehydration is advanced, it can lead to brain damage and even death.

Possible symptoms

- Dry mouth and lips.
- Lethargy.

Affected area

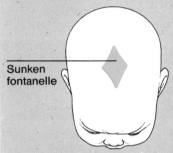

Sunken fontanelle

- Sunken fontanelle in a child under 18 months.
- Concentrated urine (dark-yellow color) or dry diapers.
- No urine output for 8 to 12 hours.

D

What should I do first?

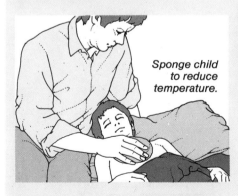

Sponge child to reduce temperature.

1 If your baby or child has diarrhea or is vomiting, check his temperature to see if he has a fever. If he does,

try to reduce it with tepid sponging (*see page 31*)

2 If your bottle-fed baby is not weaned, stop all formula. Give him only water instead for 6 hours. Continue breast-feeding your baby. If the diarrhea or vomiting hasn't stopped after this time, consult your doctor immediately.

Continued on next page ▶

Dehydration

◀ *Continued from previous page*

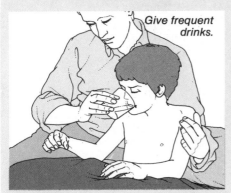

Give frequent drinks.

3 Encourage your child to take small amounts of fluids frequently— every 10 minutes or so. Don't give your child milk or undiluted fruit juices. Give your child Pedialyte, Lytren or Gatorade (diluted with equal parts water) to replace the essential minerals that have been lost. As a rough guide, your child should drink at least 3 fluid ounces (90ml) of liquid per pound of body weight in the first 24 hours of vomiting or diarrhea.

4 Never give your child over-the-counter medicines for vomiting or diarrhea unless prescribed by your doctor.

Should I consult the doctor?

Consult your doctor immediately if your baby or child has had diarrhea for an extended period of time or is vomiting and cannot keep fluids down.

What might the doctor do?

☐ In severe cases, your child may be admitted to the hospital and given essential fluids by intravenous drip.
☐ Your doctor may advise you to change your baby's formula to one that contains no sugars. Your baby may be allergic to the sugar in milk (lactose).

What can I do to help?

☐ Check the color of your child's urine. When it becomes clear and more regular, this is a good sign his body-fluid levels are getting back to normal.
☐ When the illness has passed, gradually reintroduce formula. Dilute your baby's normal formula with 3 times the usual amount of water. Gradually reduce the water in the feeding to the normal proportion over the next 2 or 3 days.
☐ If you are weaning your child to solid foods, keep his fluid intake up. Breast and formula milk have a high percentage of water. When they are replaced by solid foods, your child's fluid levels may be reduced without your realizing it.
☐ For an older child, when you reintroduce solids, do it gradually. Start with low-residue foods, such as apple sauce, bananas, rice, sugar cookies, bread, cooked carrots, eggs, ground meat, noodles, cooked peaches, cooked pears, potatoes and cooked peas.

SEE ALSO:
Diarrhea, *page 115*
Dysentery, *page 121*
Fever, *page 139*
Food poisoning, *page 141*
Gastroenteritis, *page 144*
Lactose intolerance, *see page 171*
Vomiting, *page 255*

Words in **bold** are A-Z entries

Diabetes mellitus

There are two forms of diabetes. One affects children and young adults, and one comes on in middle age. Both are due to a lack, or relative lack, of insulin in the body. Insulin is the hormone responsible for the normal metabolism of glucose in the body. (We take in glucose in our diet mainly in the form of carbohydrates.) Insulin is produced by the pancreas, and it then promotes the absorption of glucose from the blood into the cells of the body and into the liver for storage. If the body is short of insulin, glucose collects in the blood, and the body cells are deprived of their energy source. To make up for this deficiency, the body starts to break down fats and proteins to replace the lost energy. This means of energy production leads to weight loss and results in the production of poisonous waste substances, such as acetone and ketones.

Diabetes can start quite suddenly, for no known reason, though the disease may be inherited. Excess glucose spills over into the urine, so the first symptom in a child is frequent passing of large amounts of urine. Because of the loss of body fluid, your child will be very thirsty, and he may start to wet the bed because he's drinking more.

D

Possible symptoms

- Large amounts of urine passed frequently, possibly leading to bed-wetting.
- Increased thirst.
- Weight loss.
- Irritability and listlessness.
- Fruity smell on the breath, signifying presence of acetone.
- Reduced resistance to infection.

What can be done?

The diagnosis is confirmed by blood tests that show an inappropriately high blood level of glucose. Your child will be admitted to the hospital to get blood sugar under control and to learn how to administer insulin injections. The digestive juices destroy insulin taken by mouth. Many children over the age of 5 confidently give themselves injections, under parental supervision. Insulin injections must be given daily, sometimes twice a day, to keep blood glucose levels to normal limits.

Your child will need a special diet to keep the glucose steady in the blood throughout the day. No meals should be missed.

Your doctor will provide you with special equipment to use at home to test blood sugar every day. The result will help you adjust the dose of insulin to keep glucose levels normal in your child.

It is advisable for your child to wear a bracelet or medal engraved with details of his condition in case problems occur when you are not with him. Diabetic children are extremely prone to infectious illnesses, so consult your doctor as soon as your child gets any infection. Infection can change your child's insulin requirements.

Diaper rash

Diaper rash is a skin condition that affects the area normally covered by a baby's diaper. It can occur whether diapers are fabric or paper. The skin may be slightly red or broken and inflamed with pussy spots.

There are several causes of diaper rash, but it is most commonly caused by urine and stools being left in contact with the skin for too long. The bacteria in the baby's stools break down the urine and release ammonia, a strong irritant. In such cases, the rash starts around the genitals. If left untreated, the skin becomes tight and shiny, and pustules may develop. There is always a strong smell of ammonia from the diaper.

Diaper rash can also be caused by inadequate drying after bathing your baby. In such cases, the rash is usually confined to the skin creases at the top of the thighs. If the rash covers most of the diaper area, and you use fabric diapers, the rash may be due to an allergic reaction to chemicals in the laundry detergent or to fabric softener. This reaction may be an early sign of a form of **eczema**, called *atopic eczema*.

Possible symptoms

- Redness over diaper area.
- Redness that starts around the genitals and is accompanied by a strong smell of ammonia.
- Tight, papery skin with inflamed spots that have pussy centers.
- Redness that starts around the anus and moves over the buttocks and onto the thighs.

A rash that starts around the anus and moves over the buttocks and onto the thighs may not be diaper rash but a yeast infection, such as **thrush**.

Is it serious?
Diaper rash is not serious and can be easily prevented and treated at home.

What should I do first?

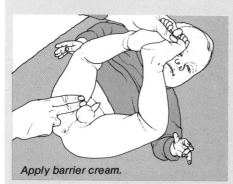

Apply barrier cream.

1 As soon as you notice any redness on your baby's bottom, wash his bottom with warm water, and dry it thoroughly. Apply liberal quantities of barrier cream, such as zinc oxide or petroleum jelly, to keep urine from irritating his skin.

2 Change diapers and wash your baby's bottom frequently (at least every 2 to 3 hours and as soon as he's had a bowel movement). Leave your baby without diapers whenever possible.

3 Use disposable diaper liners next to your baby's skin because these let urine pass through to the diaper while remaining dry next to the baby's bottom.

4 Don't use talcum powder around your baby's genitals. It cakes when wet and irritates the skin.

Continued on next page ▶

Words in **bold** are A-Z entries

Diaper rash

◀ *Continued from previous page*

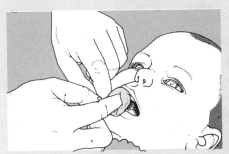

Wipe away any white patches.

5 Check inside your baby's mouth. If you notice white patches, try to wipe them off with a clean hand-kerchief. If they leave raw, red patches, your baby has oral thrush. This may have caused the diaper rash.

Should I consult the doctor?

Consult your doctor if the measures on the previous page fail to clear the rash in 2 or 3 days or if you think your baby has thrush.

What might the doctor do?

□ Your doctor will determine the cause of the rash and will make sure you've been using the most suitable home treatment. He may suggest alternatives.

□ If the diaper rash has become infected, your doctor may prescribe an antibiotic ointment.

□ If your baby has the first signs of eczema, your doctor will question you about detergents you use and may advise you to change to another brand if your present brand contains a biological component. He may pre-scribe a cortisone ointment to be used sparingly.

□ If the rash is caused by thrush, your doctor will prescribe an antifungal cream.

What can I do to help?

□ Continue to change your baby's diapers frequently, especially after a bowel movement.

□ Try to use plastic pants as little as possible. They keep air from circulating around your baby's bottom.

□ Wash your baby's fabric diapers thoroughly. Use very hot water, and rinse them 2 or 3 times to get rid of all traces of detergent and ammonia.

□ If the condition is recurrent, change the type of diapers you use from one brand of paper diapers to another or to cloth (or vice versa).

D

SEE ALSO:
Eczema, *page 126*
Thrush, *page 239*

Diarrhea

Consult your doctor if your child has loose, watery bowel movements for an extended period, especially if he's under 1 year old. Consult your doctor if diarrhea is accompanied by vomiting or fever.

D

Accompanying symptoms	Common causes
Your child has no symptoms except looser-than-normal-stools and seems perfectly happy and contented.	He has possibly eaten too much of a food high in dietary fiber, such as prunes. Unless the stools are very watery or frequent, this is not true diarrhea, and you have no need to worry.
Your child has a sudden attack of diarrhea and vomiting, with a slight fever.	He possibly has "gastric" flu, *page 144*, or a bowel infection, such as **Food poisoning**, *page 141*.
Your child has no symptoms other than the diarrhea, but he is anxious about something, for example, school.	Stress can cause attacks of diarrhea in older children. If this happens often, consult your doctor.
Your child has other symptoms, such as a cough, for which your doctor has given him medicine.	Many medicines cause diarrhea. Consult your doctor, but don't stop giving the medicine.
Your child has abdominal pain around his navel and to the lower right side of his groin.	**CONSULT YOUR DOCTOR IMMEDIATELY** Your child may have **Appendicitis**, *page 56*.
Your baby has severe abdominal cramps, is vomiting and his bowel movements are filled with blood and mucus, resembling red jelly.	**CONSULT YOUR DOCTOR IMMEDIATELY** Your baby may have a bowel blockage called **Intussusception**, *page 168*.
Your child soils his underpants involuntarily, even though he is toilet trained.	This is not true diarrhea, but possibly a condition called **Encopresis**, *page 129*.

Words in **bold** are A-Z entries

Diarrhea

Diarrhea is the frequent passage of loose, watery stools. It is a sign of an irritation of the intestines in which the intestines contract more than normal, hurrying food along. Consequently, there is not sufficient time for water from food to be absorbed into the body, and this can result in profound water loss or **dehydration**, especially in babies.

Babies on formula or breast milk pass liquid stools many times a day. This is normal. Once a baby begins to eat solid food, bowel movements become firmer and more regular. Loose, frequent stools can result when a baby or child eats too much of a certain food that is rich in fiber, such as fruit, or they may be a symptom of an infection. Infection in the intestines is commonly caused by viruses or bacteria. Food may have been contaminated with bacteria (**food poisoning**), or an infection from contaminated stools may have been spread to the mouth by unwashed hands. The infection need not be in the intestines; diarrhea can also be the symptom of a non-intestinal infection, such as an ear infection or **influenza**, when the diarrhea may be accompanied by a **fever**.

Ironically, stools similar to those of diarrhea may be caused by **constipation**. If an older child soils himself, this may be because constipation has resulted in a blockage, but the liquid stools manage to escape past it. This involuntary soiling is called **encopresis**.

Is it serious?
Diarrhea in a baby is always serious because of the dangers of dehydration. Diarrhea accompanied by **vomiting** in a young child is serious for the same reason, especially if it is accompanied by fever and sweating. Diarrhea in which stools are greasy and foul-smelling can be a symptom of a more serious, long-term condition, such as **cystic fibrosis**, in which there is a failure by the body to absorb the nutrients in food.

What should I do first?

1 If your baby is under 1 year old and has had diarrhea for 6 hours, consult your doctor.

2 Don't give your child any food or milk, but give frequent drinks of diluted fruit juice or a commercially prepared electrolyte solution, such as Pedialyte, Lytren or Gatorade.

3 Check your child's temperature to see if he has a fever. Reduce any fever with tepid sponging (*see page 31*).

4 Check the chart on page 114 to find a possible cause of your child's diarrhea.

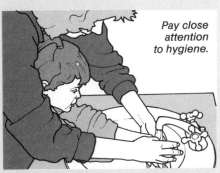

Pay close attention to hygiene.

5 Pay close attention to hygiene. Diarrhea can spread throughout the family if your child doesn't wash his hands after going to the bathroom or if you don't wash yours after changing his diapers, if he wears them.

Continued on next page ▶

Diarrhea

◀ *Continued from previous page*

Should I consult the doctor?

Consult your doctor immediately or take your baby to the emergency room if he has any symptoms of dehydration—decreased urine output, sunken eyes, listlessness. Consult your doctor immediately if your child has diarrhea with fever and vomiting or if the stools are greasy or contain mucus or blood.

What might the doctor do?

☐ After diagnosing the cause of the diarrhea, your doctor will treat the illness accordingly.

☐ As a rough guide, your child should drink at least 3 fluid ounces (85ml) of liquid per pound of his body weight in 24 hours while he has diarrhea. For a bottle-fed baby, your doctor will probably suggest you replace formula with a commercially prepared electrolyte solution, then slowly reintroduce the formula. If your baby is breast-fed, you may be advised to continue breast-feeding.

☐ If your baby is seriously ill, your doctor may admit him to the hospital so he can be given fluids intravenously.

What can I do to help?

☐ Be meticulous about hygiene. Wash your hands before preparing food and after changing your baby's diapers.

☐ Advise anyone with diarrhea to stay away from your baby.

☐ When the diarrhea has cleared up, introduce bland foods, such as yogurt, bananas, rice, cereal, carrots and soups.

SEE ALSO:
Constipation, *page 94*
Cystic fibrosis, *page 106*
Dehydration, *page 109*
Encopresis, *page 129*
Fever, *page 139*
Food poisoning, *141*
Influenza, *page 165*
Otitis media, *page 195*
Vomiting, *page 255*

Words in **bold** are A-Z entries

Diphtheria

Diphtheria is a rare bacterial infection that is very contagious. It produces a **sore throat** accompanied by a **cough**, which sounds like **croup**. If diphtheria is not treated promptly, the infection may allow **pneumonia** to develop and heart failure due to paralysis of the cardiac muscle. Muscles of the limbs may weaken and become paralyzed. A fine web of gray membrane forms over the tonsils and may make breathing difficult if the windpipe is affected. A child should be protected from the infection in the first year of life with a series of injections. Immunization has virtually eradicated the disease.

Is it serious?
Diphtheria is always serious because it is life-threatening and contagious.

Possible symptoms
- Mild fever.
- Sore throat.
- Cough and hoarseness of voice.
- Headache.

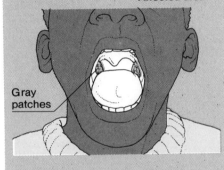

Affected area

Gray patches

- Enlarged tonsils, covered by grayish patches.

D

What should I do first?

1 Diphtheria rarely occurs spontaneously. There may be other cases in the community, so be on the alert if you hear of any outbreaks and your child has not been immunized.

2 Check to see if your child's tonsils are swollen and coated with grayish patches.

Should I consult the doctor?

Consult your doctor immediately or take your child to the emergency room if you suspect diphtheria.

What might the doctor do?

☐ Your doctor will admit your child to the hospital immediately, and your child will be given antibiotics. If there are breathing difficulties, a tracheotomy will be performed to keep airways open. This is a surgical procedure to insert a tube into the windpipe, bypassing the blockage in the throat.

What can I do to help?

☐ Help medical staff trace all known contacts of your child so they can be checked for immunity.
☐ Make sure your child is immunized, even if he's just had diphtheria, because the disease does not give immunity.

SEE ALSO:
Cough, *page 98*
Croup, *page 101*
Pneumonia, *page 201*
Sore throat, *page 222*

Dizziness

D

Dizziness is a feeling of unsteadiness and spinning around. When a child is out of breath, he may feel a bit dizzy because there is a relative lack of oxygen to his brain. Your child may also feel dizzy if he is suffering from **anemia**. A bang on the head or a **convulsion** may be preceded by dizziness. Under normal circumstances, dizziness should pass in a few minutes and your child will feel alright again.

Is it serious?
Momentary dizziness is not serious, but if dizzy spells fail to pass in 12 hours, call your doctor.

What should I do first?

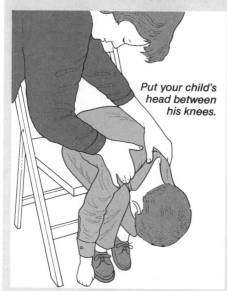

Put your child's head between his knees.

1 Sit your child down, and put his head between his knees to increase the flow of blood and oxygen to his brain. Tell him to take a few deep breaths.

2 Try to keep your child quiet and calm.

3 Note how long he says the dizzy feeling lasts.

Should I consult the doctor?

Consult your doctor immediately if your child experiences dizzy spells over a 12-hour period but has no other symptoms. Consult your doctor if your child complains of dizziness after strenuous activity.

What might the doctor do?

☐ After examining your child, your doctor will determine the cause of the dizziness. If the dizziness is a symptom of a more serious disorder, your doctor will treat it accordingly.

What can I do to help?

☐ Discourage your child from boisterous play if he complains of feeling dizzy.

SEE ALSO:
Anemia, *page 53*
Convulsion, *page 96*
Head injury, *page 151*

Words in **bold** are A-Z entries

Down's syndrome

Down's syndrome is the most common chromosomal abnormality. Children with Down's syndrome have 47 chromosomes instead of the normal 46 in each cell. The extra chromosome, chromosome 21, usually comes from the mother's egg. The incidence of Down's syndrome babies rises sharply with maternal age, but a form of screening in pregnancy, called *amniocentesis*, can identify the condition in the fetus. Termination of the pregnancy can be performed if the parents wish. An amniocentesis test, in which a sample of amniotic fluid is extracted and examined for abnormalities, is usually offered to all pregnant women 35 or over who can then choose to have the pregnancy terminated.

Children with Down's syndrome share obvious physical characteristics. The bridge of the nose is wide, and the eyes generally have an upward slant (hence the former term for this condition, *mongolism*). The hands are short and broad, there is a deep crease running across the middle of the palm and there may be a large gap between the first and second toes. In addition, Down's children may suffer some degree of mental retardation, and about 50% have a heart defect. A smaller number are born with a blockage in the intestine.

Possible symptoms

● Small, upward-slanting eyes, nose with a wide bridge, short, broad hands with a deep crease across palm, and a gap between first and second toes.

● Some degree of mental retardation.
● Often even-tempered and affectionate nature.

What can be done?

Down's children are invariably outgoing, happy and affectionate, with a love of music and rhythmic games. The degree of mental handicap varies widely, and a few children are within the normal intelligence range. Modern theories reject the idea that Down's children should all be educated in special institutions. The education of a Down's child must be determined by the mental retardation of the particular child. Excellent work in Israel has shown with a sympathetic and stimulating environment, these children can develop alongside normal children and be accepted by them and by the community as a whole.

Many Down's children need help with dressing and feeding, while others can hold down jobs and make a contribution to society if they are given the chance and encouragement. It is important that parents of a Down's child help him rise above the social stigma that used to be attached to Down's syndrome. As with all disabled children, the emphasis should be on what a Down's child can do rather than what he cannot.

Your pediatrician can refer you to local agencies for help, such as child-stimulation programs and support groups.

Drowsiness

Drowsiness in a normally alert child can be a symptom of **fever**, hypothermia (when the body temperature falls below normal) or **dehydration**. It can also occur before or after a **convulsion** or as a result of medication, such as antihistamine drugs, which commonly cause drowsiness.

Is it serious?

If a child is drowsy but contented, is eating well and has a normal temperature, there is no cause for alarm. If a child becomes drowsy while recovering from an infectious disease, such as **measles** or **chickenpox**, and he complains of headache and neck pain, it could be **encephalitis**, **meningitis**, or **Reye's syndrome**, which are serious conditions.

What should I do first?

1 Check your child's temperature. If it is over 100F (37.5C) he has a fever. If it is under 95F (35C) he will be suffering from hypothermia.

2 If drowsiness is accompanied by vomiting and diarrhea, keep your child's fluid intake up to prevent the risk of dehydration.

3 Check to see if your child has received a blow to the head.

4 Check if your child has a headache or neckache.

5 Smell your child's breath, and check the liquor cabinet—he may have drunk alcohol. Check the medicine cabinet for sleep-inducing drugs.

6 If your child has had a convulsion, let him rest after the seizure has passed.

Should I consult the doctor?

Consult your doctor if your child's temperature is over 100F (37.5C) or below 95F (35C) and he is difficult to rouse. Consult your doctor immediately if he has a headache or neckache or if he has just had measles, chickenpox or **mumps**.

What might the doctor do?

☐ After examining your child, your doctor will determine the cause of the drowsiness and will treat your child accordingly.

What can I do to help?

☐ Keep all medicines and alcohol out of your child's reach.

SEE ALSO:
Chickenpox, *page 83*
Convulsion, *page 96*
Dealing with hypothermia, *page 300*
Dehydration, *page 109*
Encephalitis, *page 128*
Fever, *page 139*
Head injury, *page 151*
Measles, *page 176*
Meningitis, *page 177*
Mumps, *page 184*
Reye's syndrome, *page 208*

Words in **bold** are A-Z entries

Dysentery

Dysentery is the inflammation of the lining of the large bowel and causes the symptoms of **diarrhea** and **fever**. The bacteria are passed with feces. If the hands are not washed after going to the bathroom, they become contaminated. The bacteria will be passed on by contact.

Is it serious?
Dysentery is especially serious in children because of the risk of **dehydration**.

Possible symptoms

- Gripping abdominal pain.
- Loose, frequent bowel movements, every hour or so, which may contain mucus, blood or pus.
- Fever.
- Nausea.
- Lethargy and weakness.
- Vomiting.

D

What should I do first?

1 If you are living or traveling in an area of poor sanitation and your child has frequent, loose stools, check the stools for blood, mucus or pus. If you notice any, consult a doctor immediately.

2 Check your child's temperature to see if he has a fever.

3 Give your child frequent drinks to keep fluid levels up.

Should I consult the doctor?

Consult a doctor immediately if you notice mucus, blood or pus in your child's loose bowel movements. Consult a doctor if your child's bowel movements are still loose after 12 hours or if his urine is infrequent and concentrated (dark-yellow color).

What might the doctor do?

☐ The doctor will treat your child for dehydration and send a sample of your child's feces to the lab for investigation.
☐ If your child has an extremely severe case of dysentery, he might be admitted to the hospital and put on an intravenous drip to counteract the dehydration.

What can I do to help?

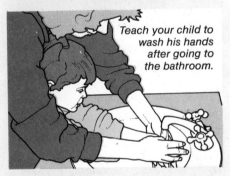
Teach your child to wash his hands after going to the bathroom.

☐ Insist on meticulous hygiene when your child goes to the bathroom.

SEE ALSO:
Dehydration, *page 109*
Diarrhea, *page 115*
Fever, *page 139*

Dyslexia

Dyslexia is a specific learning disorder concerning reading and writing. Dyslexic children have problems interpreting visual symbols. Although their hearing and vision are normal and they have the manual dexterity to form letters, they may have difficulty perceiving letters or words in their proper order or they may confuse certain letters, such as *b* and *d*, and *p* and *q*. Dyslexic children may misread words that have a similar overall configuration, and may disregard punctuation and read monotonously. They often produce incorrect spellings that reflect the sound of words (lite for light) or that transpose letters (lihgt for light).

Dyslexic children are average or above-average intelligence, though many appear clumsy. If the problem is not diagnosed and handled properly, the frustration with learning can lead to behavioral problems and unnecessary emotional strain.

Possible symptoms

- Written words that have the letters misplaced.
- Poor reading ability.
- Difficulty in visualizing words, even those just seen.

What can be done?

Dyslexia need not be educationally disabling. Provided the problem is detected early and the child is given instruction from educational psychologists and teachers (this may be done within a regular school), he should be able to overcome reading problems. Dyslexic children are helped if emphasis is given to their non-verbal skills and activities. The artistic and creative side of their development should be stressed so they never become insecure and develop behavioral problems to mask feelings of inadequacy.

Parents and teachers must persist if they believe a child has been wrongly assessed as being of low intelligence or as having some problem with sight or hearing. Dyslexic children need to be encouraged and have their confidence boosted and this is best done by parents and teachers.

Words in **bold** are A-Z entries

Ear, foreign body in

The most common foreign bodies that become stuck in a child's ear are small objects, like beads, pushed in by the child or by a playmate. Very rarely, a small insect may fly or crawl into the ear and be trapped there.

Is it serious?

Any foreign body in the ear that cannot easily be removed should be regarded as serious. It may cause an infection of the external ear canal, **otitis externa**, or damage the eardrum.

What should I do?

1 If the object is small and soft, try to remove it with a pair of tweezers. If you cannot grasp it without poking around in the ear, leave it alone and consult your doctor immediately.

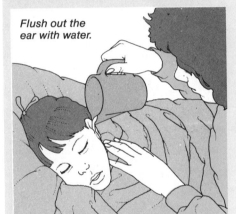

Flush out the ear with water.

2 If the foreign body is an insect, lay your child on his side with the affected ear on top. Pour warm water into the ear. The insect should float out. If it is a tic, pour warm oil into the ear to suffocate the tic. The dead tic will come out with the oil.

Should I consult the doctor?

Consult your doctor immediately if the object cannot be removed or if your child complains of pain and tenderness in his ear.

What might the doctor do?

☐ After examining your child's external ear canal, your doctor will remove the object. He will treat any damage to the skin or any infection that may have been caused by the foreign body.

What can I do to help?

☐ Don't let a child under age 4 play with small objects he could put in his nose or mouth, risking choking.

E

SEE ALSO:
Otitis externa, *page 193*

Earache

There are a number of causes of earache. The most common cause is an infection of the middle ear called **otitis media**. This is especially true in children under 6 because the tube that runs from the throat to the ear—the Eustachian tube—is relatively short. Infections of the nose and throat can be easily spread to the middle-ear cavity. A baby may not be able to isolate the site of the pain and will scratch and rub the side of his face if the pain is severe. A child may complain of earache if he is suffering from **toothache** or **tonsillitis**, when the glands in his neck are swollen or if he has been out in a cold wind without protective headgear. Earache with intense pain will result from an infection of the outer ear (**otitis externa**) if, for example, a foreign body has been poked into the ear or if a **boil** has developed or from frequent swimming.

Is it serious?
Earache, plus loss of hearing, is serious. If the condition is not diagnosed and treated, it could cause permanent damage to the middle ear. This could result in a loss of hearing that will affect your child's speech development and learning ability.

Possible symptoms
● Pain in the area around the ear.
● A temperature of over 100F (37.5C).
● Discharge of pus from the ear.
● Hearing loss.
● Inflammation of the tonsils.
● Pain when the ear is touched.
● Swollen glands.
● Rubbing and pulling of the ear in a young child.

Cross section of the ear

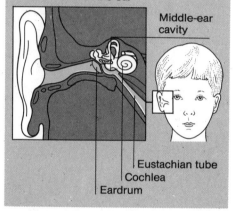

Middle-ear cavity

Eustachian tube
Cochlea
Eardrum

What should I do?

1 Take your child's temperature to see if he has a fever.

2 Check whether there is any discharge from the ear.

3 Check whether your child's hearing is diminished. To do this, call his name quietly when his head is averted. See if he turns around.

4 Examine the back of your child's throat to see if the tonsils are abnormally enlarged or red (*see page 243*). This could indicate tonsillitis.

5 Check to see if there is any inflammation in the outer ear cavity. Inflammation could be caused by a boil. Do not put anything into the ear, not even a cotton swab.

6 Never use ear drops or put anything into your child's ear, unless your doctor advises it.

Should I consult the doctor?

Consult your doctor if your child complains of earache; most earache is caused by infection. Consult your doctor immediately if your child is in pain with a high fever, especially if you notice a discharge from the ear. Consult your doctor immediately if your child is too young to tell you he's in pain but is crying, pale, irritable, not sleeping well and possibly pulling or rubbing one of his ears.

Continued on next page ▶

Words in **bold** are A-Z entries

Earache

◀ Continued from previous page

What might the doctor do?

☐ Your doctor will examine your child to determine the cause of the earache. If it is caused by a bacterial infection, your doctor will probably prescribe antibiotics.

What should I do to help?

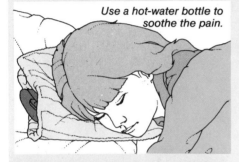

Use a hot-water bottle to soothe the pain.

☐ Place a hot-water bottle, covered by a towel, next to your child's ear to relieve pain. Do this only when the source of the earache is not a boil.
☐ Prevent water from entering the ear during bathing until the infection has cleared up.
☐ If an oral antibiotic is prescribed, be sure and give *all* medication exactly as prescribed.

SEE ALSO:
Boil, *page 71*
Ear, foreign body in, *page 123*
Otitis externa, *page 193*
Otitis media, *page 195*
Tonsillitis, *page 243*
Toothache, *page 245*

Eczema

Eczema is an allergic skin condition that produces an extremely itchy, dry, scaly, red rash on the face, neck and hands, and in the creases of the limbs.

The most common form of eczema in children is *atopic eczema*, which often develops when a baby is about 2 to 3 months old or at around 4 to 5 months, when solid foods are introduced. Certain foods, such as dairy products, eggs and wheat, and skin irritants, such as pet fur, wool or detergents, are among the main causes. An attack of eczema can also be triggered by stress or an emotional upset. It is common for eczema to be followed by other allergic complaints, such as **hay fever** and penicillin sensitivity. It is also common for a child with eczema to suffer from **asthma**. Although most children grow out of eczema by age 3, the associated allergic conditions will probably remain.

Another form of eczema, called *seborrheic eczema*, occurs where the sebaceous glands are numerous. This is most commonly found on the scalps of young babies (**cradle cap**), on the eyelashes and eyelids (**blepharitis**), in the external ear canal (**otitis externa**) and in the greasy areas around the nostrils, ears and groin. This seborrheic eczema is not as itchy as atopic eczema, and it responds well to treatment.

Is it serious?
Eczema is not serious, although it can be very irritating.

Possible symptoms

● Dry, red scaly skin that is very itchy. The rash usually starts off as minute pearly blisters beneath the skin's surface.
● Sleeplessness if the itchiness is very bad.

Affected areas

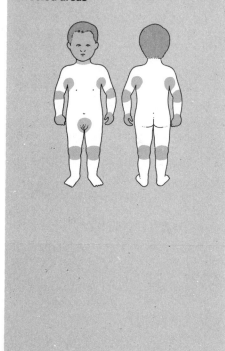

What should I do first?

1 If your child is scratching, inspect his neck, scalp, face, hands and the creases of his elbows, knees and groin for any rash.

2 Keep his fingernails short to minimize the possibility of breaking the skin. If the skin is broken, put mittens or gloves on him to prevent further scratching.

3 If you've just started weaning your breast-fed child, return to breast-feeding only until you have seen your doctor. If you have been using formula, return to that.

4 Apply an oily calamine lotion to ease irritation and soothe the skin. Don't apply any astringent lotions.

Continued on next page ▶

Words in **bold** are A-Z entries

Eczema

◀ Continued from previous page

Should I consult the doctor?

Consult your doctor if you suspect eczema.

What might the doctor do?

☐ Your doctor will question you on your family's medical history, particularly whether anyone has ever suffered from eczema-related conditions, such as asthma or hay fever.

☐ Your doctor will ask you about any changes in your child's diet, whether you have recently changed detergent, whether you have just brought a pet into the house and whether your child wears natural or synthetic fibers next to his skin.

☐ Your doctor will probably advise you to avoid foods, such as dairy products, eggs and wheat, that may have caused the reaction.

☐ If you have just started weaning your baby from the breast or bottle, your doctor may recommend that you avoid dairy products and continue breast-feeding or formula. If you don't want to do this, he may recommend that you wean your baby to soy formula.

☐ Your doctor may prescribe weak steroid creams to reduce inflammation and itchiness. These should be used only sparingly on a child's skin.

☐ Your doctor may prescribe anti-histamine medication to help your child sleep if the itching causes sleeplessness.

☐ If your child has scratched the eczema and the skin has become infected, your doctor may prescribe antibiotics.

☐ Your doctor will advise you to add bath oil to your child's bath water and stop using soap. Soap can be an irritant to the already-sensitive skin. The oil will help to keep your child's skin supple and less dry.

What can I do to help?

☐ Use an emollient cream when your child washes. This will keep his skin soft, prevent it from drying and cut down itchiness. Keep your child's skin well-lubricated with creams and lotions at all times.

☐ Keep your child's fingernails short and put gloves or mittens on his hands at night so scratching doesn't break the skin and cause infection.

☐ Make sure all your child's clothes are rinsed thoroughly to remove all traces of detergent.

☐ Consider giving your pet away if the reaction is caused by pet fur.

☐ Dress your child with cotton next to his skin when possible.

☐ Don't eliminate any foods from your child's diet without your doctor's supervision.

☐ Remove as many irritants from your child's environment as possible. For example, feather and down pillows can be a source of irritation.

E

SEE ALSO:
Asthma, *page 61*
Blepharitis, *page 69*
Cradle cap, *page 100*
Diaper rash, *112*
Hay fever, *page 150*
Itching, *page 169*
Otitis externa, *page 193*
Sleeplessness, *page 219*

Encephalitis

Encephalitis is an inflammation of the brain. The most common causes in children are viral infections, such as **chickenpox** or **mumps.** The major symptoms of encephalitis are fever, headache, pain when the neck is stretched and intolerance to bright light. Very rarely, encephalitis occurs as a severe reaction to the **whooping cough** vaccine. If your child is irritable, has a fever, and especially if he has a **convulsion**, this could be the first sign of sensitivity.

Is it serious?
Encephalitis is always serious, and in babies it can be fatal.

Possible symptoms
- Fever.
- Severe headache.
- Pain when the neck is stretched.
- Intolerance to bright light.
- Loss of appetite and perhaps vomiting.
- Drowsiness.
- Listlessness.
- Confusion, and, in later stages, convulsion and coma.

What should I do first?

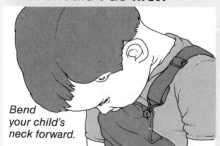

Bend your child's neck forward.

1 If your child is recovering from an infectious disease and seems unwell with a fever, ask him to bend his neck forward so his chin touches his chest. See if this causes him pain.

Should I consult the doctor?

Consult your doctor immediately if you suspect encephalitis.

What might the doctor do?

☐ Your child will be admitted to the hospital where diagnostic tests will be carried out to determine the severity of the disease. These will include a lumbar puncture in which spinal fluid is drawn under anesthesia for examination.

☐ The hospital staff will treat the accompanying symptoms of encephalitis, and your child should be better in a couple of weeks.

What can I do to help?

☐ Once your child has been discharged from the hospital, keep him comfortable and well-fed.
☐ If there has been any weakness or stiffness of your child's muscles, you may have to do exercises with him to help him regain control over them. You will be advised how to do this by a physiotherapist.

SEE ALSO:
Chickenpox, *page 83*
Convulsion, *page 94*
Drowsiness, *page 120*
Headache, *page 153*
Mumps, *page 184*
Whooping cough, *page 259*

Words in **bold** are A-Z entries

Encopresis

If a child frequently soils his underpants after he has been toilet trained, this is called encopresis. In a child of 4 or 5, uncontrollable bowel movements should be regarded as a symptom of a problem. The most common cause of encopresis is chronic **constipation**, when hard, dry stools accumulate in the bowel and loose, watery stools trickle out past them. You may even mistake this for **diarrhea**. The problem may start because of some emotional disturbance. Occasionally children persist in soiling their pants from infancy. Soiling may be a reaction against overfussy toilet training.

Is it serious?
Encopresis is not a serious problem.

Possible symptoms
- Involuntary bowel movements after the child has been toilet trained.
- Chronic constipation.

What should I do first?

1 Try to determine whether your child is constipated or not. Ask him when he last went to the bathroom.

2 Check to see if your child is affected by any obvious causes of stress, such as a new baby, moving to a new house or starting school.

Should I consult the doctor?

Consult your doctor if you think your child has chronic constipation. If you can find no reason for the involuntary soiling, your doctor may be able to uncover the tension that is affecting your child.

What might the doctor do?

☐ If your child is constipated, your doctor will prescribe a mild laxative formulated for babies and children. It is safe to give your child for short periods.
☐ If there is some emotional reason for it, your doctor will assess the situation.

If encopresis persists, it can become a vicious cycle—the bowel becomes stretched, loses tone and constipation and leakage become worse. Your doctor may refer you and your child to a psychologist.

What can I do to help?

☐ Make sure your child has a diet rich in fiber and liquids.
☐ Don't punish your child or show disgust if he soils his pants.
☐ Watch for signs of poor school performance. Your child may become a target of scorn because of the odor if he soils himself at school. Provide him with extra underpants.

SEE ALSO:
Constipation, *page 94*
Diarrhea, *page 114*

129

Epiglottitis

E

Epiglottitis is a variation of **croup** caused by bacterial infection of the epiglottis, the flap that closes over the windpipe (*trachea*) when food is swallowed to prevent it from going down into the lungs. Infection is accompanied by **fever** and a **sore throat**. Because the epiglottis and surrounding area swell, there are problems with swallowing and breathing. The condition generally occurs between the ages of 6 months and 6 years.

Is it serious?
Epiglottitis is extremely serious because complete obstruction of the airway can occur within hours of the onset of the symptoms and pose a threat to your child's life.

Possible symptoms
- Fever.
- Sore throat.
- Drooling because of the inability to swallow.
- Noisy breathing.
- Breathing difficulty—flaring nostrils, indrawing ribs.
- Inability to talk.

What should I do first?

1 If your child is drooling and having difficulty breathing, do not examine his throat. This may worsen the obstruction of the airway.

2 Take your child to the nearest emergency room immediately!

3 Stay calm. If your child senses your anxiety, he may panic and breathing will be even more difficult.

Should I consult the doctor?

Consult your doctor immediately or take your child to the nearest emergency room.

What might the doctor do?

□ If your doctor suspects epiglottitis, he will have your child taken to the hospital without delay. An X-ray of your child's neck may be taken if there is any doubt about the diagnosis, but your child will probably be taken immediately to the intensive-care unit or operating room. The epiglottis and the airway will be examined under anesthetic in a procedure called *laryngoscopy*. If epiglottitis is confirmed, a tube will be passed into the windpipe, under general anesthetic, to bypass the obstruction. Often the child is intubated for several days. A tracheotomy is a last resort. The immediate danger will be over, and your child should recover within the next few days.
□ Intravenous antibiotics will be administered to control the infection.

What can I do to help?

□ Stay with your child in the hospital if you are allowed to do so.

SEE ALSO:
Croup, *page 101*
Fever, *page 139*
Sore throat, *page 222*

Words in **bold** are A-Z entries

Epilepsy

Epilepsy is a disorder that causes periodic seizures. These occur when the normal electrical impulses in the brain are disturbed. There are two main forms of epileptic seizure. The *grand mal* form involves recurring attacks of **convulsions**. These involve a loss of consciousness and a stiff phase lasting a minute or less, followed by a series of rhythmic jerks of the limbs, clenching of the teeth (when your child might bite his tongue), involuntary urination and frothing at the mouth. The child then usually lapses into sleep.

The *petit mal* form of epilepsy has no convulsions. There is only a second or 2 of unconsciousness — like daydreaming when the child's eyes glaze over. The child appears not to see or hear anything. This form of epilepsy is often unrecognized and undiagnosed as epilepsy. Although the scale of the problem is different from grand mal convulsions, frequent petit mal seizures can interfere with a child's life, particularly school performance and certain physical activities, such as bike riding. There usually is no mental disability associated with either form of epilepsy. The disorder tends to run in families.

About 3 to 5% of children under age 6 have an occasional convulsion, but nearly

Possible symptoms

Grand mal
- Loss of consciousness.
- Clenching of teeth.
- Stiffness, followed by rhythmic jerking of the limbs.
- Involuntary urination.
- Frothing at the mouth.

Petit mal
- Daydreamlike state lasting 1 or 2 seconds, from which the child cannot be roused.

all of these are harmless febrile convulsions, when the electrical disturbance in the brain is caused by a high temperature preceding, or during, an infectious illness.

Is it serious?
Epilepsy is not a life-threatening disorder. All children grow out of the petit mal form of epilepsy by late adolescence. However, children who suffer from the grand mal form of epilepsy may need special consideration, even though the condition is controlled by drugs. They will need supervision during activities, such as swimming and bike riding.

What should I do first?

During a *grand mal* seizure

1 Protect your child from injury by placing him on the floor.

2 Loosen the clothing around his neck and chest.

3 Stay with your child until the seizure is over.

4 Don't try to hold your child's teeth apart if they are clenched or put anything in his mouth. Any injury to his tongue will occur at the beginning of the attack, so there is nothing you can do until the attack is over.

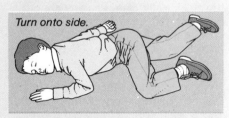
Turn onto side.

5 As soon as your child stops moving violently, turn him gently onto his side so he won't choke on his tongue or saliva.

6 Watch what happens during your child's seizure—your account will help your doctor make a diagnosis.

Continued on next page ▶

131

Epilepsy

◀ Continued from previous page
During a *petit mal* seizure

1 Guide your child to safety if he is in the street or near a stairway, for example.

2 Stay with your child until the seizure has passed.

Should I consult the doctor?

Consult your doctor as soon as the convulsion has passed, whether you think it is an epileptic seizure or a febrile convulsion. Consult your doctor as soon as possible if you think your child has petit mal seizures.

What might the doctor do?

☐ If your child has a convulsion, your doctor will examine him and question you about the attack to determine what form of seizure your child suffered from.

☐ If your child has recurrent convulsions, he may be admitted to the hospital for tests. These may include blood tests for glucose and calcium, an EEG (electroencephalogram) and possibly a brain scan to find out if an abnormal area of the brain is causing the seizures. During the scan the child is stimulated so any abnormal behavior in the brain can be picked up with the scanning equipment. Some tests are also used to diagnose petit mal seizures.

☐ Your doctor will prescribe anticonvulsant drugs to be taken daily to reduce the frequency of the seizures. There are no drugs to cure the condition but once on medication, the seizures may be under very good control. Your child may have no more seizures.

☐ Your child's condition will be reviewed periodically. If there are no seizures for a year or 2, the doctor may decide to phase out the drugs.

What can I do to help?

☐ It can be a shock to realize your child has epilepsy. You and your child will need to learn to live with the situation. Your doctor can advise you how to cope with the seizures.

☐ Make a note of the frequency of your child's petit mal seizures so you can tell your doctor.

☐ Watch your child carefully. Report any mental or personality differences that may be the result of the drugs. It's important that your child's medication be given in the proper amounts to avoid any undesirable side effects.

☐ Treat your child as normally as possible. Tell his friends and teachers about the condition so they won't be frightened if your child has a convulsion in their presence.

☐ Have a bracelet or medal engraved with information about your child's epilepsy, in case of an attack when you are not there. Make sure your child wears it all the time.

☐ If your child is prescribed anticonvulsant drugs, don't stop them without medical advice. To do so could cause a severe, prolonged convulsion after a few days.

☐ Teach your child to recognize the signs of an oncoming attack. Some sufferers experience strange sensations, such as unpleasant smells, distorted vision or an odd feeling in the stomach, just before a convulsion. This is known as an "aura," and if your child is old enough to identify these sensations as warning signs, he may be able to avoid having an accident.

SEE ALSO:
Convulsion, *page 96*

Eye, foreign body in

If a foreign body, such as a speck of dust, enters your child's eye, the eye will water and your child won't want to open it. If you can see something moving loosely over the white part of the eye, try to remove it. However, if the foreign body is embedded in the eyeball or is on the colored part of the eye (the iris), don't touch it!

Is it serious?
Small specks of dust or dirt are not serious because they are washed out naturally by tears. But if your child's eyeball is scratched, if an object has pierced it or there is a cut on the eyeball or eyelid, it is serious and should be treated as an emergency.

Possible symptoms
- Watery eye.
- Reluctance to open eye.
- Pain and irritation.
- Redness.
- A visible embedded object.

E

What should I do first?
Look closely to see whether the foreign body is moving or is embedded in the eye. Encourage your child to blink; this may dislodge the foreign body. Tears may help dislodge it if your child has been crying.

If the foreign body is not embedded in the eye

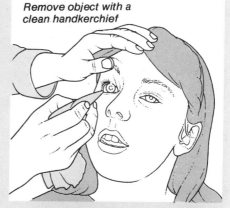

Remove object with a clean handkerchief

1 Ask your child to look up. Pull down on the lower lid to see if the object is there. If it is, remove it with the corner of a clean handkerchief.

If the foreign body is embedded in the eye

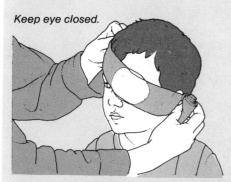

Keep eye closed.

1 Do not attempt any first aid. Keep your child's eye closed by putting a pad or clean handkerchief over the eyelid. Tape it in place. Go to the emergency room.

Continued on next page ▶

Eye, foreign body in

E

◀ Continued from previous page

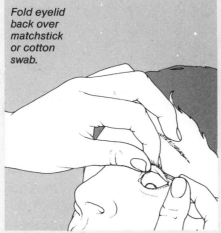

Fold eyelid back over matchstick or cotton swab.

2 To expose the area beneath the top lid, lay a matchstick or a cotton swab along the middle of the top lid. Take hold of the eyelashes, and pull them back over the matchstick or swab. Remove the object with a handkerchief. If your child won't cooperate, you'll need someone to help you. You may have to restrain your child bodily if he resists.

3 If these methods don't work, try to flush the foreign body out by pouring a glass of water across the open eye.

Should I consult the doctor?

Go to the emergency room if the eyeball is scratched or if a foreign body has pierced the eye. Consult your doctor if you fail to remove a floating foreign body from your child's eye in 1 hour. Consult your doctor if your child still complains of pain an hour or 2 after you have removed the object.

What might the doctor do?

☐ The doctor will remove any embedded foreign body from your child's eye after putting drops of a local anesthetic into the eye.
☐ If the eyeball is scratched, the doctor will prescribe antibiotic drops to guard against infection. He may bandage the eye to keep it closed for about 24 hours.
☐ If you went to your doctor because your child's eye was still sore, your doctor will examine the eye and remove any foreign object he finds.

What can I do to help?

☐ After the removal of a foreign body, pain should subside in an hour or so. If it does not, consult your doctor.

SEE ALSO:
Eye, injury to, *page 135*

Words in **bold** are A-Z entries

Eye, injury to

Treat injuries to the eye promptly because they could have long-term consequences on your child's sight. If your child receives a blow to the eye, the eye socket will probably protect the eye itself, but the surrounding area will swell and **bruise** as the tiny blood vessels beneath the skin break.

If a chemical substance is accidentally splashed into the eye, treat this as an emergency. Soap in the eye may cause your child to make a lot of fuss and in extreme cases, may cause chemical corneal abrasion. If a sharp object penetrates the eyeball or makes a **cut** near the eye or eyelid, treat it as an emergency.

Is it serious?
A black eye looks bad, but it is rarely serious. However, if a chemical substance or a sharp object injures your child's eye, it is serious. Treat it as an emergency and seek medical aid.

What should I do first?

Put a cold compress on the eye.

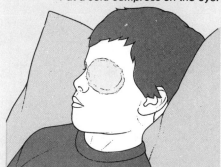

1 If your child receives a blow to his eye, place a cold compress over the eye for half an hour to limit the extent of the bruising.

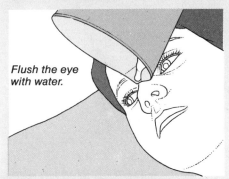

Flush the eye with water.

2 If your child's eye is injured by a chemical substance, try to flush the chemical out with water immediately, before consulting your doctor or going to the nearest emergency room. If you can, carry your child to a sink or basin, and hold his head under the cold tap with the injured eye down so chemicals do not run into the unaffected eye or down his face. Hold the eye open, and let the water run in from the inner corner. Do this for 15 minutes. Time it with a clock. If possible, have someone else call your doctor while you continue to flush. If your child is large, lay him down with his head turned to one side so the injured eye is down. Gently pour cold water from a jug, bowl or bucket into the eye. Apply a pad or clean handkerchief, held in place with tape, to the eyelid to keep it closed.

3 If there are chemical particles sticking to the eyeball, don't attempt to remove them. Apply a pad or clean handkerchief, held in place with tape, to the eyelid to keep it closed. Take your child to the nearest emergency room.

Continued on next page ▶

Eye, injury to

◀ *Continued from previous page*

Cover the injured eye.

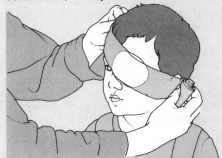

4 If the injury is caused by a sharp object, cover the injured eye with a pad or clean handkerchief. Tape it in place, and go immediately to the emergency room.

5 If there is blood coming from the wound, hold a pad firmly against the cut to stem the blood flow, and take your child to the nearest emergency room.

Should I consult the doctor?

Consult your doctor immediately or go to the emergency room after flushing the chemicals from your child's eye. Go to the emergency room immediately if your child suffers any other injury to his eye, other than a black eye or minor cut.

What might the doctor do?

☐ How the doctor treats the eye depends on the cause of the injury. If the problem was caused by a chemical substance, take the bottle containing the chemical with you. Otherwise note what caused the damage, and tell the doctor.
☐ If your child's eyelid was cut, the doctor will stitch it to reduce scarring, if this is necessary.

What can I do to help?

☐ Keep a clean pad or handkerchief taped over the injured eye to keep your child from rubbing it. Buy him a pirate patch to make him feel special.

SEE ALSO:
Bruise, *page 78*
Cuts and scrapes, *page 104*
Eye, foreign body in, *page 133*

Words in **bold** are A-Z entries

Failure to thrive

If a child fails to develop and grow normally, this is usually due to malnutrition. It may be the result of social factors, such as poor parenting, to a chronic illness, such as heart or kidney disease, to a genetic disorder, such as **cystic fibrosis**, or to inadequate production of growth hormone by the pituitary gland.

Is it serious?
Failure to thrive is always serious.

Possible symptoms

● Height, weight and head circumference do not increase normally.
● Physical skills are slow to develop.

F

What should I do first?

1 If you think your child is small for his age and you are both average or above-average height and weight, keep a regular check on his growth pattern. As long as your child is growing steadily, he is normal.

2 Take a critical look at your child's diet. Is it adequate and well-balanced? Most children eat a varied diet, but children who develop fads and eat only a small number of foods may not get enough essential nutrients.

3 Take your baby to the doctor regularly for a "well-baby" checkup.

4 If your child is unhappy and disturbed, this may result in a failure to thrive. Try to find out if there is any psychological reason for his condition.

Should I consult the doctor?

Consult your doctor if your child seems to be below-average height and weight for his age, if he is not eating well or if he seems disturbed and unhappy.

What might the doctor do?

□ Your doctor will treat any underlying physical illness that may be causing the malnutrition. Your child may be hospitalized for a short time if complicated diagnostic procedures are necessary or your child's food intake needs to be monitored or verified.

□ Your doctor may arrange for laboratory blood tests, including hormone studies, to check for any hormonal disorder.

□ Your doctor may do psychological tests, such as the Denver developmental test, to measure growth and development.

□ If your child seems unhappy and disturbed, you and your child may be referred to a psychologist for counseling.

What can I do to help?

□ If your doctor prescribes a special diet for your child, make sure your child sticks to it. The rest of the family can eat the same meals so your child doesn't feel different.

□ Provide as much love and support as possible for your child. Examine your feelings and behavior toward him, and seek help if you don't think they are what they should be.

□ Read books and pamphlets, attend parenting classes or ask a visiting nurse to come to your home.

SEE ALSO:
Cystic fibrosis, *page 106*

Fever

A fever is a temperature of 100F (37.5C) or over. Consult your doctor if your baby's temperature remains high despite tepid sponging (*see page 31*). Consult your doctor immediately if your child's temperature is as high as 104F (40C).

F

Accompanying symptoms	Common causes
Your child has a cough and a runny nose.	He possibly has a **Common cold**, *page 91*.
Your child has a cough, sore throat and aches and pains.	He possibly has **Influenza**, *page 165*.
Your child has a sore throat and difficulty swallowing.	He may have **Tonsillitis**, *page 243*. If his voice is hoarse, he may have **Laryngitis**, *page 172*. If his neck glands are swollen, he may have **Mononucleosis**, *page 179*.
Your child has a rash of itchy, red spots starting on the trunk.	He may have **Chickenpox**, *page 83*.
Your child passes urine frequently, and, if he is old enough, complains of a burning sensation.	He may have a **Urinary-tract infection**, *page 250*.
Your child had a runny nose and sore eyes and now has a brown-red rash.	He possibly has **Measles**, *page 176*.
The sides of your child's face and the area under his chin are swollen.	He possibly has **Mumps**, *page 184*.
Your child has an earache or, if he is too young to tell you, he cries and tugs at his ear.	He could have a middle ear infection, **Otitis media**, *page 195*.
Your child has diarrhea.	He could have "gastric" flu, *page 144*, or a bowel infection, such as **Food poisoning**, *page 141*.
Your baby or child is breathing rapidly and with great difficulty.	**CONSULT YOUR DOCTOR IMMEDIATELY** Your child may have **Bronchitis**, *page 76*, **Bronchiolitis**, *page 75*, **Pneumonia**, *page 201*, or **Croup**, *page 101*.
Your child cannot bend his neck without pain and turns away from bright light.	**CONSULT YOUR DOCTOR IMMEDIATELY** Your child may have **Meningitis**, *page 177*.

Words in **bold** are A-Z entries

Fever

The range of normal body temperature is 96.8 to 98.6F (36 to 37C). Anything over 100F (37.5C) is a fever, although the height a temperature reaches is not necessarily an accurate reflection of the seriousness of the illness. A fever is not in itself an illness but a symptom of one (*see page 138*). Apart from any illness, your child's temperature will reflect the time of day and activity level. After a very strenuous game of football, for example, the temperature could temporarily be over 100F (37.5C).

Is it serious?
A temperature of over 100F (37.5C) is always cause for concern in a baby under 6 months old.

What should I do first?

1 If you suspect your child has a fever, take his temperature.

2 Put your child to bed, and remove most of his clothing, even if the room is cool. A child with a fever need only be covered by a light sheet.

3 Lower a temperature of over 104F (40C) by sponging your child all over with tepid water (*see page 31*).

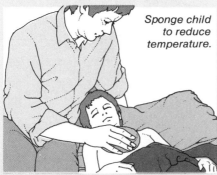

Sponge child to reduce temperature.

Stop tepid sponging when the temperature drops to 100F (37.5C). If your child shivers, add a little more hot water. Never use cold water because it causes the blood vessels to constrict, preventing heat loss and driving the temperature up. Never use alcohol.

4 Give acetaminophen. Never give aspirin to a child with the symptoms of **chickenpox** or **influenza** because aspirin use has been linked to the development of **Reye's syndrome**.

5 Encourage your child to drink as much liquid as possible by offering small amounts of fluid at regular intervals.

6 If your child is not uncomfortable with the fever, don't treat him with

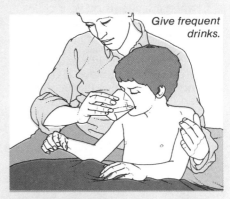

Give frequent drinks.

anything more than increased fluid. There is no degree of fever in a normal person that will cause brain damage. A certain degree of fever is beneficial because it helps the body fight infection.

Should I consult the doctor?

Consult your doctor if your child is under 6 months old, if your child has a **convulsion**, if he has had a convulsion in the past or if febrile convulsions run in the family. Consult your doctor if the fever lasts for more than 24 hours or if you are worried about any of the accompanying symptoms.

Continued on next page ▶

Fever

◀ *Continued from previous page*

What might the doctor do?

□ The course of treatment depends on the underlying cause of the fever. If the cause is bacterial infection, antibiotics will probably be prescribed. If the cause is an ailment like chickenpox, a **common cold** or other viral illness, then most likely no medication will be given, just advice on how to make your child comfortable.

What can I do to help?

□ Change the sheets on your child's bed frequently, and cover him with a sheet only.
□ Place a cold compress or a wet face cloth on your child's forehead.
□ Don't wake your child to take his temperature or to give him acetaminophen. Sleep is more important.

SEE ALSO:
Chickenpox, *page 83*
Common cold, *page 91*
Convulsion, *page 96*
Influenza, *page 165*
Measles, *page 176*
Reye's syndrome, *page 208*

Words in **bold** are A-Z entries

Food poisoning

Food poisoning is a form of **gastroenteritis** caused by eating food that is contaminated with poisons, usually bacteria. Within 3 to 24 hours, depending on the poison, the symptoms of abdominal cramps, **fever**, **vomiting** and **diarrhea** occur with unpleasant ferocity. If the food was contaminated with bacteria, they release their own poisons, called *toxins*, which have a direct effect on the lining of the bowel, causing inflammation. There are many types of bacterium that cause food poisoning, but the most common are *salmonella, shigella, staphylococcii* and *E. coli,* which is the bacterium most commonly responsible for food poisoning among babies, usually in bottle-fed babies. Of the non-bacterial types of food poisoning, symptoms can arise from eating chemicals, insecticides or certain plants.

Is it serious?
In a baby, this condition is serious because the symptoms can rapidly lead to **dehydration**.

Possible symptoms

- Abdominal cramps.
- Fever.
- Vomiting.
- Frequent, loose stools that may contain blood, pus or mucus.
- Muscular weakness and chills.
- Loss of appetite.

F

What should I do first?

1 If your child is vomiting and has diarrhea, check his temperature to see if he has a fever.

2 Check your child's stools for mucus or blood.

3 Put your child to bed, and stop all foods. Keep up his fluid levels by offering frequent small drinks of water or commercially prepared electrolyte solution, such as Gatorade or Pedialyte.

4 Try to determine what your child could have eaten to cause the symptoms.

Should I consult the doctor?

Consult your doctor immediately or take your baby to the emergency room if vomiting and diarrhea continue for more than 6 hours and you cannot bring them under control with a fluids-only diet. Consult your doctor immediately if your child's condition has not improved within 24 hours or if you suspect your child has drunk an insecticide or eaten a poisonous plant. Take your child to the nearest emergency room and take the suspected poison with you.

What might the doctor do?

□ In most cases, there is no special treatment for food poisoning except to replace the fluid and salts that have been lost through diarrhea and vomiting. Your doctor will probably prescribe an electrolyte solution.
□ If your baby or child is in danger of dehydration, your doctor will admit
Continued on next page ▶

Food poisoning

◀ *Continued from previous page*
him to the hospital to be given fluids intravenously. If vomiting is very severe, your doctor may give your child an injection of an anti-emetic drug to stop the vomiting.

What can I do to help?

☐ Place a pan next to your child's bed, so he doesn't have to run to the bathroom to vomit.

Cool your child's forehead.

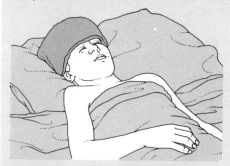

☐ Keep him cool and refreshed with an icepack or damp face cloth if he has a fever.
☐ Have your child rinse his mouth out with water after he has vomited.
☐ Be meticulous about hygiene. Food poisoning is infectious, so make sure your child washes his hands after going to the bathroom. Wash your own hands after changing diapers.
☐ To prevent food poisoning, refrigerate all cooked food. If you reheat it, do so thoroughly. Salmonella thrives in warmed food but is killed by high temperatures.
☐ If your child refuses to drink enough fluids or doesn't like the taste of the electrolyte solution, give him cubes of melon to suck.
☐ Defrost foods well before cooking, particularly poultry and pork. Make sure they are thoroughly cooked.

☐ Check back over what your child has eaten in the previous 24 hours. Throw out any cooked meats, fish, dairy products or pastries that you suspect may have caused the illness.
☐ Reintroduce foods that are easily digested, such as soups, yogurt, jellies and non-fatty foods, as soon as your child asks for something to eat. The effects of the illness usually pass within a week.
☐ Follow your doctor's instructions for reintroducing formula for a bottle-fed baby.

Dehydration, *page 109*
Diarrhea, *page 115*
Fever, *page 139*
Gastroenteritis, *page 144*
Vomiting, *page 255*

Words in **bold** are A-Z entries

Frostbite

Frostbite occurs after exposure to extreme cold when the blood flow to the exposed area stops and the affected area of skin becomes frozen. Typically, the skin first becomes red, then shiny, then a dull, gray color. Occasionally, blisters may form. The fingers, toes, nose and ears are most often affected.

Is it serious?
Frostbite is serious and should be treated as an emergency. There is a first-aid routine (see below) to carry out immediately. If treated quickly, frostbite has no lasting effect, but severe cases can lead to gangrene and amputation of the affected part.

Possible symptoms

- Hard, red, cold skin, usually on the hands, toes, nose or ears, that becomes shiny then a dull, gray color.
- Tiny blisters on the affected area.
- Numbness in the affected area.

What should I do first?

1 Get your child out of the cold immediately. If you can, get someone else to call the doctor. If you are on your own, call a doctor after you have followed the first-aid procedure.

2 Do *not* apply direct heat or rub the affected part. If the fingers or toes are frostbitten, immerse them in warm water. Keep adding warm water so the temperature remains constant. If you have no access to warm water, keep the affected part warm by putting your child's hands or feet under your armpits or holding his face against your body.

3 Wrap your child in blankets, and give him hot drinks. Feed the drinks to him yourself if his hands are affected. Don't let your child walk on frostbitten feet.

4 When the affected part becomes pink, stop warming it. Wrap it in gauze, cotton or any soft, warm fabric you have, and go immediately to the emergency room.

5 While you are traveling to the hospital, keep the affected part level with your child's chest to encourage blood flow. For example, raise his feet or put his hands across his chest.

Should I consult the doctor?

Take your child to the emergency room as soon as you have restored pinkness to the affected skin.

What might the doctor do?

☐ The doctor will check to see if circulation has returned to the frostbitten area. Drugs to improve blood circulation may be necessary if the blood flow has not returned to normal.

What can I do to help?

☐ Always wrap your child up warmly in cold weather.
☐ Keep an eye on him when he's outside, playing in cold weather. Don't let him get too cold.

Gastroenteritis

Gastroenteritis is an inflammation of the stomach and intestines. The symptoms include **vomiting**, nausea, **diarrhea**, abdominal cramps and loss of appetite. The most common cause of gastro-enteritis in children is the *rotavirus,* which can be inhaled and tends to spread easily through a community. It may also be caused by direct infection of the intestines with bacteria, usually from contaminated food, when it is called **food poisoning**, or by a parasite, when the condition is sometimes called **dysentery**.

Gastroenteritis may also be a symptom of another infection, such as **influenza**, when the infecting bacteria may spread to the bowel through the bloodstream. When vomiting and diarrhea accompany flu symptoms, this is often referred to as "gastric flu."

Symptoms of gastroenteritis in babies and young children may be caused by **lactose intolerance**, when the sugar (lactose) in cow's milk is poorly digested.

Is it serious?

Gastroenteritis can be serious in children, especially babies, because the symptoms of vomiting and diarrhea can rapidly lead to **dehydration**.

Possible symptoms

- Vomiting.
- Nausea.
- Diarrhea.
- Abdominal cramps.
- Loss of appetite.
- Raised temperature.

What should I do first?

1 Stop all food and milk, and give your child only clear liquids, such as soda or slightly sweetened tea, in small amounts every 15 minutes.

2 Put your child to bed with a bowl by the bed in case he vomits.

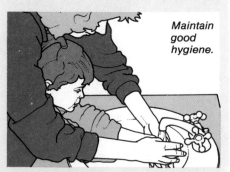

Maintain good hygiene.

3 Make sure your child washes his hands after going to the bathroom to prevent spread of infection.

Continued on next page ▶

Words in **bold** are A-Z entries

Gastroenteritis

◀ *Continued from previous page*

Should I consult the doctor?

Consult your doctor if your child has diarrhea and vomiting that cannot be brought under control with a fluid-only diet within 24 hours.

What might the doctor do?

□ Your doctor will determine the cause of the vomiting and diarrhea if it is not gastroenteritis. He will determine the extent of dehydration and recommend feeding methods. To avoid dehydration, your child should be given 3½ fluid ounces (91ml) of water for every pound of his body weight in the first 24 hours of diarrhea and vomiting.
□ Your doctor may recommend bed rest and a liquid diet until the vomiting and diarrhea have subsided.
□ For a bottle-fed baby, your doctor may recommend that you replace all formula with an electrolyte-and-glucose solution, such as Lytren or Pedialyte. He will then provide you with a regime for reintroducing formula.
□ If your baby is seriously ill, your doctor may admit him to the hospital so he can be given fluid intravenously to counteract dehydration.

What can I do to help?

□ If your child is admitted to the hospital, try to stay with him. Most hospital authorities now encourage parents to do this.
□ Be meticulous about hygiene. Wash your hands before preparing any food or formula for your child and after changing diapers.
□ Avoid giving your child acidic drinks, such as orange and grapefruit juice. They may irritate his stomach further.
□ Reintroduce foods slowly when your child seems interested. Start with bland, easily digested foods, such as jellies, yogurt, soups and non-fatty foods.
□ If your child refuses to drink enough fluids, try Popsicles or Jello.

SEE ALSO:
Appetite, loss of, *page 58*
Dehydration, *page 109*
Diarrhea, *page 114*
Dysentery, *page 121*
Food poisoning, *page 141*
Influenza, *page 165*
Lactose intolerance, *page 171*
Vomiting, *page 254*

German measles

German measles, or rubella, is a mild, infectious disease caused by a virus. It is contagious and has an incubation period of 14 to 21 days. The rash usually starts behind the ears, then spreads to the forehead and the rest of the body. It looks more like a large patch of redness than a series of spots. The rash lasts 2 to 3 days and is rarely accompanied by serious symptoms, just a mild fever and enlarged glands at the back of the neck. The main danger with German measles is not to your infected child but to any pregnant woman who may contract the disease from your child. Rubella can cause birth defects, such as blindness and deafness.

Is it serious?
Rubella is not a serious childhood illness. However, keep your child isolated for 5 days after the rash appears. Like other infectious childhood diseases, rubella carries a slight risk of **encephalitis**.

Possible symptoms
● Slightly raised temperature.
● Tiny pink or red spots, starting behind the ears and spreading to the forehead, then the rest of the body.

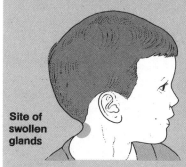

Site of swollen glands

● Enlarged, swollen glands at the back of the neck.

What should I do first?

1 Make sure any woman who might be pregnant and has been in contact with your child is informed of your child's infection.

2 Keep your child away from school and from public places.

3 If your child's temperature rises above 103F (39.5C) give him acetaminophen.

4 If your child is feeling ill, put him to bed.

Should I consult the doctor?

Call your doctor to confirm your child has German measles. Consult your doctor immediately if your child complains of a stiff neck or is intolerant of bright light.

What might the doctor do?

☐ There is no treatment for German measles, but your doctor will advise you to alert any women you know who might be pregnant.

What can I do to help?

☐ You don't need to give your child any special treatment for German measles. He can return to school as soon as he is active.

☐ Vaccinate your children against the disease at 15 months.

SEE ALSO:
Encephalitis, *page 128*
Rash, *page 206*

Words in **bold** are A-Z entries

Growing pain

A growing pain is a dull, vague ache in a limb; it doesn't last long. The child can usually be distracted from it. One in six school-age children suffers from some kind of growing pain. These pains can occur when your child is going through a growth spurt. The muscles and bones grow at slightly different rates, leading to an aching soreness that is worse in the evening. Pains can also occur after strenuous activity. It's important to distinguish a growing pain from a joint pain. A growing pain is felt between the joints of a limb; joint pain is specific to the joint area. In a child, a joint pain can be a symptom of **rheumatic fever** or **arthritis**.

Is it serious?
A growing pain is not serious, but any pain in the joint may be, particularly if it is accompanied by a fever. It might be septic arthritis.

Possible symptoms
● Aches and pains in the arms or legs, most often in the legs.
● Disturbed sleep if pain is severe.
● Painful muscles after strenuous activity.

What should I do first?

1 Check your child's joints for swelling and tenderness by pressing on and around them. If there is no swelling or tenderness, check muscles the same way.

2 See if your child limps when he walks.

3 Ask your child when the pain started and how long it lasts.

Should I consult the doctor?

Consult your doctor if the pain is over a joint and is accompanied by a fever or if it lasts longer than 24 hours.

What might the doctor do?

☐ After excluding other possible causes of pain, your doctor will reassure you and your child that there is no cause for concern.

What can I do to help?

☐ Show sympathetic interest in the pain—it may be sufficient to relax your child.
☐ Give your child a warm bath or a heating pad set on low. These can be soothing if your child has trouble sleeping.
☐ Gently massage the affected muscles to relax tension.

SEE ALSO:
Arthritis, *page 59*
Limp, *page 175*
Rheumatic fever, *page 209*

Hair loss

Children rarely lose their hair. However, in newborn babies, the first fluffy hair is often lost just after birth, and the second growth may be slow, so your baby will appear to be bald for several months. Babies also lose hair through friction. Simply by the pressure of their heads on the crib sheet, they may have large bald patches on the back or sides of their heads. This is because newborn baby hair is not very firmly embedded in the skin, and only a small amount of friction is needed to rub it loose.

By far the most common cause of hair loss in older children is the fungal infection of the scalp called **ringworm**. This produces circular patches of pink or gray scaly baldness in the scalp, and it is extremely itchy. Another cause of temporary baldness in children is a condition called *alopecia areata*. Round, bald patches appear suddenly, and within a few months fine, white hairs break through into the bald area, followed by normal hair. Some children can actually inflict hair loss on themselves with a nervous **tic** or mannerism, compulsively pulling, twisting and breaking their hair. This condition, which is called *trichotillomania*, is often worse when your child is concentrating on something.

Is it serious?

Hair loss is not normally serious, though your child may feel self-conscious until the hair grows back again.

What should I do first?

1 Check any patches of baldness on your child's scalp. If the skin is pink or gray and scaly, this indicates ringworm. If not, your child could be suffering from alopecia areata.

2 Watch and see if your child pulls and tugs at his hair while concentrating.

Should I consult the doctor?

Consult your doctor as soon as possible if you suspect ringworm. This is infectious but can be easily cleared up with medication. Consult your doctor if you are unsure about the cause of the patches of baldness on your child's head or if you are worried about the tic.

What might the doctor do?

☐ Your doctor will treat the underlying cause. If your child has ringworm, he will prescribe an anti-fungal ointment for the skin and tablets to take.
☐ If alopecia areata is the cause, your doctor will advise you that there is no treatment and that the condition is only temporary.

What can I do to help?

☐ Let your child wear a hat if he feels self-conscious about the bald patches.
☐ Try not to make a fuss about the baldness. Treat it as a normal condition. Inform your child's teacher about the problem.
☐ If your child fiddles with his hair, try not to let him see it annoys you. Discourage him gently, and make sure he doesn't get overtired or anxious because this can make tics worse.
☐ Check for regrowth regularly, and encourage your child not to be disheartened.

SEE ALSO:
Ringworm, *page 210*
Tic, *page 242*

Words in **bold** are A-Z entries

Hay fever

Hay fever is similar to **asthma** except the allergic reaction occurs in the mucous membranes of the nose and eyelids, not the chest. The condition is also called *allergic rhinitis* and causes sneezing, a runny nose and itchy, watery eyes. It occurs seasonally and is usually due to a reaction to pollen from flowers, grasses, trees or molds. Most hay-fever sufferers are sensitive to more than one pollen and, short of isolation in an air-conditioned room, it is difficult to avoid the symptoms. Children who suffer from hay fever can become mouth-breathers because the nose is so blocked. Hay fever tends not to occcur before age 5, but it can start or stop at any time and tends to run in families. Some children who are allergic to animals and house dust, as well as pollens, suffer all year round from hay fever. This condition is called *perennial allergic rhinitis*.

Is it serious?
Hay fever is periodically troublesome, but it has no serious consequences.

Possible symptoms
- Sneezing.
- Runny nose with clear discharge.
- Itchy, watery, red-rimmed eyes.

What should I do first?

1 If your child is sneezing a lot, check his temperature to make sure he isn't ill with an infection, such as **influenza** or a **common cold**.

2 Discourage your child from rubbing his eyes. This will make them worse. Bathe his eyes with cool water to ease the irritation.

Should I consult the doctor?

Consult your doctor if you think your child may be suffering from a more serious infection or if the hay fever is making your child miserable.

What might the doctor do?

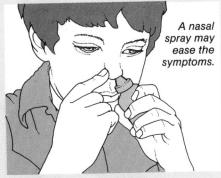

A nasal spray may ease the symptoms.

☐ Your doctor will probably prescribe decongestant nasal drops or anti-histamine spray, elixir or tablets to relieve the symptoms.

Continued on next page ▶

Hay fever

◀ *Continued from previous page*
☐ If your child's condition is severe,
your doctor may arrange for your
child to have a series of skin tests to
track down the allergen that is causing
the symptoms of hay fever. After one or
more allergens have been determined,
a special vaccine can be made for your
child and a course of desensitizing
injections given over a period of weeks
or months to protect him. These don't
always work, however, and have to be
given during the winter.

What can I do to help?

☐ Watch the pollen count each day.
If one type of plant or weed is particularly
high, this may give you an idea of what
your child is allergic to.
☐ Avoid feathers in your child's bedding
and fluff in his clothing.
☐ Keep your house as dustfree as
possible. Even if your child isn't allergic
to dust, a dusty atmosphere makes
hay fever worse.

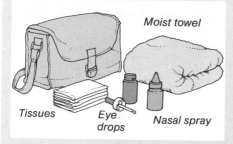

Moist towel

Tissues   Eye drops   Nasal spray

☐ Prepare an emergency pack for
outings. It should contain tissues, eye
drops to reduce eye irritation, a moist
towel to soothe your child's eyes and
whatever medication has been
prescribed.

SEE ALSO:
Asthma, *page 61*
Common cold, *page 91*
Influenza, *page 165*

Words in **bold** are A-Z entries

Head injury

Children hit their heads frequently. In the majority of cases, the child has stopped crying and is playing normally within 10 to 15 minutes of the accident. With some harder bumps on the head, there is **headache** and local swelling. If the skin is broken, the blood flow may be alarming from even a small cut.

When there is no outward sign of injury, a mild headache is probably all your child will complain about. However, if he lapses into unconsciousness, complains of **dizziness** or appears stunned and vomits, this may be concussion, when the brain is shaken inside the skull. The symptoms of concussion may not appear for several hours.

Is it serious?
A head injury resulting in unconsciousness, dizziness or **vomiting** should always be treated as serious. If your child has any bleeding or straw-colored discharge from his nose or ear after a blow to his head, treat it as an emergency because it indicates a skull fracture. If there is a fracture and an open wound or any bleeding into the brain, the chances of brain damage are higher.

Possible symptoms
- Headache.
- Stunned and dazed state.
- Drowsiness.
- Period of unconsciousness.
- Irritability.
- Vomiting.
- Discharge of blood or straw-colored fluid from nose and ears.
- Indentation on skull.

What should I do first?

1 If your child has fallen on his head or suffered a blow to his head, check for any of the symptoms of concussion or a fracture of the skull. Treat any symptoms other than a mild headache as an emergency. Take your child to the emergency room.

2 If your child complains of a headache but seems alert, let him lie down for an hour in a dark room. But watch him to be sure he doesn't lose consciousness.

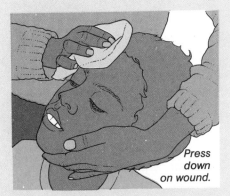

Press down on wound.

3 If the wound is bleeding, press a clean pad or handkerchief on it for about 10 minutes or until the

Continued on next page ▶

Head injury

◀ *Continued from previous page*
bleeding has stopped. If it is a small wound, clean the area with soap and water, and place a clean bandage over it to keep pressure on the wound.
If the wound is jagged or long, take your child to the emergency room for stitching.

4 If there is discharge coming from ears or nose, do not try to stop the flow—put a pad against the ear or nose to absorb it. Take your child to the nearest emergency room.

Should I consult the doctor?

Consult your doctor immediately or take your child to the emergency room if he loses consciousness, even for a short time, if he complains of a severe headache and dizziness, if he vomits or if there is any discharge from his nose or ears. Take your child to the emer-gency room if a cut needs stitching. Consult your doctor immediately if you are worried about your child's behaviour, even hours after a head injury, particularly if he is pale, un-naturally quiet and has lost interest in food. Tell the doctor what sort of fall or incident caused the injury.

What might the doctor do?

☐ If there is any likelihood of a skull fracture, your child will have a skull X-ray.
☐ If there is a cut, the doctor will stitch it under local anesthetic.
☐ If there are no signs of a fracture, but your child is dizzy and has a headache, the doctor may admit him to the hospital for overnight observation.

SEE ALSO:
Cuts and scrapes, *page 104*
Dizziness, *page 118*
Headache, *page 153*
Vomiting, *page 255*

Words in **bold** are A-Z entries

Headache

About one in five children suffers from recurrent headaches, although a serious physical cause is hardly ever found. Usually children complain of pain in their heads after sitting in a hot, stuffy room, if they are worried or anxious about something, if they have a **fever** or if they have a **toothache** or visual changes. Some children complain frequently of headache and tummy ache. Such pain is called *abdominal migraine*.

Is it serious?

Headaches are rarely serious but if a single headache is accompanied by a temperature, neck stiffness, confusion or an intolerance to bright light, this may be a symptom of a more serious illness, such as **encephalitis** or **meningitis**. Seek medical advice immediately. Similarly, if your child has had a recent injury to his head, you should get immediate medical attention.

What should I do first?

1 Ask your child if he has pain anywhere else. Run your hands over the area around his cheeks, jaw and ears to see if toothache or **earache** are the problem.

2 Check your child's temperature to see if he has a fever. Headache and fever could be among the first symptoms of an infectious illness.

3 Check to see if your child has any injury to his head.

4 If headaches are frequent, see if your child is worried about anything.

5 If your child complains of nausea or vomits, this could be a migraine headache. These headaches are usually quite severe. They may be preceded by an aura. Migraines tend to run in families.

6 If your child has no other symptoms to concern you, give him a drink and a single dose of acetaminophen to relieve the pain, and put him to bed in a darkened room for half an hour.

Should I consult the doctor?

Consult your doctor immediately if the headache is accompanied by a temperature of 100F (37.5C) with vomiting, neck stiffness and drowsiness or if your child has recently had a bump on his head. Consult your doctor if the headaches persist.

What might the doctor do?

☐ Your doctor will examine your child to try to determine the cause of the headache. The examination may include taking your child's blood pressure and a visual screening. Further tests will be carried out only if your doctor finds something wrong in addition to the headaches.

☐ If the headache is a symptom of a more serious condition, such as meningitis, your doctor will treat the condition accordingly.

What can I do to help?

☐ If your child complains of headaches at the end of the school day, give him a drink and a nutritious snack. Encourage him to go outside and play in the fresh air.

SEE ALSO:
Earache, *page 124*
Encephalitis, *page 128*
Fever, *page 139*
Head injury, *page 151*
Meningitis, *page 177*
Toothache, *page 245*

Heat exhaustion

Heat exhaustion results when too much body fluid is lost through sweating. It occurs when the body becomes over-heated by excessive exposure to sunshine, excessive humidity or through overexertion. Although a strenuous game can raise the body's temperature to over 100F (37.5C), the rise is usually tem-porary, and the temperature rapidly returns to normal. However, if it doesn't, your child will develop the symptoms of heat exhaustion and become pale and clammy and may complain of **dizziness**, nausea and **headache**.

Is it serious?
Heat exhaustion isn't serious as long as you recognize the problem and cool your child down and prevent **heatstroke**.

Possible symptoms
- Temperature over 100F (37.5C).
- Pale and clammy skin.
- Dizziness.
- Nausea.
- Headache.
- Rapid pulse rate.
- Muscle cramps.

What should I do first?

1 Lay your child down in a cool place with his feet raised. Remove most of his clothing.

2 Use tepid sponging (*see page 31*) to cool the skin down quickly.

3 Keep the air in the room as cool as possible.

4 Give your child plenty of fluids.

5 Take your child's temperature to make sure it is coming down.

Should I consult the doctor?

You should not need to consult your doctor if your child is suffering only from heat exhaustion and is cool and feels better in an hour. Consult your doctor immediately or take your child to the emergency room if, after an hour, your child is still extremely hot but his skin is dry. He could be suffering from heatstroke. Consult your doctor if your child's temperature fails to come down after an hour. He may be suffering from some other illness.

What might the doctor do?

☐ If your child is suffering from heat-stroke or an infection, your doctor will deal with this accordingly.

☐ Your doctor may advise you to keep your child inside during the heat of the day or until he is acclimatized.

What can I do to help?

☐ Discourage your child from playing active games in the heat.

☐ Watch your child if he has a tendency to become exhausted in hot weather.

SEE ALSO:
Dizziness, *page 118*
Headache, *page 153*
Heatstroke, *page 156*

Words in **bold** are A-Z entries

Heat rash

Heat rash is a faint red **rash** in the areas of the body where the sweat glands are most numerous—on the face, neck, shoulders and in the skin creases, such as the elbows, groin and behind the knees. It is common in babies because their sweat glands are still undeveloped and not efficient at regulating body temperature. Heat rash is not due to exposure to sunlight but occurs when the body becomes overheated and the skin responds with excessive production of sweat.

Is it serious?
Heat rash is never serious.

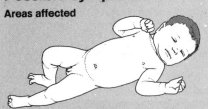

Possible symptoms
Areas affected

● Faint, red rash over the face, neck, shoulders and in the creases, such as the elbows, groin and knees.
● Flushed, hot appearance.

H

What should I do first?

1 Check your baby's clothing. He may be wearing too many clothes.

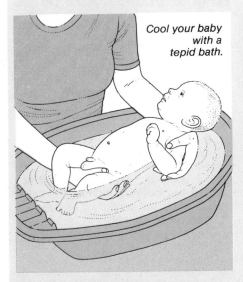

Cool your baby with a tepid bath.

2 Undress your baby, and bathe him in tepid water. Pat him dry to remove most of the moisture. Allow the rest to evaporate—this will cool his skin.

Should I consult the doctor?

There is no need to consult the doctor for a heat rash unless it gets worse or you have doubts or questions.

What might the doctor do?

☐ Your doctor will examine your baby to exclude any other reason for the rash. He will probably advise you to dress your baby in natural fibers that do not trap perspiration.

What can I do to help?

☐ Keep the temperature in your baby's room cool. Keep air flowing by opening a window slightly or with a fan.
☐ Don't overdress your child in hot weather.
☐ Don't put wool or manmade fibers next to your baby's skin. Dress him in a cotton undershirt first.
☐ Sprinkle your baby's neck, armpits and groin with cornstarch.

SEE ALSO:
Rash, *page 206*

155

Heatstroke

Heatstroke, or sunstroke, is due to exposure to extreme heat, which causes the body's temperature-regulating mechanism to break down. Sweat glands fail to work, and the body cannot cool itself in the normal way by producing sweat. Your child's skin will remain dry instead of sweaty, and he may become drowsy with a rapid pulse. He may then become confused and lapse into unconsciousness. If your child is not first acclimatized to the sun and heat, **heat exhaustion** and heatstroke can easily result.

Is it serious?
Heatstroke is very serious and may even be fatal. It should be treated as an emergency, and there are first-aid procedures to follow.

Possible symptoms
- Temperature as high as 104F (40C).
- Hot skin that remains dry, not sweaty.
- Drowsiness.
- Rapid pulse.
- Confusion followed by unconsciousness.

What should I do first?

1 Undress your child completely, and lay him down in a cool room.

2 Check his pulse (*see page 26*), and take his temperature to see if he has a fever. If his temperature is as high as 104F (40C), consult your doctor immediately or take your child to the emergency room.

3 Try to bring your child's temperature down slowly. Fan him, and sponge his whole body with tepid water (*see page 31*).

4 Place an icepack on your child's forehead, and give him plenty of cool drinks.

5 Take your child's temperature to make sure it is dropping.

Should I consult the doctor?

Consult your doctor immediately, or take your child to the emergency room if his temperature is as high as 104F (40C).

What might the doctor do?

□ The doctor will continue to cool your child's body. There are special drugs that can be given in emergencies to bring the body temperature down.

What can I do to help?

□ Apply a sunblock cream to your child's skin before he is exposed to the sun. Get him to wear a hat.

□ Watch your child when he plays in very hot or sunny conditions. A young child is often incapable of exercising caution, so you must monitor the time he spends in full sunlight if he has not been acclimatized.

□ Limit amount of time babies are in the heat.

□ Offer extra fluids when your child plays outside in the heat.

SEE ALSO:
Heat exhaustion, *page 154*

Words in **bold** are A-Z entries

Hemophilia

Hemophilia is an inherited disease of the blood, caused by a faulty gene. It is carried by some females, in whom the disease does not show. A carrier female may pass it to her daughter, who then becomes a carrier herself, or to her son, who will be a hemophiliac.

Hemophiliacs lack a substance called *antihemophilic globulin (AHG)* that is essential for making blood clot. A hemophiliac therefore bleeds profusely from even small wounds, and the blood flow does not stop. In a normal person, a trivial knock produces a little bleeding into the tissues, which results in a bruise; in a hemophiliac, it produces deep bruising, swelling and pain in the affected area for several days.

Possible symptoms

- Profuse and prolonged bleeding from any open wound.
- Heavy bruising, pain and swelling after even a light knock.
- Stiff joints or muscles due to internal bleeding.

What can be done?

Most hemophiliac families are aware the disorder exists. Boys in these families should be tested after birth to see if hemophilia is present. Women in such families are advised to consult their doctor and a genetic counselor before conceiving, to assess the risks involved. During pregnancy, amniocentesis—a process in which amniotic fluid is drawn from around the fetus through a needle—can determine the sex of the baby. If it is a boy, and the mother is a carrier of the hemophiliac gene, termination of the pregnancy will be offered.

In unsuspected cases, the symptoms tend to show themselves when the baby boy is several months old and is becoming more active, learning to crawl and walk.

The main treatment for hemophilia is replacement of the missing AHG by intravenous injection, as soon as possible after bruising, swelling or injury, or before dental and surgical procedures. In the case of injury, this injection may have to be repeated daily until the bleeding or swelling has ceased. Many older boys can insert the needle themselves, with the help of a parent or telephone supervision by a doctor.

Be swift to apply the correct first-aid techniques if your child is injured. Bleeding must be staunched at once with firm pressure and the affected part raised to reduce blood flow. Keep your child very still while waiting for medical assistance.

A hemophiliac should wear a disk that states he has the disease, his blood group and what to do and whom to call in an emergency.

The doctor or nurse may also pass on advice on how to protect your son against injury. For example, your child should sleep on a low bed, be careful on slippery floors and avoid playing with hazardous toys that may lead to physical injury.

Hepatitis

Hepatitis is an infection that causes inflammation of the liver. The most common form of the illness in children is acute hepatitis A, caused by the type-A virus. It is highly contagious. The virus is found in the stools of a sufferer, and if the hands are not washed after going to the bathroom, the infection can be passed to others by contaminated food and drink. The virus is also found in blood and saliva. The first symptom is loss of appetite. **Influenza**like symptoms then develop, followed by **jaundice**, with its associated symptoms of yellowing of the skin and whites of the eyes, dark-brown urine and abnormally pale stools.

Is it serious?
Hepatitis itself is rarely a very serious illness in children; they usually make a recovery. However, because it is contagious and can spread quickly through a household or school, it should be treated promptly.

Possible symptoms
● Loss of appetite.
● Influenzalike symptoms of headache, fever, aching joints.
● Jaundice (yellow skin), dark-brown urine and pale stools.

What should I do first?

1 If your child loses interest in food and has flulike symptoms, keep a check on his skin, urine and stools for any changes in color.

2 If your child won't eat, give him frequent drinks of diluted fruit juice, soda or Popsicles.

3 If you suspect hepatitis, keep your child home from school.

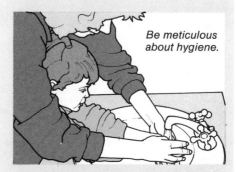

Be meticulous about hygiene.

4 Be meticulous about your child's hygiene—make sure he washes his hands after going to the bathroom. Keep his towel, face cloth and eating and drinking utensils separate from the rest of the family's.

Continued on next page ▶

Words in **bold** are A-Z entries

Hepatitis

◀ *Continued from previous page*

Should I consult the doctor?

Consult your doctor immediately if you suspect your child has hepatitis, especially if jaundice develops.

What might the doctor do?

□ Your doctor will take a blood sample to test for hepatitis.
□ Your doctor will recommend bed rest and isolation measures for at least 2 weeks, until the flu symptoms have passed. After another 2 weeks your child will probably feel well enough to return to school.
□ Although there is no specific treatment for hepatitis, other than bed rest, some doctors advise a high-calorie, low-fat diet to reduce the strain on the liver. However, others don't consider this worthwhile.
□ Your doctor may suggest the rest of the family have gamma globulin injections to minimize the risk of their contracting the infection.

What can I do to help?

□ Observe the isolation measures for at least 2 weeks or until your doctor says otherwise. Nurse your child in his own room. Restrict physical contact with others, and keep his eating utensils, toys and other objects separate from those of the rest of household.
□ Maintain high standards of hygiene. Wash out the toilet bowl with disinfectant after your child has used it. Wash his eating things separately from those of the family, and continue to keep his face cloth and towel separate.
□ Despite these measures, try not to make your child feel left out.
□ Check with your doctor before you reduce isolation measures and before you send your child back to school.

□ Post-hepatitis symptoms, such as lethargy, difficulty in concentrating and moodiness, may persist for up to 6 months, so be patient and understanding with your child.

SEE ALSO:
Appetite, loss of, *page 58*
Influenza, *page 165*
Jaundice, *page 170*
Rash, *page 206*

Hernia

A hernia results when a small defect in the muscular wall of the abdomen allows soft tissue to protrude through it. This appears as a slight bulge in the skin and can be seen even more clearly if your child coughs or strains. The most common hernia in children is the *umbilical hernia*. It appears near the navel and results from a weakness that occurs in the abdominal wall at birth. An *inguinal hernia* appears lower down in the groin and is most common in boys. The defect occurs after the testicles have descended into the scrotum. Umbilical hernias rarely need any treatment; they heal spontaneously. Inguinal hernias may also heal themselves, but if a small part of the bowel becomes trapped in the hernia, it will have to be corrected by minor surgery.

Is it serious?
A hernia is not usually serious unless the bowel is trapped.

Possible symptoms

Areas affected

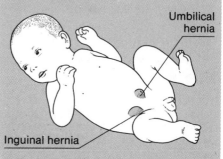

Umbilical hernia

Inguinal hernia

● Painless bulge in the skin's surface near the navel or in the groin. The bulge increases in size when the child coughs, sneezes or cries.
● Vomiting, with sharp abdominal pain, if the bowel has become trapped.

What should I do first?

Try to push the hernia gently inward. Most hernias respond to gentle pressure by sliding back inside the muscular wall.

Should I consult the doctor?

Consult your doctor if you notice a bulge in your baby's abdomen before he is 6 months old. Consult your doctor if a hernia becomes hard, the bulge won't go back with the application of gentle pressure and there is accompanying abdominal pain and vomiting.

What might the doctor do?

☐ If the hernia is hard or won't go back, your doctor will refer you to a pediatric surgeon because the hernia will probably have to be repaired

surgically. The operation for a hernia repair is simple. If your child is under 6 months old and has an inguinal hernia, your doctor may recommend surgical repair to avoid trapping the bowel.

What can I do to help?

☐ As long as the umbilical hernia is there, check periodically, such as at bathtime, to make sure it is not enlarging, it is not hard and it goes back when gently pushed.
☐ Discuss future action with your doctor, and decide together whether or not you are going to let the hernia heal by itself or whether it should be operated on.
☐ Take your child for a checkup at regular intervals, as determined by your doctor.

Words in **bold** are A-Z entries

Hiccups

Hiccups are involuntary, uncontrollable contractions of the diaphragm. The sound of the hiccup is produced when the spasm of the diaphragm causes the glottis at the back of the throat to close during inhalation. A newborn baby hiccups often. This is normal and will not bother him. The cause of these short hiccup episodes is not known. Prolonged or recurrent episodes may be caused by swallowing a hot or irritating substance.

Are they serious?
Hiccups are not usually serious.

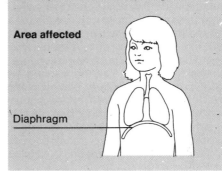

Possible symptoms

● Characteristic "hic" sound with each spasm of the diaphragm.

Area affected

Diaphragm

What should I do first?

1 If your baby has short episodes of hiccups—do nothing. They will go away naturally.

2 If your older child is irritated by hiccups, the best remedies involve making the lungs work harder. Have your child hold his breath to the count of 10, or have him breathe into a paper bag, then rebreathe the air from the bag (don't use a plastic bag), or have your child drink a glass of water rapidly. Other remedies include having your child swallow dry bread, crushed ice or a teaspoon of dry sugar.

Should I consult the doctor?

Consult your doctor if your child's hiccups persist longer than 8 hours.

What might the doctor do?

☐ Your doctor will examine your child, and he may prescribe a mild tranquilizer or sedative to ease recurrent attacks of hiccups.

What can I do to help?

☐ Don't fuss if your baby has hiccups. They will not upset him.

Hives

Hives, also called *urticaria* or *nettle rash*, is a skin condition. The **rash** that results is easy to recognize: the skin erupts into white lumps on a red base. These are called *wheals*. The wheals can be as small as pimples or an inch across. Hives can be caused by skin contact with an allergen, such as primrose, or it can result from eating certain foods, such as strawberries or shellfish. Hives can be caused by certain drugs, particularly penicillin and aspirin, or by viral illness. Hives is most common after a nettle sting. Each crop of wheals is extremely itchy and lasts up to an hour. It then disappears and is replaced by more wheals elsewhere on your child's face or body.

Is it serious?

Hives is not serious, but if it appears on the face, especially in or around the mouth, and is accompanied by swelling, seek medical assistance immediately. This allergic reaction is known as *angio-neurotic edema.* If swelling spreads to the tongue or the throat, it can cause severe breathing problems.

Possible symptoms

Classic appearance of rash

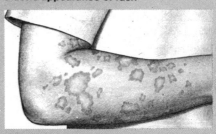

- White lumps on a red base.
- Extremely itchy rash.
- Wheals that disappear in an hour or so to be replaced elsewhere by other wheals.
- Swelling on the face.

What should I do first?

1 Apply calamine lotion to the wheals to soothe the skin.

2 Give your child a warm bath to relieve itching.

Should I consult the doctor?

Consult your doctor immediately if hives on your child's face causes swelling, particularly in and around the mouth. Consult your doctor if the wheals are not gone after several days or if your child is miserable with the itchiness.

What might the doctor do?

☐ Your doctor may prescribe anti-histamine tablets or medicine to relieve the itchiness of your child's skin.
☐ Your doctor may give your child an injection of adrenalin if the swelling causes breathing problems.

What can I do to help?

☐ If your child has frequent attacks, make a note of any new foods he might have eaten. Provided it is not an essential food for a growing child, exclude the suspected allergen for a week or two, then reintroduce it and watch for a reaction.

SEE ALSO:
Itching, *page 169*
Rash, *page 206*

Words in **bold** are A-Z entries

Hyperactivity

The word "hyperactive" is often used as a label for children with minor behavioral problems, such as disruptive behavior, poor attention span, **sleeplessness** and excitability. Most hyperactive children are simply extremely active and normal.

Although research in the United States has found that certain food colorings and flavorings contribute to patterns of hyperactive behavior in children, proper handling and tolerance by parents can solve many of the problems of individual behavior in a child.

Is it serious?
There are few degrees of hyperactivity in children that are abnormal or serious.

Possible symptoms
- Disruptive behavior.
- Restlessness.
- Short attention span.
- Sleeplessness.
- Foolhardiness and unpredictability.

What should I do first?

1 Try to determine whether your child is bored or restless for some reason. Intelligent children need a lot of stimulation.

2 Don't exaggerate the problem. Most parents agree their preschool child is hyperactive some of the time.

Should I consult the doctor?

Consult your doctor for advice if you find your child is difficult to live with or if his behavior is interfering with his schoolwork.

What might the doctor do?

☐ It is difficult to find two doctors who agree on the origin, features or even the fact of hyperactivity. If minor behavioral problems are combined with learning disability, such as **dyslexia**, the confusion is compounded. Your doctor may refer your child to a child psychologist for assessment if there is learning disability.

☐ Your doctor may prescribe medication, such as stimulants. These have a calming effect on children. Children on these drugs need to be monitored carefully for adequate growth, appetite and sleeping habits.

What can I do to help?

☐ The essential approach for parents with hyperactive children is proper handling. Adopt the same approach together so your child cannot manipulate either of you.

☐ Learn to live with your child by treating him as an exciting, unpredictable, but nevertheless normal, child. By the time he goes to school, he should have learned, with your help, to concentrate.

☐ You will need to be more vigilant if your child is careless and more inventive at providing games, so he won't get bored.

SEE ALSO:
Dyslexia, *page 122*
Sleeplessness, *page 219*

Impetigo

Impetigo is a bacterial skin infection most often seen around the lips, nose and ears, but it can be anywhere on the body. It is caused by common skin organisms (*streptococcus* and *staphylococcus*), which are carried in the nose and on the skin. The rash starts as small **blisters**, which break and crust over to become yellow-brown scabs that look like brown sugar.

Is it serious?
Impetigo rarely has serious effects, but because it is highly contagious, it should be treated immediately.

Possible symptoms

Common sites

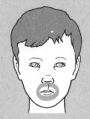

● Tiny blisters around the nose and mouth or ears, which ooze and harden to form crusty, yellow-brown scabs.

What should I do first?

1 If the rash on your child's face starts to weep, don't let him touch it. Wash away crusts with warm water. Pat dry with a paper towel.

2 Keep your child away from school until you have seen the doctor.

Should I consult the doctor?

Call your doctor and he will tell you whether he wants to see your child.

What might the doctor do?

□ Your doctor will prescribe an antibiotic cream that should clear up the impetigo in 5 days.
□ Your doctor may prescribe a course of antibiotics to be taken by mouth to eradicate the infection from your child's body.

What can I do to help?

□ Before applying any ointment, wash away yellow crusts with warm water, and pat dry with a paper towel.
□ Be meticulous about hygiene. Wash your hands before and after administering the treatment. Encourage your child to keep his hands away from the outbreak. Keep his fingernails short to reduce the risk of spreading the infection to other parts of the body.
□ Be strict with your child if he sucks his thumb, bites his nails or picks his nose. This can spread the infection.
□ When the infection has cleared, keep the area moist with lotion or cream.
□ Keep your child's face cloth and towel separate from the rest of the family's to avoid spreading the infection.

SEE ALSO:
Blister, *page 70*

Words in **bold** are A-Z entries

Influenza

Influenza (flu), like the **common cold**, is caused by a virus and has similar symptoms, such as a runny nose, **sore throat**, **cough**, **fever**, shivering and aches and pains all over the body. Because it is a viral infection, there is no cure for flu, and it usually lasts about 3 to 4 days. Unless there is a secondary infection, treatment of the symptoms is all that is necessary in most cases.

Is it serious?

Even if influenza is accompanied by a high temperature, it is rare for serious complications to occur. However, as with any viral infection, natural resistance is reduced, and a secondary infection, such as **pneumonia**, **bronchitis** or **otitis media**, may result. Influenza is always serious in a child who has lungs weakened by **asthma** or another serious condition, such as **diabetes mellitus**.

Possible symptoms

- Runny nose.
- Sore throat.
- Cough.
- Temperature above 100F (37.5C).
- Aches and pains.
- Shivering.
- Diarrhea, vomiting or nausea.
- Weakness and lethargy.

Areas affected

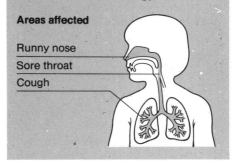

Runny nose

Sore throat

Cough

What should I do first?

1 Check your child's temperature, and if it doesn't come down within 36 hours, consult your doctor.

2 Give your child acetaminophen to reduce the fever and the aches and pains, and put him to bed.

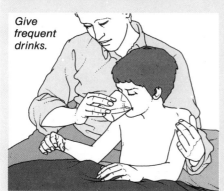

Give frequent drinks.

3 Don't force your child to eat. Make sure he gets plenty to drink, but

don't give him milk if he has diarrhea. Small quantities of diluted fruit juice or water taken often are the best way to replace fluids lost through sweating and fever, or use an electrolyte solution.

4 Do **not** give aspirin to any child under age 19. It could lead to a condition called **Reye's syndrome**.

Should I consult the doctor?

Consult your doctor immediately if your child's temperature fails to come down within 36 hours. Consult your doctor immediately if you notice a deterioration in your child's condition after 48 hours. Watch for a worsening cough, which suggests the infection has gone to your child's chest, or an earache, which may suggest otitis media.

Continued on next page ▶

Influenza

◀ *Continued from previous page*

What might the doctor do?

□ Your doctor will confirm whether or not there is a secondary infection. If there is, he will prescribe an antibiotic to eradicate the infection. If not, your doctor will advise you to continue with acetaminophen elixir and bed rest. If your child has a persistent cough, your doctor may prescribe an appropriate cough mixture.

What can I do to help?

□ Your child should rest in a room with a constant temperature. If he is bored, make a bed in the den or living room so he can be near you during the day.
□ As soon as he wants to be active, let him. But if his temperature rises again, make him rest.

□ Don't leave used tissues lying around. Encourage your child to throw them away as soon as they are used. If he uses handkerchiefs, wash them in boiling water to prevent the spread of the virus through the household.
□ Protect your child each winter with an injection of influenza vaccine if he has a chronic illness, such as asthma or diabetes. This has been shown to protect some children. However, every year a different strain of the virus appears. Immunity, whether from a vaccine or contracting the virus, is only short-lived.
□ If, after your child should have recovered, his temperature rises and he vomits, consult your doctor immediately. The rare, but serious, childhood illness, Reye's syndrome, could be the cause of his deterioration.

SEE ALSO:
Asthma, *page 61*
Bronchitis, *page 76*
Common cold, *page 91*
Cough, *page 98*
Diabetes mellitus, *page 111*
Fever, *page 139*
Measles, *page 176*
Otitis media, *page 195*
Pneumonia, *page 201*
Reye's syndrome, *page 208*
Sore throat, *page 221*

Words in **bold** are A-Z entries

Ingrown toenail

When a toenail fails to grow straight out from the nailbed and curves over into the sides of the toe, it is called an ingrown toenail. This occurs most often to the nail of the big toe, and it causes pain and discomfort. An ingrown toenail is more likely to occur if the toe is broad and plump, if the toenail is cut down at the sides instead of straight across, if the toenail is small or if tight shoes and socks push the nail into the skin. If untreated, the nail will penetrate the skin, possibly become infected, and cause inflammation and a pussy discharge around the edges of the nail.

Is it serious?
An ingrown toenail is painful but not serious.

What should I do first?

1 Examine the skin around the nail to see if it has penetrated the skin.

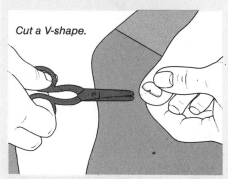
Cut a V-shape.

2 Cut a tiny V-shape in the top edge of the nail to relieve pressure on the sides of the nail.

3 Apply an antiseptic ointment to the sides of the nail to prevent infection.

4 If there is any sign of redness or pus, have your child lie down with his foot propped up. Apply a sterile dressing to the toe.

Should I consult the doctor?

Consult your doctor if the nail has penetrated the skin, if you notice any redness or pus around your child's toenail or if ingrown toenails are a recurrent problem.

What might the doctor do?

☐ Your doctor may prescribe antibiotic tablets and cream to clear up the infection. Your doctor may also prescribe an astringent lotion to toughen up the skin around the toenail.
☐ If the problem is recurrent, your doctor may refer your child to a surgeon to see whether the ingrown edge of the toenail should be removed. This is a minor operation and is usually done in the doctor's office.

What can I do to help?

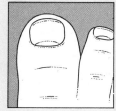 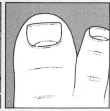
Incorrect   *Correct*

☐ Cut your child's toenails straight across and not too short. Cut them regularly; don't let them get too long.
☐ Make sure your child's shoes and socks are not too tight. Allow him enough space to wiggle his toes.
☐ If your child's toenail becomes infected, don't put socks on him. Cut the toe out of an old shoe, or let him wear sandals while the infection is healing.

Intussusception

Intussusception is a condition that occurs when part of the small intestine telescopes inside the intestine ahead of it, sort of like a finger in a glove being turned inside out. The twisted intestine swells, and this causes a blockage. In an effort to overcome this blockage, the affected intestine goes into spasm. There is no known cause for intussusception, and it can happen at any age. However, it most often affects baby boys under 12 months old who have previously been in excellent health. The baby may suddenly cry out as the muscular spasms begin and may vomit and be pale and feverish. In between spasms, he may appear quite normal and have normal bowel movements for the first few hours. However, as the attacks continue, bowel movements characteristically look like red-currant jelly because they contain mostly blood and mucus.

Is it serious?

Though rare, intussusception is a serious condition. If left untreated, it can be fatal.

Possible symptoms

● Severe abdominal pain, possibly accompanied by screaming.
● Vomiting.
● Paleness.
● Slight fever.
● Bowel movements, containing blood and mucus, that resemble red-currant jelly.

Affected area

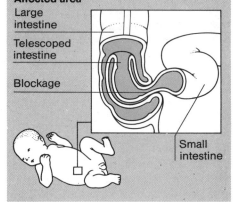

Large intestine

Telescoped intestine

Blockage

Small intestine

What should I do first?

1 If your baby has a number of spasmodic attacks when he screams and pulls his legs up to his stomach in pain, yet he appears quite well in between attacks, consult your doctor immediately.

2 Check your baby's bowel movements for blood or mucus.

3 In between attacks, take your baby's temperature to see if he has a fever.

Should I consult the doctor?

Consult your doctor immediately if your baby has a number of attacks of abdominal cramps or if you notice any blood or mucus in your baby's bowel movements.

What might the doctor do?

☐ Your doctor may order a barium enema to confirm the diagnosis of intussusception. This is a painless investigation in which fluid is pumped into the intestines through your baby's rectum. The condition of the intestines can then be seen on X-ray. The barium enema sometimes causes the condition to clear up. If it does not, your baby will have an operation to push the intestine back into its normal position.

SEE ALSO:
Colic, *page 89*
Vomiting, *page 254*

Words in **bold** are A-Z entries

Itching

Itching is usually a symptom of some underlying skin problem (**eczema, ringworm**), the result of an infestation (**scabies,** fleas or **worms**), sensitivity to some food or drug, dry skin, skin contact with an irritant (**hives**) or the result of an infectious disease (**chickenpox**). Sometimes nervous tension and worry can cause itching, and scratching can make the itchiness even worse.

Is it serious?
Itching is rarely serious, but you shouldn't ignore it.

What should I do first?

1 Try to determine the cause of the itching. The site may give you a clue. For example, itching around the anus and genitals could indicate worms or **thrush**, itchiness in the hair, ringworm, on the feet, **athlete's foot**, or between the fingers, scabies.

2 Check any pets your child comes into contact with for fleas.

3 Check to see if your child has eaten any new foods recently.

4 Note whether your child is taking any new medicines, especially if itching is accompanied by a rash.

5 Try soothing the itching with lots of calamine lotion, or give your child a cool bath with baking soda dissolved in the water.

Should I consult the doctor?

Consult your doctor if you can find no apparent reason for the itching or if your child is having difficulty sleeping because of constant itchiness.

What might the doctor do?

☐ Your doctor will examine your child and determine the cause of the itching. If itching is a symptom of another condition, he will treat this accordingly. He may prescribe antihistamine tablets, elixir or cream to curb the itching.
☐ If your child is having difficulty sleeping, your doctor may prescribe a mild sedative.

What can I do to help?

☐ Dress your child in cotton underwear so fabrics, such as wool and nylon, that irritate do not touch his skin.
☐ If you have recently changed your laundry detergent or fabric softener, use the old brand, and see if the irritation subsides. Rinse clothes well.
☐ Use a mild soap and shampoo for your child.

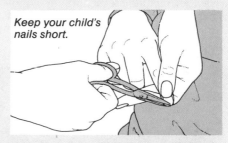
Keep your child's nails short.

☐ To keep your child from scratching, put mittens on him when possible. Keep his nails short to prevent infection if he breaks the skin by scratching too hard.

SEE ALSO:
Athlete's foot, *page 63*
Chickenpox, *page 83*
Chilblains, *page 84*
Eczema, *page 126*
Hives, *page 162*
Ringworm, *page 210*
Scabies, *page 212*
Thrush, *page 239*
Worms, *page 261*

Jaundice

Jaundice is a symptom of an underlying disease, and it causes a yellow coloration of the skin and whites of the eyes.

The condition is due to the presence of yellow bile pigment, *bilirubin,* in the blood. Bile pigment is made during the normal breakdown of old red blood cells. When certain illnesses are present, the bile pigment accumulates in the blood, tinging the skin yellow. Possible causes include **hepatitis** (liver infection), a blockage or malformation of the bile duct and certain types of **anemia**. The yellow skin coloration is often accompanied by dark-brown urine because bile pigment overflows from the blood into the urine. There may also be pale stools because the pigment is no longer present in the intestinal contents to darken their color.

Newborn jaundice occurs in ⅓ of all babies during the week after birth and is also called *physiological jaundice.* In nearly all cases, there is no underlying disease. The condition is due to the baby's liver and digestive system adapting to life outside the womb.

Is it serious?

Jaundice may be serious because it can be a symptom of an underlying complaint.

Possible symptoms

- Yellow coloration of the skin and the whites of the eyes.
- Dark-brown urine.
- Pale-colored stools.
- Nausea and loss of appetite.

What should I do first?

1 See if your child's urine is a darker color, and see if his stools are abnormally pale.

2 If your child feels sick and will not eat, give him frequent drinks to prevent dehydration.

3 Be meticulous about hygiene until you have consulted your doctor. Your child may have hepatitis, which is contagious.

Should I consult the doctor?

Consult your doctor immediately if you suspect your child is jaundiced or if your baby seems yellow or unusually suntanned. A baby who is jaundiced must be checked by a doctor because excess bilirubin can damage internal organs. Your child must also be checked for any underlying disease.

What might the doctor do?

☐ The underlying disease will be identified and treated as necessary. If it is hepatitis, your child may need to be isolated.
☐ Your child will need regular checkups even after the problem has cleared up to ensure there are no aftereffects.

What can I do to help?

☐ Keep your child on any special diets and treatments.
☐ Be sympathetic. Your child may feel tired and depressed for some weeks.

SEE ALSO:
Anemia, *page 53*
Hepatitis, *page 158*

Words in **bold** are A-Z entries

Lactose intolerance

Lactose intolerance is difficulty digesting cow's milk. The enzyme *lactase* is necessary for the digestion of all milk, except breast milk. It breaks down the sugar in the milk, called *lactose.* If there is a deficiency of this enzyme, the lactose will not be absorbed into the bloodstream. It stays in the intestine, ferments and causes symptoms of **gastroenteritis**, such as foamy diarrhea and vomiting.

Temporary lactose intolerance can occur in a baby after a severe attack of gastroenteritis that damages the intestinal lining. The enzyme lactase disappears in adulthood in all but the white races, so many Black and Oriental people develop a permanent lactose intolerance later in life. In some instances, the condition is inherited, and the baby will be born with the disorder.

Is it serious?
Lactose intolerance is serious, but it is easily treated with a change in diet. If left untreated, your child may fail to thrive.

Possible symptoms
- Foamy, explosive diarrhea.
- Vomiting
- Slow weight gain, growth and development.

What should I do first?
If your baby has the symptoms of gastroenteritis, give him only water and consult your doctor.

Should I consult the doctor?
Consult your doctor if your baby has foamy, explosive diarrhea and vomiting or if the symptoms return when milk is reintroduced to the diet after an attack of diarrhea and vomiting.

What might the doctor do?
☐ If the lactose intolerance is temporary and caused by gastroenteritis, your doctor will advise you to substitute synthetic formula, free from lactose. After a short time on a milk-free diet, symptoms should disappear. Your doctor will advise you to reintroduce cow's milk and watch for a recurrence of the symptoms. When symptoms cease to appear, the condition is cured.
☐ If the condition is present at birth, your doctor will probably advise an infant formula that contains little lactose.

What can I do to help?
☐ Symptoms can be relieved or controlled in permanent cases of lactose intolerance with a diet free of milk and milk products.
☐ If your baby has had a temporary intolerance, and vomiting and diarrhea reappear, consult your doctor.

SEE ALSO:
Failure to thrive, *page 137*
Gastroenteritis, *page 144*

Laryngitis

Laryngitis is an inflammation of the larynx or voice box. Many minor viruses, and occasionally bacteria, enter the body through the throat and quickly infect the larynx. The most obvious symptoms of laryngitis are hoarseness, a dry **cough** and sometimes **fever**.

Is it serious?

Laryngitis is rarely serious and lasts less than 7 days, even if it is part of a more serious infection, such as **tonsillitis** or **bronchitis**. However, in young children a swollen larynx can obstruct the passage of air, causing breathing difficulties and **croup**, which is a serious complication. If laryngitis develops into croup, seek medical treatment immediately.

Possible symptoms

- Hoarseness or loss of voice.
- Dry cough.
- Slight fever.
- Sore throat.
- Croup (a barking type of cough).

Cross section of the throat

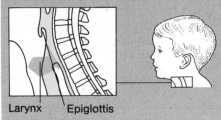

Larynx   Epiglottis

What should I do first?

1 If the hoarseness is not accompanied by any other symptoms of a respiratory-tract infection, such as bronchitis, keep a check on your child's temperature. If it rises above 100F (37.5C), there may be another infection present.

2 Listen closely for the barking cough of croup.

3 Keep the air in your child's room moist if possible. Use a cool-mist humidifier or vaporizer.

Should I consult the doctor?

Consult your doctor immediately if you think your child has croup. Consult your doctor if your child has a fever or you think he has contracted another infection.

What might the doctor do?

☐ If there is a bacterial infection, such as bronchitis or tonsillitis, your doctor will prescribe antibiotics.

What can I do to help?

☐ Discourage your child from talking out loud. Make a game of it, and have the whole family talk in whispers.

☐ Give your child plenty of warm liquid to soothe his throat. Try hot lemon and honey, or heat any fruit juice drink by diluting it with hot water.

SEE ALSO:
Bronchitis, *page 76*
Cough, *page 98*
Croup, *page 101*
Fever, *page 139*
Tonsillitis, *page 243*

Words in **bold** are A-Z entries

Leukemia

Leukemia is a rare form of cancer caused by the rapid overgrowth of millions of primitive white blood cells. The cancerous white blood cells prevent the normal growth of red blood cells, leading to anemia. They cause a lack of mature white blood cells, which reduces immunity to infection. Leukemia prevents the growth of platelets, which help in the blood-clotting mechanism of the body. Often the first indication of leukemia is the anemic condition of the child and his failure to recover quickly from an infectious illness.

Possible symptoms

- Anemia—paleness, tiredness and shortness of breath.
- Susceptibility to infection.
- Pain in the limbs; if in the legs, perhaps seen as a limp.
- Purpura—a purple-red rash that doesn't disappear with pressure.
- Tendency to bruise easily.
- Recurrent nosebleeds.

What can be done?

At one time, the outlook for children with leukemia was not good. But over the last 10 years, therapy has improved the chances of a complete cure for many children suffering from the most common type of childhood leukemia.

A child with the disease will be treated by a pediatrician who specializes in childhood leukemic diseases. Several drugs are given at the same time, some by mouth and some by injection. In the most common type of childhood leukemia, X-ray therapy and special drugs may be used to kill the cancer cells in the brain. A blood transfusion may be given at the beginning of the treatment. If the number of white blood cells falls to a very low level, your child will be isolated against infection, and visitors will need to wear masks and gowns. After several weeks, your child should be allowed to return home to lead as normal a life as possible. Regular checkups will be necessary to keep track of the condition.

The important role for you as parents is to support your child through the long, arduous treatment by keeping up his morale with the prospect of an eventual cure. Children with leukemia must not be exposed to common childhood infectious diseases, such as chickenpox, unless they are already immune, so make sure your child has all his immunizations and screen his friends carefully.

L

Lice

The head louse is a tiny insect that infests the hair on the human head. The adult louse lays its eggs (nits) at the root of the hair, to which they become firmly attached. This distinguishes them from **dandruff**, which can be flaked off easily with a fingernail. Eggs hatch after 2 weeks, and the lice bite the scalp to get blood. Your child's head will be itchy where the lice bite, particularly after strenuous exercise when he is hot and perspiring. Your child can become infested by contact with another infested person.

Are they serious?
Lice and nits are irritating, but they can be easily eradicated and are not serious.

Possible symptoms

● Itchy scalp, particularly when the head is hot.

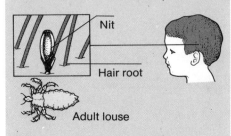

Nit

Hair root

Adult louse

● Tiny, pearl-white eggs covering the roots of the hair.

What should I do first?

1 If your child scratches his head, inspect the roots of the hair for nits.

2 If you find them, keep your child home until you have administered the treatment. Inform the teacher of the outbreak.

3 Ask your druggist to recommend a shampoo for removing nits. Follow the directions for use.

4 Examine the heads of the rest of the family to check for nits. Treat the other members of your family with the appropriate shampoo. Contact for less than 1 second with someone who has lice is sufficient to transfer the lice.

5 After treatment, remove any dead eggs with a fine-toothed comb.

Should I consult the doctor?

Consult your doctor if the treatment doesn't work. You may not have administered the treatment properly.

What might the doctor do?

☐ Your doctor will question you about any self-help treatment you have used. He may prescribe another shampoo.

What can I do to help?

☐ Repeat the treatment in 7 days in case any eggs remain.
☐ Clean any headgear, brushes or combs that have been used by your child with the anti-louse shampoo.

SEE ALSO:
Dandruff, *page 107*
Itching, *page 169*

L

Words in **bold** are A-Z entries

Limp

Your child is limping if he doesn't take the full weight of his body on one leg as he walks. The cause, on investigation, may be obvious, such as a **cut**, a **blister** or a **splinter** on the sole of the foot or the heel, a protruding toenail, an **ingrown toenail**, tight shoes, wrinkling of the inner sole in his shoes or a pebble in a shoe. A persistent limp that has no obvious cause may be a symptom of some other, more serious, problem.

Is it serious?

Limping for no apparent reason should always be treated seriously in a child. An unexplained limp can be a symptom of the rare form of blood cancer, **leukemia**. If the limp is accompanied by swelling or tenderness of the joints, it may be caused by **rheumatic fever**, **arthritis** or **osteomyelitis**. These could have long-term complications and should be treated seriously.

What should I do first?

1 Look for obvious injuries, and examine any areas that your child claims are painful.

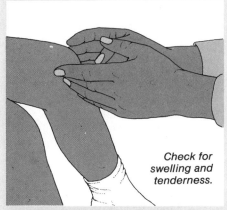

Check for swelling and tenderness.

2 Check to see if the joints are swollen and inflamed.

3 If you suspect your child may have a **broken bone**, don't hesitate to get medical attention. The injury may not always be obvious.

Should I consult the doctor?

Consult your doctor immediately for a thorough investigation of the limp if you can't find a reason for it or if you suspect a broken bone. Consult your doctor immediately if any of your child's joints are swollen or tender.

What might the doctor do?

□ Your doctor will examine your child's leg thoroughly and may refer him to an orthopedic surgeon to find the cause of the problem.

What can I do to help?

□ Never give up if your child has a limp. Continue taking your child to your doctor for investigation. Be persistent until the cause is found.

L

SEE ALSO:
Arthritis, *page 59*
Blister, *page 70*
Broken bone, *page 73*
Cuts and scrapes, *page 104*
Ingrown toenail, *page 167*
Leukemia, *page 173*
Osteomyelitis, *page 192*
Rheumatic fever, *page 209*
Splinter, *page 224*

Measles

Measles is an infectious disease caused by a virus. It is very contagious and has an incubation period of between 8 and 14 days. The first indication of measles is usually symptoms similar to those of a **common cold**, with a **fever** that gets increasingly higher and small, white spots inside the mouth, on the linings of the cheeks (Koplik's spots). Sometimes your child's eyes will be red and sore. The initial symptoms are followed about 3 days later by small, brown-red spots behind the ears that merge together to form a rash over the face and body.

Is it serious?
Measles is an unpleasant childhood disease, but it is not usually serious. However, in rare cases your child may develop complications, such as **otitis media**, **pneumonia** or **encephalitis**.

Possible symptoms
- Runny nose and dry cough.
- Headache.
- Fever, rising as high as 104F (40C).
- Small, white spots inside the mouth.
- Red, sore eyes, intolerant of bright light.
- Brown-red rash of small spots starting behind the ears and spreading to the rest of the body.

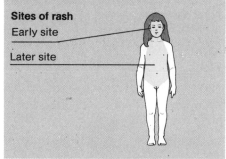

Sites of rash
Early site
Later site

What should I do first?

1 If your child has a fever, bring it down with tepid sponging (*see page 31*).

2 If his eyes are sore, bathe them with cool water.

3 Make sure he has plenty of fluid by offering small amounts regularly.

Should I consult the doctor?

Consult your doctor to confirm the diagnosis. Measles is not common and needs to be reported to the health department. Consult your doctor immediately if your child gets worse after recovering or he complains of **earache**.

What might the doctor do?

□ Your doctor will advise you to keep your child in bed for as long as his temperature remains high. He will examine your child's ears to see if there is an ear infection. If there is, he will prescribe antibiotics.

□ Your doctor may prescribe eye drops for your child's eyes if they are sore.

What can I do to help?

□ Don't send your child back to school until the rash has faded.

□ Have all children inoculated against measles at 15 months of age. Measles inoculation is required by many school districts before your child will be allowed to attend school.

> **SEE ALSO:**
> **Common cold,** *page 91*
> **Earache,** *page 124*
> **Encephalitis,** *page 128*
> **Fever,** *page 138*
> **Otitis media,** *page 195*
> **Pneumonia,** *page 201*

Words in **bold** are A-Z entries

Meningitis

Meningitis is an inflammation of the membranes (*meninges*) that cover the brain and spinal cord. It most frequently results from viral or bacterial infection. Viral meningitis is usually not a very serious illness.

Bacterial meningitis is serious but can be treated successfully with antibiotics if it is diagnosed early enough. Meningitis can be difficult to diagnose in babies and children whose inability to communicate what they feel may lead to a delay in diagnosis. Under age 2, the fontanelle will bulge slightly.

Is it serious?
Bacterial meningitis is a very serious disease. If it is left untreated, it can be fatal.

Possible symptoms
- Fever as high as 102F (38.9C).
- Stiff neck.
- Lethargy.
- Headache.
- Inability to tolerate bright light.
- Bulging fontanelle.
- Drowsiness and confusion.
- Vomiting.
- Purple-red rash over most of the body.

Cross section of the meninges

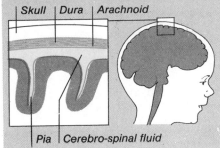

Skull | Dura | Arachnoid

Pia | Cerebro-spinal fluid

M

What should I do first?

1 If you suspect meningitis, bend your child's head forward so his chin touches his chest. See if there is any stiffness or pain in his neck.

2 See if your child screws his eyes up in bright light. If he is under 2, feel the fontanelle to see if it bulges.

Should I consult the doctor?

Consult your doctor immediately if you suspect meningitis.

What might the doctor do?

☐ Your doctor will refer your child to the hospital for lumbar puncture. This involves taking a sample of spinal fluid from your child for testing and is done under local anesthetic. It causes little pain.

☐ If your child is suffering from bacterial meningitis, he will be given high doses of antibiotics intravenously. Viral meningitis clears up on its own, but your child will be observed in the hospital for several days.

What can I do to help?

☐ Recently a vaccine has been introduced to protect children against bacterial meningitis caused by hemophilus influenza Type B. Have any child between 2 and 5 inoculated.

SEE ALSO:
Drowsiness, *page 120*
Fever, *page 138*
Headache, *page 153*

Milia

Milia is a rash of tiny white- or yellow-headed spots that may appear on the nose and cheeks of a newborn baby within the first 3 weeks of life. The spots appear because the baby's sweat glands are not developed well enough to function properly. Spots remain until the sweat glands mature, usually within the first 3 months. The spots are not itchy and cause no unpleasant symptoms in the baby.

Is it serious?
Milia is never serious and resolves itself naturally without treatment.

Possible symptoms

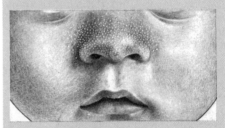

● Tiny white or yellow spots, usually over the nose and cheeks.

What should I do first?

1 Do not squeeze the spots. Though they may appear to have heads of pus, they are not infected. The skin of a baby is too fragile to take any pressure or squeezing.

2 Don't put any creams or lotions on the spots.

Should I consult the doctor?

There should be no need to consult your doctor unless you are concerned about the cause of the rash.

What might the doctor do?

☐ Your doctor will reassure you and will not interfere with the milia.

What can I do to help?

☐ Ignore the milia. The spots will disappear in time.
☐ Milia is very common in newborn babies, so relax and wait until they disappear.

M

Words in **bold** are A-Z entries

Mononucleosis

Infectious mononucleosis is a viral infection. It begins in much the same way as **influenza**, with a runny nose, **sore throat**, aches, pains, and tiredness. In a small number of cases, it begins with a rash like **German measles**. It is a fairly common disease mostly affecting teenagers and young adults. Children can also contract it, but they tend to be less severely affected by the disease.

There is no known cure for mononucleosis. It has to run its course—generally at least a month. As part of the body's reaction to the infection, the glands become swollen and the spleen may become enlarged. This does not in itself give rise to unpleasant symptoms, and the spleen, which is part of the lymphatic gland system, returns to normal once the infection is gone.

Is it serious?

Although debilitating, mononucleosis is not usually serious. Many of its symptoms are similar to those of other illnesses so you should consult your doctor for a diagnosis.

Possible symptoms

- Swollen glands, most commonly in the neck, accompanied by fever.
- Depression and lethargy.

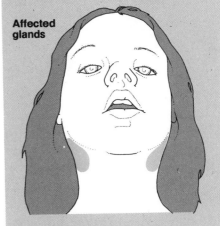

Affected glands

- Runny nose.
- Sore throat.
- Aches and pains.
- Rash that starts behind the ears and spreads to the forehead.

What should I do first?

1 While many of the early symptoms of mononucleosis are similar to those of other ailments, be alerted if the neck glands are swollen and there is a **fever**. Check your child's temperature regularly if his glands are swollen. If it remains high, give him a dose of acetaminophen.

2 Keep your child isolated until you have a definite diagnosis. The virus is infectious and is passed on by intimate contact, such as kissing.

Should I consult the doctor?

Consult your doctor immediately if you suspect your child is not just suffering from flu or a **common cold**.

What might the doctor do?

☐ Your doctor will take a blood sample for analysis. Mononucleosis can be diagnosed with certainty only by finding the virus in the blood. You will be advised to keep your child indoors and to make sure he has plenty of rest. No further treatment is required.

What can I do to help?

☐ Your child will not be able to return to school without your doctor's permission. Arrange for school work to be sent home for him once he feels up to doing it.

Continued on next page ▶

Mononucleosis

◀ Continued from previous page
☐ If your child wants to stay in bed, let him. If he doesn't, keep him indoors until the fever subsides.

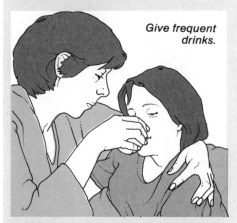

Give frequent drinks.

☐ If your child has a temperature, offer him plenty of fluid to prevent dehydration.
☐ Mononucleosis is debilitating, and it may be 6 months before your child is completely fit and his old self again.
☐ Keep him entertained and cheerful. The length of time the disease takes to run its course can lead to boredom and depression. So, although your child needs plenty of rest, keep him busy in quiet ways with books, puzzles and television.
☐ The virus may reappear during the 2 years after the first attack, so watch for a recurrence of the symptoms. Consult your doctor if you are concerned.

SEE ALSO:
Common cold, *page 91*
Fever, *page 140*
German measles, *page 146*
Influenza, *page 165*
Sore throat, *page 222*

Words in **bold** are A-Z entries

Motion sickness

Motion sickness occurs when the balance organs in the ear are upset by movement. When this sensation of movement doesn't correspond with what the eyes see, it causes confusion in the brain. The problem can result if a child rides a roller coaster or swings at a playground or rides in a car, boat or plane. Symptoms range from slight queasiness to **vomiting** and faintness. Children tend to suffer from motion sickness more than adults, though why is not known. Most children outgrow it by adolescence.

Is it serious?
Motion sickness is not serious, but it is inconvenient. With a young child there is a slight risk that prolonged vomiting could cause **dehydration**.

Possible symptoms
- Nausea.
- Vomiting.
- Pale, clammy forehead.
- Weakness or dizziness.
- Fainting.

What should I do first?

1 If your child complains of feeling sick, looks pale or becomes abnormally quiet while you are traveling, see if his forehead feels cold and clammy.

2 Tell your child to close his eyes, and lay him down if possible. This should minimize the confusing signals being received by the brain.

Should I consult the doctor?

Consult your doctor if your child suffers from motion sickness on even short trips or if over-the-counter brands of motion-sickness medicine do not help.

What might the doctor do?

☐ After questioning you about symptoms and their frequency, your doctor may prescribe a drug, such as an antihistamine, though some antihistamines can have side effects such as **drowsiness**.

What can I do to help?

☐ Don't make a fuss before you travel. This can make your child more excited and apprehensive, and he may be sick as a result.
☐ Prevent motion sickness by giving your child medicine *before* you start the trip. There are several good over-the-counter medications available at the drugstore.
☐ Give your child a small snack before leaving. Don't let him travel on either an empty or a full stomach.
☐ Take plenty of drinks with you, or see if they will be available along the way to prevent the possibility of dehydration through vomiting. Drinks can also reduce the feeling of nausea.
☐ Carry strong brown paper bags in case of vomiting.

SEE ALSO:
Dehydration, *page 109*
Drowsiness, *page 120*
Vomiting, *page 255*

Mouth sores

Children may suffer from many mouth sores that are painful, though most are relatively harmless. *Aphthous ulcers* are usually small and creamy-white and appear on the tongue, gums or lining of the mouth. These ulcers are sometimes associated with stress.

A *traumatic ulcer* is larger and usually starts as a sore patch on the inside of the cheeks, possibly after injury by biting or by rubbing of a rough tooth. It enlarges to form a painful yellow crater. It heals very slowly and, regardless of treatment, takes 10 to 14 days to clear. White, painful blisters on the roof of the mouth, on the gums and inside the cheeks can be the result of a primary infection with the **cold sore** virus. White, curdlike blisters could indicate a **thrush** infection.

Small white **blisters** on cheeks, gums, tongue and throat, often accompanied by fever, are symptoms of a viral infection. It is sometimes called *hand, foot and mouth disease* because there may be a rash on palms and soles.

Are they serious?
Mouth sores are rarely serious.

Possible symptoms

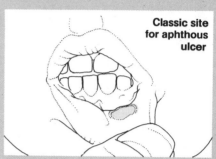

Classic site for aphthous ulcer

● Small, creamy-white, painful areas anywhere on the tongue, gums or lining of the mouth.
● Large red area with a yellow center, particularly inside the cheeks.
● White blisterlike spots inside the mouth, sometimes accompanied by fever.
● Loss of appetite because eating is painful.

What should I do first?

1 If your child complains of a sore mouth or tongue, check to see if there are any areas of soreness.

2 If the sore is large and is inside the cheek, check for a jagged tooth that might be rubbing the cheek lining and causing the injury.

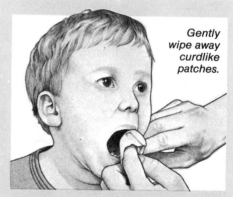

Gently wipe away curdlike patches.

3 If the sores resemble white curds, try to wipe them off with a handkerchief. If this leaves red, raw patches, the sores could be caused by thrush.

Continued on next page ▶

Words in **bold** are A-Z entries

Mouth sores

◀ *Continued from previous page*

4 If your bottle-fed baby has a traumatic ulcer on the roof of his mouth, check the nipple. It may be too hard for your baby's tender mouth.

Should I consult the doctor?

Consult your doctor if the sores are very painful. Consult your doctor if the mouth sores are recurrent. If the ulceration is caused by a jagged tooth, take your child to the dentist to have the tooth repaired.

What might the doctor do?

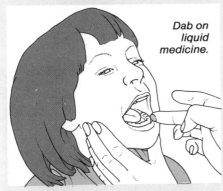

Dab on liquid medicine.

□ Your doctor will reassure you that your child will be all right.
□ He may give you a liquid medicine to dab on the sores to numb the pain.

What can I do to help?

□ Purée foods to minimize chewing when the sores are most painful. Let your child eat through a straw if he wants.
□ Give Popsicles and ice cream. Avoid hard, crunchy, salty foods and citrus fruit.
□ Discourage your child from biting his lips or cheeks. This can lead to injury of the mouth and lip lining and eventually to ulceration.
□ Give your child acetaminophen for pain if your doctor advises.

SEE ALSO:
Blister, *page 70*
Cold sore, *page 88*
Thrush, *page 239*

Mumps

Mumps is an infectious childhood disease, mostly affecting children over the age of 2. It is caused by a virus and has an incubation period of 17 to 28 days. Your child will seem generally unwell for a day or 2 before the major symptoms appear. The salivary glands in front of, and beneath, the ears and chin swell up, and there may be **fever**. The swelling will change the shape of your child's face. It can appear first on one side of the face, then the other or on both sides at once. The swelling causes pain when swallowing, and your child will complain of a dry mouth because the salivary glands have stopped producing saliva. A less common symptom is swelling of the testes or ovaries, causing local pain in boys and abdominal pain and tenderness in girls.

Is it serious?

Mumps is a mild disease. However, if after 10 days your child has a severe headache and a stiff neck, this could be **encephalitis** or **meningitis**, which are serious complications.

Possible symptoms

Affected areas

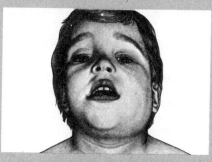

● Swelling of the glands on either or both sides of the face just below the ears and beneath the chin.
● Pain when swallowing.
● Dry mouth.
● Fever.
● Headache.
● Swollen, painful testes in boys or lower abdominal pain in girls.

What should I do first?

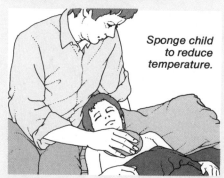

Sponge child to reduce temperature.

1 Check your child's temperature to see if he has a fever. If he has, try to bring it down with tepid sponging (*see page 31*).

2 Purée your child's food, and feed him through a straw if he is having difficulty eating.

3 Give him plenty to drink. Encourage him to rinse out his mouth to alleviate dryness.

4 Put your child to bed with a hot-water bottle wrapped in a towel to hold against the affected side.

Should I consult the doctor?

Consult your doctor to confirm the diagnosis of mumps or if your son's testes are very painful or your daughter is suffering abdominal pain. Consult your doctor immediately if, after 10 days, your child's condition has worsened and he has a headache and a stiff neck.

Continued on next page ▶

Words in **bold** are A-Z entries

Mumps

◀ Continued from previous page

What might the doctor do?

☐ There is no specific treatment for mumps. Your doctor will advise you to keep your child away from school until 5 days after the swelling has gone down.

☐ If the testes are swollen, your doctor will advise complete bed rest until the swelling has subsided. He will probably prescribe acetaminophen for the pain of your son's swollen testes or if your daughter has abdominal pain from swollen ovaries.

What can I do to help?

Egg-enriched milkshake.

Yogurt.

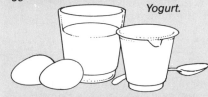

☐ Be inventive with liquid foods, such as egg-enriched milkshakes, soups and yogurt, which go down easily.

☐ Immunize your child against mumps at 15 months.

SEE ALSO:
Encephalitis, *page 128*
Fever, *139*
Meningitis, *page 177*

Muscular dystrophy

Muscular dystrophy is the term given to a group of disorders that is usually inherited and results in a gradual wasting and weakening of the muscle fibers. The most common form of the disease in children is Duchenne muscular dystrophy, which affects only boys. The boy will be slow at developing muscular power. He will be late for his age to sit, walk and run. But only about 25% of all boys suffering from this form of muscular dystrophy have any mental handicap. The disorder is usually diagnosed by the time the child is 3 years old.

As mobility deteriorates, your child will walk with a waddling gait and an arched back because of the weakness of the pelvic muscles. He will have difficulty climbing stairs. His calf muscles, though weakened, will appear overdeveloped, and the muscles in the upper arm will also be abnormally large. Walking becomes impossible by the age of about 12. Because there is no known treatment, 75% of all sufferers die by age 20.

The cardiac muscles of muscular dystrophy sufferers also weaken, so this increases the risk of serious or persistent chest infections, which can result in sudden death.

Possible symptoms

- Late development in ability to sit, walk and run.
- Waddling gait.
- Difficulty getting upright.
- Difficulty climbing stairs.
- Overdeveloped muscles, particularly noticeable in the calves.
- Deformation of the spine.

What can be done?

There is no effective treatment for muscular dystrophy. The child should be kept active and walking as long as possible, without strenuous exercise because this hastens the muscle deterioration. The use of lightweight splints and braces can prolong walking. Too much bed rest is not advisable because it speeds up muscular disintegration. Physiotherapy treatment may be used to limit physical disability.

Duchenne muscular dystrophy is carried by women, so seek genetic counseling before deciding to have a baby if there is any family history of muscular dystrophy. If a pattern of inheritance can be found, there is a 50% chance of a male child being affected and the same chance of a female child being a carrier. Early in pregnancy, amniocentesis, in which a sample of amniotic fluid is extracted and examined for defective cells, will determine the child's sex. A pregnant woman can then decide whether to terminate her pregnancy if the fetus is a male child and at a 50% risk of being affected. In the near future, more precise tests for muscular dystrophy will be available early in pregnancy.

Nightmares

Everyone dreams, and most children have occasional unpleasant dreams or nightmares. Your child may wake up screaming in panic or sobbing uncontrollably. He will seem to be in a state halfway between consciousness and sleep, with his eyes open, though he will not be in touch with reality. He may not even recognize you or understand what you are saying to him.

Nightmares can occur for a number of reasons. If your child has a high temperature or is uncomfortable because of illness, he may wake hot and frightened in the night. If he has gone to bed over-tired, he may wake crying within an hour or two of going to sleep. He may have seen a frightening television program just before going to bed. Or he may be scared of the dark or dislike being alone in his bedroom. In normal children, if nightmares occur with frequency, the underlying cause is usually anxiety about school or home life, such as the arrival of a new baby.

Are they serious?
Nightmares are not serious and don't require medical attention unless they occur very frequently.

What should I do first?

Go to your child immediately. Don't let him get too hysterical. Turn on the light, hold him close to you and speak quietly to soothe him. Don't raise your voice and scold him; this may make him hysterical. Don't ask him why he woke up frightened or what his dream was about.

Should I consult the doctor?

Consult your doctor for advice if the nightmares are frequent (every night, for example) and your child is losing sleep because of them.

What might the doctor do?

☐ Your doctor will probably do nothing but reassure you your child will outgrow the habit.
☐ If your child is losing sleep, your doctor may prescribe a mild sedative to help him sleep.

What can I do to help?

☐ Stay with your child until he drifts back to sleep.
☐ If he is old enough to explain, ask him what he thinks might have caused the nightmare but wait till the following day to do so.
☐ Try to reduce your child's anxiety by reassuring him. If you can guess the cause of his tension, such as the arrival of a new baby, do your best to allay his fears.

N

Nose, foreign body in

If there is a foreign body in your child's nose, it was probably pushed in by your child or a playmate. The problem may not be noticed by you or your child at first, but after 2 or 3 days there will be a **nosebleed**, or a blood-stained, foul-smelling discharge from the affected nostril.

Is it serious?
If the foreign body can be easily removed from the nose, it is not serious and should have no aftereffects. The situation becomes serious if your child inhales the object into his lungs. This may partially block the air passages and cause **croup**, breathing difficulties or **choking**.

Possible symptoms

- Nosebleeds.
- Smelly, blood-stained discharge from the nostril.
- Red, swollen, tender area over the nose.
- Peculiar odor on your child's breath, sometimes said to smell like ripe cheese.

What should I do first?

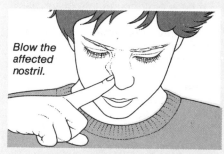

Blow the affected nostril.

1 If your child is old enough to understand, ask him to hold a finger against the good nostril (or do this for him) and blow the affected one. This may dislodge the foreign body. Don't ask a young child to do this—he might sniff the object back into his air passages.

2 Lay your child on his back on a flat surface, and shine a light on his face. If the object can be seen near the entrance to the nose, and if it is soft, remove it with tweezers. If it moves farther up the nostril as you attempt this, leave it alone. If your child has breathing problems, treat this as an emergency.

Should I consult the doctor?

Consult your doctor immediately, or take your child to the emergency room if you cannot easily remove the foreign body from your child's nose.

What might the doctor do?

☐ Your doctor will remove the foreign body with a pair of forceps. If your child is very young or refuses to stay still, he may have to be taken to the hospital and have the foreign body removed under general anesthetic.

What can I do to help?

☐ Try not to allow a child under age 3 to play with toys or objects small enough to swallow or put up his nose, such as peanuts, popcorn kernels, peas or beans.

SEE ALSO:
Choking, *page 85*
Croup, *page 101*
Nosebleed, *page 189*

Words in **bold** are A-Z entries

Nosebleed

A nosebleed occurs when a small area of blood vessels on the inner surface of the nose ruptures. This can be caused by hard nose blowing or sneezing when your child has a **common cold** or **hay fever**, by a bump on the nose, by picking the nose or by a foreign body in the nose. The blood loss from a nosebleed can look dramatic but it is usually very little.

Is it serious?
A nosebleed is hardly ever serious. If your child has frequent nosebleeds which don't stop easily or if his nose bleeds after a bump on the head, call your doctor.

What should I do first?

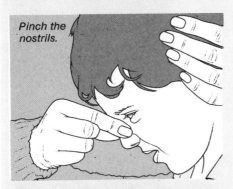

Pinch the nostrils.

Don't try to stop the blood by pushing anything into the nostrils. Sit your child down with his head forward over a basin or sink. Apply firm pressure to both nostrils, gripping his nose between your thumb and forefinger where the bone ends. Squeeze for 10 minutes or until bleeding stops. Don't let your child put his head back during a nosebleed. This allows blood to go into the stomach and can cause irritation and vomiting.

Should I consult the doctor?

Consult your doctor immediately if the nosebleed fails to stop after 30 minutes and your child is dizzy and pale. Consult your doctor as soon as possible if you think there may be a foreign body in your child's nose, or if the nosebleeds are frequent.

What might the doctor do?

☐ If your child has suffered a bump on the head, your doctor will probably X-ray the head to discount the possibility of a fractured skull.
☐ If the nosebleed doesn't stop, your doctor will pack your child's nose with gauze to stem the blood flow. This will be done under a local anesthetic. The gauze can be removed after a couple of hours.
☐ If your child has a foreign object stuck in his nose, your doctor will remove it under general anesthetic.
☐ If nosebleeds are frequent, your doctor may refer you to an ear, nose and throat specialist for assessment. If the recurrent nosebleeds are caused by a fragile blood vessel, the specialist may cauterize it. This involves burning off the end of the vessel.
☐ If nosebleeds are caused by drainage from allergies, your doctor may prescribe an antihistamine.

What can I do to help?

☐ Don't let your child blow his nose for 3 hours after a nosebleed.
☐ Use a cool-mist vaporizer in your child's bedroom if you live in a dry area.

SEE ALSO:
Common cold, *page 91*
Hay fever, *page 149*
Nose, foreign body in, *page 188*

N

Obesity

A child is termed "obese" or "overweight" if he is 20% heavier than the average for his height and age. A child is not obese if he merely has a protruding tummy or a round, chubby-cheeked face, which are quite common in children under age 5. The best test for obesity is to look at the upper arms and thighs of your child; if there are rolls of fat, your child probably has a weight problem.

Obesity in babies and children is rarely due to any kind of family trait or hormonal disease. It is nearly always due to poor eating habits, usually overfeeding by parents. It's for this reason that parents of a fat child rarely understand there's a weight problem.

Is it serious?

Obesity in children is serious. There will be an emotional strain on the child when he is teased by his friends. More importantly, fat children may grow into fat adults who run higher-than-normal risks of heart disease, high blood pressure and joint disorders.

Possible symptoms

Overweight baby   Normal-weight baby

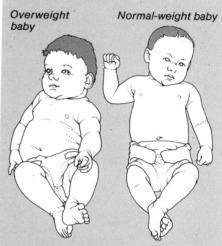

- 20% or more above-average weight for height and age.
- Rolls of fat around the thighs, upper arms, breasts and chin.
- Breathlessness on exertion.

What should I do first?

1 Weigh your child, and check the charts on page 304 to see if he is heavier than normal for his age.

2 Examine your child for rolls of fat around his upper arms and thighs. See if he has overdeveloped breasts.

3 Look at his diet. Do you give him high-calorie foods, such as soft drinks, lots of white flour and sugar products?

4 Compare your child with his playmates—is he as physically active?

Should I consult the doctor?

Consult your doctor if you think your child has a weight problem. If you are overweight yourself, you may be confusing your child's natural plump-ness with the more serious problem of obesity. Your doctor can advise you.

What might the doctor do?

☐ Your doctor will examine your child. In the rare cases in which obesity is due to a glandular disorder, your doctor will refer your child to an endocrinologist (a specialist in hormonal disorders) for investigation.

☐ If no disease is suspected, your doctor will give you advice on diet and advise you to encourage your child to use up more energy.

Continued on next page ▶

Words in **bold** are A-Z entries

Obesity

◄ *Continued from previous page*

What can I do to help?

☐ Consider whether obesity is a family problem. If you plan changes in your child's diet, adopt these yourself to set an example. Find out about eating in a healthful way.

Fresh fruit and vegetables

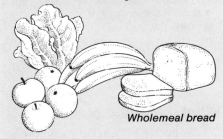

Wholemeal bread

☐ Don't put your child on a special diet to lose weight. Change his diet to include more unrefined, fiber-rich foods, such as whole-wheat flour, brown rice, fresh fruit and vegetables. Cut out refined flours and sugar in cooking, and avoid cakes, cookies, sweets and sugary drinks.
☐ Try not to fry food; grill or steam it instead. Cut the fat off the meat before cooking.
☐ Don't give your child cockies, which are full of sugar. Give him dried whole-wheat toast or pieces of celery or apple instead.
☐ Dilute fresh fruit juice with water, and avoid carbonated drinks.
☐ Encourage your child to be active. Don't confine a toddler to a playpen or stroller. Let him use up his energy by crawling or walking. Play lively games with him.

O

Osteomyelitis

Osteomyelitis is a rare bacterial infection of the bone. Although it can affect any bone in the body, arm and leg bones are most commonly affected. The infection may arise because of an injury to the bone itself, or it may be carried in the blood from an infected cut elsewhere in the body. Pus forms in the bone, and the area becomes tender and painful. Within a day or 2 the skin over the bone swells; if left untreated, a pus-filled abscess forms on the skin's surface.

Is it serious?
Osteomyelitis is always serious and can result in bone deformity or stiffness.

Possible symptoms
● Extreme pain and tenderness over an affected bone, usually in the arms or legs.
● Red, swollen area after a day or 2, which may develop into a pus-filled abscess.
● Reluctance to use or move the affected part.
● Limping if the infection is in a leg.
● High temperature.
● Loss of appetite.

What should I do first?

1 If your child suddenly complains of pain in a limb, try to find out whether he has bumped himself or suffered an injury to the affected part.

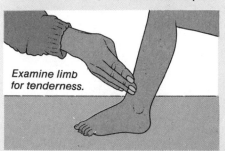
Examine limb for tenderness.

2 Try to determine how painful the area is by pressing it gently and noting your child's reaction.

3 Take your child's temperature to see if he has a fever.

4 Put your child to bed to rest the affected part.

Should I consult the doctor?

Consult your doctor immediately if your child has a fever and is in great pain for no apparent reason.

What might the doctor do?

☐ Your doctor will probably admit your child to the hospital for blood tests and X-rays to make a definite diagnosis. If osteomyelitis is confirmed, your child will be given antibiotics.
☐ If an abscess has formed, the infected bone and skin will be cleaned out surgically under an anesthetic. The cavity left behind may take some time to heal completely, but new bone usually forms within 6 months.

What can I do to help?

☐ If possible, try to stay with your child in the hospital. When he is discharged, help him exercise the affected limb.

SEE ALSO:
Limp, *page 175*

Words in **bold** are A-Z entries

Otitis externa

Otitis externa is an infection of the external ear canal—the passage that leads from the ear flap (*pinna*) to the eardrum. Infection may be caused by a foreign body in the ear, by a **boil** in the canal or as the result of damage to the skin from overvigorous cleaning or scratching. The infection is more common in children who swim a great deal. Symptoms of the infection are **earache**, inflammation, swelling, itchiness, dry, scaly skin or a discharge.

Is it serious?
The external ear canal does not contain the ear's delicate hearing mechanisms, so the infection is relatively minor. However, otitis externa should always be treated because the infection could spread to the bones of the skull and possibly the brain. Any discharge from the ear should be treated seriously because this could be a symptom of the serious middle ear infection, **otitis media**.

Possible symptoms
- Earache.
- Redness and tenderness of the ear flap and external ear canal.
- Pus-filled boil in the canal.

Area affected

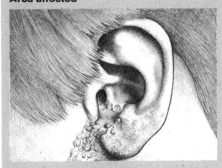

- Discharge from the ear.
- Itchy, dry, scaly ear.

What should I do first?

1 Look at the ear and into the external ear canal to check for any signs of infection or foreign objects.

2 Do not push or poke anything into your child's ear. Discourage him from touching or scratching it if it's sore.

3 Ask your child to open his mouth as wide as possible to see if this causes pain.

4 Pull back gently on the ear flap to see if this causes pain.

5 Clean away any discharge with warm water and soap.

6 Give your child acetaminophen to relieve pain. Put a piece of cotton over the ear to absorb any discharge.

Should I consult the doctor?

Consult your doctor if you notice any discharge from your child's ear or if you suspect infection of the external ear canal.

What might the doctor do?

☐ Your doctor will examine your child's ear with an otoscope and may clean out the ear with a probe. He will probably prescribe antibiotics or antibiotic ear drops to clear up the infection.

☐ If there is still a foreign body in your child's ear, your doctor will remove it or refer your child to the hospital for its removal.

☐ If the pain is the result of a boil, your doctor may lance it and drain the pus away. This relieves the pain almost immediately.

Continued on next page ▶

Otitis externa

◀ Continued from previous page

What can I do to help?

☐ Give your child acetaminophen on the advice of your doctor if the condition is still painful.

☐ Prevent water from entering the ear during bathing until the infection has cleared up. Don't let your child go swimming.

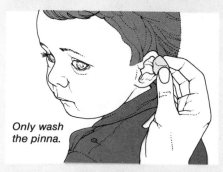

Only wash the pinna.

☐ Don't interfere with your child's external ear canal. Wash around the pinna but never poke cotton swabs into the area to clear wax. Wax is not abnormal. It is a natural lubricant, keeping infection at bay. A cotton swab or a twisted piece of face cloth only pushes wax farther into the canal or damages the lining, increasing the chances of infection.

☐ Never use over-the-counter ear drops unless your doctor advises them.

SEE ALSO:
Boil, *page 71*
Ear, foreign body in, *page 123*
Earache, *page 124*
Otitis media, *page 195*

Words in **bold** are A-Z entries

Otitis media

Otitis media is an infection of the middle ear. The infection causes fluid to build in the middle ear, producing **earache** and sometimes **deafness**. It is common in young children because the tube connecting the throat with the ear, the Eustachian tube, is relatively short, and children spend a lot of time lying down. This means any bacteria or viruses that invade the nose or throat can make a short journey and reach the middle ear. Infection may also result when enlarged adenoids block the entrance to the Eustachian tube. If the tube is blocked, mucus will not be able to drain away and may become sticky and gluelike, leading to **serous otitis**.

Is it serious?

Otitis media is painful and serious. If left untreated, it can result in permanent loss of hearing.

Possible symptoms

● Severe pain in the ear. In a baby, the pulling or rubbing of an ear accompanied by crying.
● Temperature of over 102F (38.6C).
● Vomiting.
● Partial deafness.
● Pussy discharge from the ear.

Cross section of the ear

Middle-ear cavity

Eustachian tube

What should I do first?

1 Take your child's temperature to see if he has a fever.

2 Keep your child comfortable and cool. If the pain in the ear is severe, a well-wrapped hot-water bottle placed against it may help relieve pain.

3 Give your child acetaminophen to relieve the earache.

4 Check for any discharge from the ear.

Should I consult the doctor?

Consult your doctor immediately if you suspect a middle ear infection. Consult your doctor if you suspect any hearing loss.

What might the doctor do?

□ Your doctor will examine your child's ear with an otoscope and will probably prescribe antibiotics to clear up the infection. If there is any fluid in the Eustachian tube, your doctor may also prescribe a drug to reduce swelling so the fluid can drain down the throat.
□ If the attacks are recurrent, your doctor may refer your child to an ear, nose and throat (ENT) specialist for assessment.

What can I do to help?

□ Check your child's hearing regularly (*see page 108*).

O

SEE ALSO:
Deafness, *page 108*
Earache, *page 124*
Serous otitis, *page 216*
Tonsillitis, *page 243*

Paronychia

Paronychia is an infection of the fold of the skin at the side of a fingernail or toenail. The bacteria that cause the infection are able to enter the skin if it is soggy because of prolonged immersion in water or if the nail or adjacent skin is constantly picked at or bitten. While pus is building up in the nail fold, the area will be painful.

Is it serious?
Paronychia is not serious and can be easily treated. Sometimes a yeast, such as monilia, can complicate a paronychia and cause a chronic condition that has a greater risk of deformity and requires prolonged treatment.

Possible symptoms

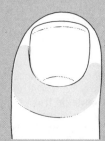

Area
affected

- Redness and swelling around the nail fold.
- Pus under or next to the nail.
- Throbbing pain.

What should I do first?

1 If your child complains of a throbbing pain around a nail and you can see pus has collected under the skin, don't try to let the pus out yourself. You may damage the nail bed.

2 Apply a warm compress or a pad of cotton soaked in warm water to bring the pus to a head. Or soak the finger or toe in warm, soapy water. It should burst or drain away naturally.

3 Protect the finger or toe from bumps with a thick pad of cotton and tape.

Should I consult the doctor?

Consult your doctor if the pus does not drain within a few hours of coming to a head or if the pain is severe.

What might the doctor do?

☐ If pus has collected, your doctor will probably lance it and let the pus drain away. This is usually done under local anesthetic. Sometimes, if the condition is severe, a small piece of nail is removed under anesthetic

to allow the pus to drain. This relieves the pain immediately

☐ If there is an acute Infection, your doctor will prescribe antibiotics to be taken by mouth or in a cream form to be spread on the nail to eradicate the bacterial infection.

☐ If the paronychia fails to improve, your doctor may refer you to a dermatologist to see whether or not there is a yeast infection. If so, your child may be prescribed anti-fungal cream.

What can I do to help?

☐ Keep your child's nails short, and file any rough pieces that your child may bite to make smooth.
☐ Discourage your child from biting or picking at his nails or at the skin around the edge of the nail.
☐ Cut toenails straight across.

Words in **bold** are A-Z entries

Penis caught in zipper

This situation may arise if your son is hurrying after going to the bathroom or is not paying attention to what he's doing when he gets dressed and catches both skin and fabric in the teeth of a zipper.

Is it serious?
There should be no serious complications, but the pain your child will be suffering means you should treat it as an emergency.

What should I do first?

1 Don't touch the penis or the zipper unless you're sure you can separate the two quickly and easily. Use a pair of pliers or metal cutters if you have them to cut off the bottom end of the zipper.

2 It you can't cut through the zipper and if your child will let you, place a cold compress or pieces of ice tied in a clean cloth over the zipper and penis. This should numb the area and relieve the pain while you get medical attention.

Should I consult the doctor?

Consult your doctor immediately or take your child to the emergency room.

What might the doctor do?

Your doctor will inject a local anesthetic into your child's penis. This can be painful. When the penis is thoroughly numb, your doctor will be able to undo the zipper.

What can I do to help?

☐ Apply antiseptic cream to the damaged penis three or four times a day to soothe the area and prevent infection. Let your child do it if he wants to.
☐ Leave the skin open to the air as much as possible to promote healing and prevent rubbing.
☐ Give your child a bowl of warm water to pour over his penis as he urinates to stop stinging. He will probably complain it is painful to pass urine for about 48 hours.
☐ Keep your child quiet and calm so he doesn't accidentally bump himself. There will be bruising and swelling for 4 or 5 days.
☐ Give your child acetaminophen if he's in pain.

Phenylketonuria

Phenylketonuria (PKU) is a rare, inherited disease that affects the body's ability to break down the amino acid *phenylalanine.* (Amino acids are the chemicals that make up proteins.) PKU sufferers lack the enzyme necessary to break down phenylalanine; if allowed to accumulate in the body, phenylalanine damages the nervous system and results in mental retardation.

PKU will be inherited *only* if both parents carry the PKU gene. However, PKU is entirely preventable with early diagnosis and a special diet low in phenylalanine. At 2 to 3 days of age (just before discharge from the hospital), all babies are given a simple blood test, called the *Guthrie test.* By this time, the baby's level of phenylalanine will be apparent, and PKU can be detected.

Possible symptoms
● Mental retardation.
● Convulsions.

What can be done?
If the initial blood test shows a raised level of phenylalanine, this does not prove your baby has PKU. The test will be repeated and further investigation carried out before a definite conclusion can be drawn. If the diagnosis is confirmed, a low phenylalanine diet will be started. This may begin with a special-formula milk, although some breast milk may be allowed. Regular blood samples will be taken to monitor the levels of phenylalanine and control the intake sufficiently to keep it from rising to toxic levels. Phenylalanine cannot be eliminated entirely from the diet because it is essential for normal growth so enough phenylalanine must be given to allow normal growth. Once your child is weaned off the special formula, his diet will consist mainly of vegetables and salads. It is a fairly dull diet and will require imagination on your part to make it interesting for your child. The diet will also include supplements of special foods. However, your child will be able to live a normal life, and there is some optimism that at 10 to 12 years of age (possibly even earlier), the body becomes resistant to damage from high levels of phenylalanine and the diet may be relaxed. Seek help and advice from the dietician your doctor recommends.

PKU diet is also prescribed for pregnant women, so the fetus is not damaged.

Words in **bold** are A-Z entries

Pigeon toes

A child has pigeon toes if the toes of each foot point in toward each other by more than a few degrees. Most toddlers have some degree of transient pigeon toes. Pigeon toes may be due to an inturning of the forefeet, in which case the other parts of the leg will be normal and the knees will face forward. However, pigeon toes more commonly result because the whole leg, from the hip down (including the knee), is turned inward. The cause is generally irrelevant because the condition usually rights itself with time (by age 3 if the forefeet are affected and by age 6 if the hip is affected). A slight inturning of the feet is normal and usually noticed when your child starts to walk.

Is it serious?

This is not a serious condition and does not stop your child from walking.

Possible symptoms

Classic appearance

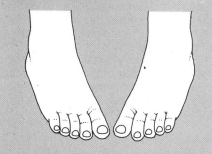

● Exaggerated inturning of the toes.

What should I do first?

1 With your child standing up straight, with no shoes or socks on, check to see that the line of the toes and feet is straight.

2 If your child's feet point inward, check to see if his knees turn in toward each other.

Should I consult the doctor?

Consult your doctor if your child's feet persistently turn inward. Consult your doctor if the inturning of your child's feet causes him to have difficulty running.

What might the doctor do?

☐ Your doctor will examine your child's legs, noting the alignment of the hips, thighs, knees, lower legs and feet. If necessary, your doctor will arrange for your child to have X-rays.

☐ If there is a significant inturning of your child's feet, your doctor may give your child a series of exercises or have an orthopedic specialist look at him.

☐ If the feet are only slightly inturned, your doctor will probably not recommend any action.

What can I do to help?

☐ If your child has been given exercises, help him with them.

☐ Even if you've been given no specific exercises, you can help your child with passive stretching exercises. Sit at his feet, facing him, and hold his heel in the palm of your hand. With the other hand, gently turn the foot out. Repeat for the other foot.

Plantar wart

A plantar wart is a **wart** on the sole of the foot that has been pushed up into the foot by the pressure of walking. It is highly infectious and is spread by direct contact with surfaces where infected feet have been, such as swimming pools, showers and gyms. It takes about 2 years for the body to build up resistance to the wart virus (warts usually disappear naturally). But because a plantar wart can be spread easily and because it can be painful, treatment is advisable.

Is it serious?
A plantar wart is never serious but it can cause pain and discomfort, depending on where it appears on the sole of the foot.

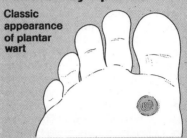

Possible symptoms

Classic appearance of plantar wart

- White or brown flat lump on the sole of the foot.
- Pain when walking or standing on the foot.

What should I do first?

1 Wash your child's feet and let them soak in warm water to soften the skin.

2 With an emery board, file away thin layers of the softened wart very gently. It is always wiser to file off too little rather than too much.

3 Apply an over-the counter-wart treatment, obtainable from the drugstore. Don't apply the wart treatment to healthy skin. To avoid this, use a corn plaster or a piece of ordinary plaster with a hole the size of the wart cut out of it, to protect the surrounding areas. After putting on the lotion, cover the wart with a Band-aid.

4 Repeat the procedure every day until the wart has disappeared.

Should I consult the doctor?

Consult your doctor if the wart is painful, if the warts are increasing in number or if self-help treatment fails.

What might the doctor do?

☐ Your doctor may refer you to a dermatologist or he may remove the wart himself. The wart will be removed by treatment with a freezing agent, such as liquid nitrogen, or by being burned off or scraped out under local anesthetic.

What can I do to help?

☐ Cover the wart with a Band-aid when your child goes barefoot. This should prevent the spread of the virus.
☐ Discourage your child from scratching the wart. He could infect himself elsewhere.

SEE ALSO:
Warts, *page 257*

Words in **bold** are A-Z entries

Pneumonia

Pneumonia is the term used to describe inflammation of the lungs. It may be caused by viral, bacterial or fungal infection or by a foreign body that has been inhaled into the lungs. In young children, pneumonia is nearly always due to an upper-respiratory infection, such as a **common cold** or **influenza**, spreading to the lungs. It can also be caused by **bronchitis** (called *broncho-pneumonia*). Certain underlying conditions predispose to bronchopneumonia; these include **asthma** and **cystic fibrosis**.

Older children may contract a type of pneumonia called *lobar pneumonia*, where one or more of the lobes of the lungs may be infected by the *pneumococcus bacterium*. This form of pneumonia can start without warning, even when there is no other infection present.

The common symptom of all types of pneumonia is difficulty breathing. With bronchopneumonia there will also be a noticeable deterioration of an existing illness and a high temperature.

Is it serious?
Pneumonia is always serious.

Possible symptoms

- Difficulty breathing; the nostrils flare, the chest wall sinks with every breath and efforts to breathe produce grunting sounds.
- Dry cough.
- Fever, up to 102F (38.6C).
- Vomiting and diarrhea.
- Pain in the chest, made worse by deep breathing.

What should I do first?

1 If your child has an upper-respiratory infection or an infectious illness and his condition worsens, look for a dry cough and breathing difficulty.

2 Take your child's temperature to see if he has a fever. If he has, try to bring his temperature down with tepid sponging (*see page 31*).

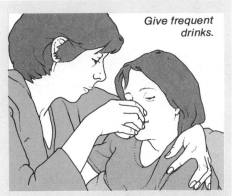

Give frequent drinks.

3 Give your child plenty of fluid to prevent him becoming dehydrated.

Continued on next page ▶

201

Pneumonia

◀ Continued from previous page

Should I consult the doctor?

Consult your doctor immediately if your child's condition worsens and breathing becomes difficult. Any breathing problems in a child warrant *immediate* medical attention.

What might the doctor do?

☐ Your doctor will examine your child and may prescribe antibiotics. If your doctor is in any doubt about the presence of pneumonia, your child may have to have a chest X-ray.
☐ Your doctor will advise you about nursing procedures to treat your child at home.

What can I do to help?

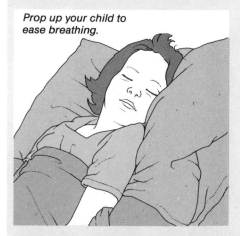

Prop up your child to ease breathing.

☐ If he is feverish and too lethargic to take a bath, give him a sponge-bath to refresh him.

☐ Prop your child up in bed; this may help his breathing.
☐ Keep the room well-ventilated but not hot and stuffy.
☐ Give your child plenty of fluid. When he feels like eating, give him foods that are easy to digest, such as yogurt, fruits and soups.

SEE ALSO:
Asthma, *page 61*
Bronchitis, *page 76*
Common cold, *page 91*
Cystic fibrosis, *page 106*
Influenza, *page 165*

Words in **bold** are A-Z entries

Poliomyelitis

Poliomyelitis (polio) is a viral infection of the spinal cord and nerves. It has the same symptoms as many other viral infections, with a **fever, sore throat, headache** and stiff neck. Often the disease does not progress to paralysis, and there is complete recovery without polio even being suspected. If it does progress, most commonly there is paralysis of the lower limbs, making walking difficult or even impossible. The disease is carried in the stools of an infected person and can quickly reach epidemic proportions. It is now entirely preventable with an immunization course of three doses of a vaccine taken by mouth followed by two booster doses.

Is it serious?
Polio is always serious. If it is not diagnosed and the disease progresses, permanent paralysis may occur.

Possible symptoms
- High temperature, rising to 102F (38.6C).
- Sore throat.
- Headache.
- Pain and stiffness in the neck.
- Vomiting.
- Weakness.
- Paralysis of muscles, usually in the lower limbs or in the chest, causing breathlessness.

What should I do first?
If you know of any cases of polio in your community, and for some reason your child has not been immunized, be on the alert if you notice your child has a stiff and painful neck and a fever.

Should I consult the doctor?
Consult your doctor immediately if your child has flulike symptoms then has difficulty in moving his limbs or becomes breathless—even if he has been immunized against polio.

What might the doctor do?
☐ Your doctor will admit your child to the hospital for assessment if polio is suspected. Absolute quiet and bed rest are the only treatment for polio because antibiotics have no effect on a viral illness. Your child may return home if you can manage the special nursing he will require.

☐ If your child is nursed at home, your doctor and physiotherapist will advise you about the diet and exercise regime your child should follow.

What can I do to help?
☐ Immunize your baby against polio within the first year of life, and follow this with booster doses. (The polio vaccine is given with DTP on the standard immunization schedule.) Even though polio is no longer the menace it once was, there is no reason for complacency. Risks from the vaccine are virtually unknown.

P

SEE ALSO:
Fever, page 139
Headache, page 153
Sore throat, page 222

Psoriasis

Psoriasis is a chronic, recurrent skin disorder. With this condition the rate of cell production is faster than normal, leading to layers of dry, flaky skin with red patches underneath. Psoriasis is most commonly found on the knees, elbows and scalp, and occasionally under the arms and around the anus and genitals. Psoriasis is more often seen in girls than boys but rarely occurs before age 6. It is common and tends to run in families. There is no known cure, but treatment can clear up each outbreak as it occurs. The first and only sign of the condition for some time may be pitted fingernails.

Is it serious?
Psoriasis is not serious. It does not affect general health, but because of its chronic and unesthetic nature, it can cause unhappiness.

Possible symptoms
- Pitted fingernails.
- Small, red patches of skin covered by dry, flaky scales, most commonly on the knees, elbows and scalp.

What should I do first?
If you notice red, scaly patches on your child's body, particularly on those parts exposed to friction, such as elbows and knees, consult your doctor.

Should I consult the doctor?
Consult your doctor if you suspect psoriasis and there is some family history of the condition.

What might the doctor do?
☐ Your doctor will examine your child and question you about the incidence of skin disorders in your family. Your doctor may refer your child to a dermatologist to confirm diagnosis.
☐ Your child will be prescribed tar-containing shampoos or lotions or salicylic acid ointments to rub into the affected areas. Many cases of psoriasis respond to a regime of tar baths, ultraviolet light treatment and ointments.

What can I do to help?
☐ Unless your child has sensitive skin, encourage him to play out in the sun because careful exposure to sunlight can help clear up the condition.
☐ Try to keep up your child's morale.
☐ If your child scratches, keep his fingernails short and his hands clean to prevent him breaking the skin, which increases the likelihood of infection.
☐ Cover the affected areas of skin to help keep your child from feeling self-conscious.

Words in **bold** are A-Z entries

Pyloric stenosis

Pyloric stenosis is a congenital condition—it is present at birth. The ring of muscle (*pylorus*) that links the stomach to the duodenum thickens and narrows, preventing the contents of the stomach from passing through it to the intestine. The cause is unknown, but when the baby is about 1 month old, symptoms begin. Food builds up in the stomach, which contracts powerfully in an attempt to force the food through the thickened pylorus. Because this is impossible, milk is vomited up violently after a feeding. This is called projectile **vomiting**, and the unpleasant-smelling milk curds and mucus can be thrown as far as 6 feet (2m) away. Projectile vomiting should not be confused with spitting up, in which a baby naturally regurgitates milk after feeding.

Is it serious?
Pyloric stenosis is serious. The vomiting eventually leads to **dehydration** and **failure to thrive**.

Possible symptoms

- Projectile vomiting after a feeding, beginning at around 4 weeks of age.
- Failure to thrive.
- Weakness and listlessness.
- Lack of bowel movements.

Cross section of the pylorus

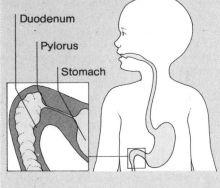

Duodenum

Pylorus

Stomach

What should I do first?

1 If your baby vomits violently after three consecutive feedings, consult your doctor immediately.

2 While you are waiting for medical attention, feed your baby frequent, small amounts of milk to keep his fluid levels up.

Should I consult the doctor?

Consult your doctor immediately if your baby vomits violently after every feeding.

What might the doctor do?

☐ If pyloric stenosis is suspected, your doctor will refer your baby to the hospital. He will examine your baby's abdomen during a feeding to see if the enlarged pylorus can be felt.

☐ A simple surgical operation to widen the thickened pylorus will be performed, affecting a complete cure.

What can I do to help?

☐ Stay with your baby in the hospital. After the operation, you will be advised to feed your baby gradually increasing amounts of milk. Forty-eight hours after the operation, his feeding routine should be back to normal.

P

SEE ALSO:
Dehydration, *page 109*
Failure to thrive, *page 137*
Vomiting, *page 255*

Rash

A skin rash can be a symptom of infection, either in the skin or elsewhere. It can also be an allergic reaction to something on the skin or the body's reaction to an irritating chemical or to physical damage.

Many childhood infectious diseases have a rash as one of their main symptoms, among them **chickenpox**, **German measles** and **measles**. Localized rashes may be the result of a skin infestation by **scabies** mites or **ringworm** fungus. A child who is allergic to a drug may break out in a rash when he takes the drug. Nettles and other plants cause a rash when touched.

The skin condition called *purpura* looks like a rash but is the result of a blood disorder. If there is a problem with the blood's clotting mechanism, tiny areas of bleeding tend to occur in the skin, looking like small spidery "spots". These marks do not itch, and there are no other skin changes. Purpuric marks can be distinguished from other rashes by pressing the side of a drinking glass gently on them. If the marks are still visible, this indicates purpura. A purpuric rash may be brought on by infection or sensitivity to certain drugs.

Is it serious?

Skin rashes are hardly ever serious, though they may be irritating. However, you should never ignore a rash because it may indicate a serious underlying illness. Purpuric rash, in particular, may be a symptom of a serious disorder, such as **leukemia**, **hepatitis** or **meningitis**.

What should I do first?

1 Note where the rash is on your child and whether it has spread from one part of his body to another. He could have one of the common infections, such as chickenpox.

2 Take his temperature to see if he has a fever.

3 Check whether your child has eaten something new (like shellfish or strawberries) or whether he has started a course of medicine (for example, penicillin).

4 Check whether your child has any symptoms of infestation, especially if his skin is very itchy between the fingers. This could indicate scabies.

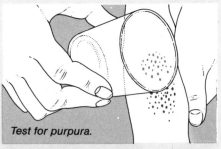
Test for purpura.

5 Press a drinking glass against your child's skin to see if the rash remains visible. The rash could be purpuric.

6 If the rash is itchy, use calamine lotion to relieve the irritation.

Should I consult the doctor?

Consult your doctor for an accurate diagnosis of your child's rash. Consult your doctor immediately if the rash is purpuric and your child has a fever; these two symptoms could indicate meningitis.

Continued on next page ▶

206

Rash

◀ *Continued from previous page*

What might the doctor do?

☐ Your doctor will examine your child
to determine the cause of the rash,
which will then be treated accordingly.
☐ If the rash is purpuric, your doctor
will arrange for a blood test to determine the cause.

What can I do to help?

☐ If the rash is itchy, add a handful
of baking soda to the bath water to ease
the irritation.
☐ Keep your child's skin cool to
reduce irritation.

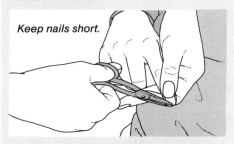

Keep nails short.

☐ Discourage your child from scratching the rash. Keep his hands clean
and his nails short to prevent damage
to the skin if he does scratch it.

SEE ALSO:
Chickenpox, *page 83*
German measles, *page 146*
Hepatitis, *page 158*
Leukemia, *page 173*
Measles, *page 176*
Meningitis, *page 177*
Ringworm, *page 210*
Scabies, *page 212*

Reye's syndrome

Reye's syndrome is a childhood illness in which a child suddenly becomes ill with **vomiting** and **fever**. The body's reaction to the illness causes the brain to become inflamed, so your child may also become delirious and even lapse into a coma. Reye's syndrome usually occurs a few days after a child has had a mild viral infection, such as **chickenpox** or **influenza**. It is particularly associated with illnesses in which aspirin was used to relieve symptoms or reduce temperature. The cause of Reye's syndrome is only now becoming clear—a virus or some other poisonous agent damages cells in various parts of the body. However, only certain children seem susceptible. It is believed that susceptibility may be related to the body's inability to deal with certain chemical substances, especially fats.

Possible symptoms

- Uncontrollable vomiting.
- Delirium.
- Drowsiness or unconsciouness.
- Fever.

Is it serious?

Reye's syndrome is very serious and can result in death if it is not identified quickly. However, it is rare.

What should I do first?

1 If your child is recovering from an infectious disease and he starts to vomit, take his temperature to see if he has a fever.

2 If he does have a fever, consult your doctor immediately. *Do not* give him any form of aspirin. Try tepid sponging (*see page 31*) to lower his temperature.

3 Consult your doctor immediately if your child has been vomiting then becomes drowsy or difficult to rouse.

Should I consult the doctor?

Consult your doctor immediately, or call an ambulance if there is any delay, or if your child has become drowsy and difficult to rouse.

What might the doctor do?

☐ If your doctor suspects Reye's syndrome, he will admit your child to the hospital immediately. Usually a physical examination is all that is necessary to confirm the diagnosis, but if there is any doubt, the doctor will remove a tiny piece of liver under local anesthetic, using a hollow needle (a procedure called *liver biopsy*). This sample will be analyzed for abnormal fat distribution, which is characteristic of the illness.

☐ Your child will be treated in an intensive-care unit and given intravenous glucose. Various measures will be taken to control swelling of the brain.

What can I do to help?

☐ Stay with your child in the hospital if possible.

☐ Be prepared for a long convalescence. Ask about any special precautions that should be taken to avoid a recurrence of the syndrome.

> **SEE ALSO:**
> **Chickenpox,** *page 83*
> **Fever,** *page 139*
> **Influenza,** *page 165*
> **Vomiting,** *page 254*

Words in **bold** are A-Z entries

Rheumatic fever

Rheumatic fever is a rare disease characterized by inflammation of the joints and the heart. It usually follows a streptococcal bacteria infection, such as **tonsillitis**. However, most children have many strep infections without rheumatic fever.

Rheumatic fever usually begins within a week or 2 of the infection and produces symptoms of general ill health, fever and aching joints. In some cases, there may be a circular, blotchy, red rash on the trunk and limbs. Rheumatic fever is now less common because streptococcal infections are usually treated with antibiotics at an early stage and living conditions have improved.

Is it serious?
Rheumatic fever can have serious consequences. The earlier the treatment, the less likelihood there is of any heart disease in later life.

Possible symptoms

- Fever.
- Swollen, painful joints.
- Blotchy, circular red rash on the trunk and limbs.
- Chest pain.
- Listlessness.
- Loss of appetite.

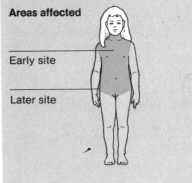

Areas affected

Early site

Later site

What should I do first?

1 If your child has recently had tonsillitis and complains of pain in his joints when he should be getting better, see if he has a fever.

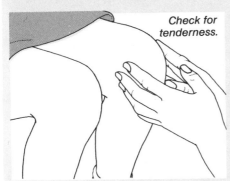

Check for tenderness.

2 Feel for swelling and tenderness by pressing on and around major joints.

3 Look for a circular rash on your child's trunk and limbs.

Should I consult the doctor?

Consult your doctor immediately.

What might the doctor do?

☐ Your doctor will admit your child to the hospital for bed rest and medication. This usually takes the form of large doses of aspirin.

What can I do to help?

☐ Administer prescribed medication as directed by your doctor. For many years after he has recovered, your child will need penicillin to prevent a recurrence.

SEE ALSO:
Tonsillitis, *page 243*

Ringworm

Ringworm is a fungal infection of the skin and hair that shows itself as bald patches in the hair and as round, red or gray scaly patches on the skin. As the infection spreads, the edges of the ring remain scaly, and the center begins to look more like normal skin. Ringworm is usually contracted from animals, such as a household pet, or from other infected humans.

Is it serious?
Though not a serious disorder, ringworm is unattractive and irritating. It is also contagious and must therefore be treated promptly.

Possible symptoms
● Red or gray scaly rings on any part of the body, particularly warm, moist areas, and on the scalp, where they produce bald patches.
● Itchiness in the ringed areas.

What should I do first?
1 If your child is scratching, check his body for the distinctive rings of ringworm.
2 Don't try to treat it yourself. Wash your hands after examining your child. Discourage him from touching the infected areas.

Should I consult the doctor?
Consult your doctor about the problem.

What might the doctor do?
☐ Your doctor will prescribe an anti-fungal cream for the skin and antibiotic tablets to take for problems on the scalp. Pills will have to be taken for at least 4 weeks.

What can I do to help?
☐ Throw out any brushes, combs or headgear your child may have used while infected. Disinfectant will not destroy the fungi.
☐ Keep your child's face cloth and towel separate from the rest of the family's to avoid spreading the infection.
☐ If your pet is a possible source of ringworm, take it to the vet for treatment as soon as possible.
☐ Ringworm on the skin clears up quickly, but treatment of the scalp may take a couple of weeks.
☐ Be sure you and your child wash your hands carefully before and after touching affected areas.

SEE ALSO:
Hair loss, *page 148*
Itching, *page 169*

Words in **bold** are A-Z entries

Roseola infantum

Roseola infantum is a common viral infection that causes **fever** and **rash** in young children. It is contagious and has symptoms that may be mistaken for **scarlet fever**. It starts with the sudden onset of a high fever that lasts for 3 days, usually without any other symptoms. As the fever subsides, a rash of flat red or pink spots appears, first on the trunk, then spreading to the limbs and neck. The rash fades after about 48 hours, with no other side effects.

Is it serious?
Roseola infantum is not serious, though the temperature can be high.

Possible symptoms

● Fever with temperature of 102 to 104F (38.6 to 40C) for 3 days, with no apparent symptoms.

Areas affected

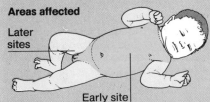

Later sites

Early site

● Rash of separate, flat, red or pink spots that appear first on the trunk—they are not itchy.

What should I do first?

1 Check your child's temperature. If it is high, try to reduce it with tepid sponging (*see page 31*).
2 Note where the rash starts and what part of the body it spreads to, if any.

Should I consult the doctor?

Consult your doctor for a definite diagnosis of the condition. Consult your doctor immediately if your child has a febrile **convulsion**.

What might the doctor do?

☐ There is no specific treatment for viral illnesses, only treatment for the symptoms. Your doctor will advise you on how to reduce your child's fever and will recommend you keep your child in bed until the rash appears.
☐ If your child has had a febrile convulsion before, a doctor may occasionally prescribe drugs to prevent possible convulsions. This depends on many variables.

What can I do to help?

☐ Take your child's temperature at regular intervals. If it rises, try to bring it down, first by tepid sponging, then with acetaminophen.
☐ Don't give your child aspirin because of the danger of **Reye's syndrome**.

SEE ALSO:
Convulsion, *page 96*
Fever, *page 139*
Rash, *page 206*
Reye's syndrome, *page 208*
Scarlet fever, *page 213*

Scabies

Scabies is an irritating, itchy rash caused by a tiny mite. The burrowing and egg-laying of these mites produce a rash that nearly always affects the hands and fingers, particularly the clefts between the fingers. It may also affect the ankles, underarms, feet, toes, elbows and the area around the genitals. When eggs hatch, they are easily passed to another person by direct contact. People can also pick them up from bedding or linen that is infested with the mites.

Is it serious?
Scabies is not serious, but it is contagious and could infect a family or school class if not treated promptly.

Possible symptoms
● Intense itchiness.

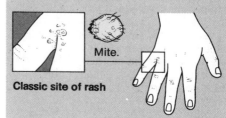

Mite.

Classic site of rash

● Fine, short lines that end in a black spot the size of a pinhead, most often found between the fingers.
● Scabs on itchy areas.

What should I do first?

1 If your child is scratching a lot, look for the fine lines of the mites' burrows.

2 If you suspect scabies, keep your child away from school until you have administered treatment.

3 Try to discourage your child from scratching. This may hinder the doctor's diagnosis and cause sores that could become infected.

Should I consult the doctor?

Consult your doctor if you suspect scabies or if your child is scratching a lot.

What might the doctor do?

☐ Your doctor will prescribe a lotion.

What can I do to help?

☐ After thorough washing, paint the whole body below the neck with the lotion, and let it dry. Don't wash it off for 8 to 12 hours.
☐ Carry out the treatment for everyone in the family simultaneously.

☐ Wash or air all bedding and clothing to eradicate the mite. The mite cannot live longer than a few hours after it is removed from human skin.

SEE ALSO:
Itching, *page 169*
Rash, *page 206*

Words in **bold** are A-Z entries

Scarlet fever

Scarlet fever is one of the less common infectious diseases of childhood, even though it is caused by the widespread *streptococcus* bacterium (the same bacterium that causes **tonsillitis**). It is similar to tonsillitis, except that it produces a rash and a **sore throat**. The incubation period is 1 to 5 days, after which the symptoms manifest themselves. After 3 days of a sore throat, inflamed tonsils, **fever**, **vomiting** and possibly abdominal pains (because of swollen glands near the bowel), a rash of small spots that merge with one another appears on the chest and neck, then the whole body. The rash may be itchy but is distinctive because it does not affect the area surrounding the mouth. The tongue may also be red and furry. The rash fades after 5 days, but the skin flakes off for up to 2 weeks.

Is it serious?

Scarlet fever is rarely serious. However, if your child is sensitive to the bacterium, the infection can cause inflammation of the kidneys or the joints and heart (**rheumatic fever**). However, these complications are rare.

Possible symptoms

- Sore throat.
- Inflamed tonsils.
- Fever, as high as 104F (40C).
- Vomiting.
- Abdominal pains.

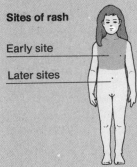

Sites of rash

Early site

Later sites

- Rash of small spots starting on the chest and neck, then merging together over the whole body, except the area around the mouth.
- Strawberry-red patches on a furry tongue.

What should I do first?

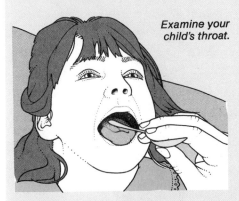

Examine your child's throat.

1 Check your child's throat to see if the tonsils are red and swollen

(*see page 243*). Check his tongue to see if it is furry with bright red patches.

2 Check your child's temperature to see if he has a fever. If he has, put him to bed and try to bring his temperature down with tepid sponging (*see page 31*).

3 Give your child plenty of cool drinks and acetaminophen to soothe his throat if he is in pain.

Should I consult the doctor?

Consult your doctor if you suspect scarlet fever.

Continued on next page ▶

Scarlet fever

◀ Continued from previous page

What might the doctor do?

☐ Your doctor will prescribe antibiotics to minimize the severity of the illness and prevent complications.

What can I do to help?

☐ Bed rest is not usually necessary, but keep your child warm and quiet.
☐ Scarlet fever is not generally a severe illness. Your child should be well enough to return to school 7 days after the onset of the symptoms.

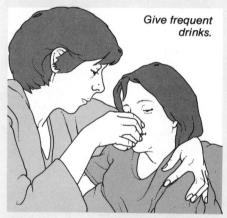

Give frequent drinks.

☐ Give your child plenty of fluids if he has lost his appetite or if he has a sore throat that makes swallowing painful.
☐ Purée his foods if this makes swallowing easier for him.

SEE ALSO:
Fever, *page 139*
Rheumatic fever, *page 209*
Sore throat, *page 222*
Tonsillitis, *page 243*
Vomiting, *page 255*

Words in **bold** are A-Z entries

Scoliosis

Scoliosis is a sideways curvature of the spine, often slight. It is noticed at adolescence because of the child's growth spurt. The spinal deformity may be present from birth or it may be the result of injury to, or a weakness of, muscles in the back, such as that caused by **muscular dystrophy**.

Scoliosis can also develop at any time in healthy children. It may be triggered by a fast growth spurt or by one leg being longer than the other. The condition is much more common in girls than in boys.

Is it serious?

Scoliosis should always be treated seriously. Early diagnosis is necessary to prevent deformity. If left untreated, the condition can also affect the lungs, resulting in breathing difficulties.

Possible symptoms

● Looked at from behind, one shoulder is slightly lower than other.
● Lopsidedness when your child bends forward.
● Shirts don't hang evenly.

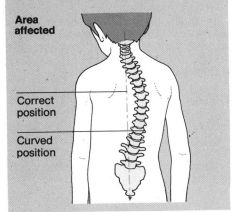

Area affected

Correct position

Curved position

What should I do first?

Ask your child to stand up straight with his heels together, then bend forward from the waist. If there is a curvature, one shoulder will appear higher.

Should I consult the doctor?

Consult your doctor if you suspect scoliosis.

What might the doctor do?

☐ Your doctor will first take X-rays, then refer your child to a specialist if necessary. The orthopedic specialist will monitor the curvature. Depending on the severity of the condition, the specialist may decide that it is necessary for your child to wear a back brace until he has stopped growing.
☐ Physiotherapy may be used to correct posture.

What can I do to help?

☐ Seek help from a scoliosis self-help group in your area. Your doctor will be able to give you an address. If your child has to wear a brace, this can be a frightening experience. Communication with other parents experienced in coping with the problem may help.
☐ Treat the condition as casually as possible. Don't draw attention to it.

S

SEE ALSO:
Muscular dystrophy, *page 186*

Serous otitis

Serous otitis is the term for a condition that results when the Eustachian tube and middle ear fill with fluid as a result of infection. The Eustachian tube, which runs from the throat to the ear, produces large quantities of fluid as a response to chronic infections, such as enlarged adenoids, **tonsillitus** or, most commonly, **otitis media**.If the tube in either ear is blocked by inflammation, the fluid cannot drain. It becomes sticky, impeding the efficient vibration of sound, causing loss of hearing.

Is it serious?

Although painless, serous otitis should be treated seriously because it can lead to **deafness** and eventually permanent loss of hearing in the affected ear. If undetected, it can cause problems with speech development and learning.

Possible symptoms

- A feeling of fullness in the ear.
- Partial loss of hearing or deafness in one or both ears.

What should I do first?

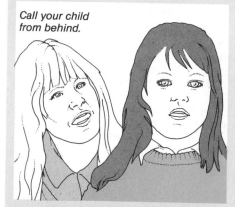

Call your child from behind.

1 If your child seems inattentive and has recently had upper-respiratory tract infection, such as otitis media or a **common cold**, do a hearing test. Call quietly when the head is averted, and see if there is a response. Even if your child can hear you, the hearing may be impaired so he cannot tell where you're calling from.

Should I consult the doctor?

Consult your doctor if you suspect your child's hearing has deteriorated in any way.

What might the doctor do?

☐ Your doctor will examine your child's ears with a special instrument (an otoscope) and treat the serous otitis according to the severity of the blockage.

☐ In mild cases, your doctor will prescribe antibiotics to clear up the infection. He may also prescribe vaso-constrictor drugs, which promote drainage by reducing swelling in the Eustachian tubes.

Continued on next page ▶

S

Words in **bold** are A-Z entries

Serous otitis

◀ Continued from previous page

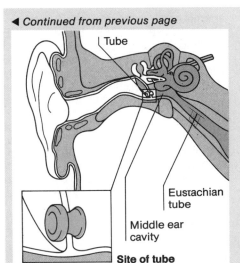

Tube

Eustachian tube

Middle ear cavity

Site of tube

☐ In severe, recurrent cases, your child will probably be referred to an ear, nose and throat specialist. The specialist may decide to insert tubes in the affected ear(s). These tiny plastic tubes allow mucus to drain away, thus preventing further buildup of the sticky secretions. The tubes either fall out after several months when the ears are healthy again or can be removed by the pediatrician at a regular checkup. If serous otitis is a result of repeated infections or enlarged adenoids, the underlying problem will also be treated to prevent recurrences.

What can I do to help?

☐ If your child has had tubes inserted, he may have to wear earplugs when swimming or bathing. A few ear, nose and throat specialists advise against swimming when tubes are in place. Your pediatrician will determine this.
☐ Keep the ear as dry as possible at all times.

S

SEE ALSO:
Common cold, *page 91*
Deafness, *page 108*
Otitis media, *page 195*
Tonsillitis, *page 243*

Sickle cell anemia

Sickle cell anemia is an inherited condition caused by an abnormal form of hemoglobin in the blood. The inheritance is recessive; that is, both parents carry an abnormal gene but are themselves healthy. The risk of a child having sickle cell anemia in such a family is 1 in 4. The anemia that results from the blood condition is not present at birth but develops in the first 6 months.

Hemoglobin is the protein contained in red cells in the blood. It picks up oxygen from the blood and carries it to various parts of the body. Sickle cell anemia occurs when the inherited hemoglobin causes the red blood cells to become sickle-shaped as a result of abnormally low oxygen levels. In a child with this condition, blood is less likely to clot efficiently, and it flows through the blood vessels less smoothly than in a normal child. If it clogs the vessels, your child will experience pain in the area of the blockage and a worsening of anemia, jaundice and an increased susceptibility to infections, such as coughs and colds. It is almost exclusively people of African descent who are affected by this disease.

Possible symptoms

- Anemia.
- Fatigue.
- Mild jaundice—yellowing of the whites of the eyes.
- Pain in the limbs and abdomen, wherever blockages occur in the blood vessels.
- Susceptibility to infection.

What can be done to help?

Sickle cell anemia does not affect a child's intelligence, and most children with this condition can attend ordinary schools. However, your child may suffer an acute attack (called a *crisis*) at school and have severe joint and abdominal pain. His teachers should be alerted to the need to get immediate medical attention for him. The crisis will be treated with painkilling drugs, and any infection will be treated promptly with antibiotics.

A sickle crisis can be precipitated by strenuous activity, particularly if it is cold and damp. It is essential for your child to be fully immunized against all infectious diseases and to take any prescribed vitamin supplements. Because the condition is inherited, it is important for potential carriers to seek genetic counseling before deciding to have a baby. A blood test will show if the prospective parents are carriers of the disease.

Words in **bold** are A-Z entries

Sleeplessness

Sleeplessness may be a problem for parents when their child is very young. Your baby may sleep a less-than-normal amount from the first weeks of life; 12 hours instead of the accepted norm of 16 to 20 out of 24. These 12 hours may be taken in short, unpredictable bursts so you never have more than a few hours consecutive sleep yourself. Sleepless babies are usually full of life, interested in everything that's going on, affectionate and sociable. As long as your baby is happy and cheerful when he's awake, he is normal and does not need medical attention.

The sleep patterns of toddlers can be very different. Some need to sleep for an hour or 2 during the day until they are 4 or 5 years old, while others need no daytime nap, sleep only 8 hours at night and wake early in the morning. Usually, a child that needed little sleep as a baby needs little sleep as a toddler. Providing a child can cope with school work and normal daily routine and is cheerful and bright, the sleep he takes is the amount of sleep he needs.

Is it serious?
Sleeplessness—that is, less than 8 hours in a 24-hour day—is hardly ever serious, though it may seem serious and disruptive to parents.

What should I do first?

1 Realize your baby's relative sleeplessness, and sort out a shift system for the first months so both parents don't become overtired.

2 If your baby wakes and cries in the night, go to him, comfort him and be cheerful. Try not to pick him up and take him into bed with you. If he continues to cry or call out, stay with him awhile so he doesn't feel you are deserting him.

3 Have plenty of toys and books and a drink by your toddler's bed so he can entertain himself if he wakes early.

Should I consult the doctor?

Consult your doctor if you are exhausted and the sleepless nights are affecting you or your baby's health.

What might the doctor do?

☐ If your baby is fit and well, but you are not, your doctor may prescribe a sedative for your baby to give you a break and to try to get him into a sleep routine.

What can I do to help?

☐ Make sure your baby's room is warm and snug.
☐ Try not to become resentful about your baby's wakefulness. Accept it as a fact of life and take practical steps to make sure you get enough sleep yourself. Sleep whenever your baby sleeps, get friends to help look after the baby and look for support groups in your area.
☐ Never use bed as a punishment with an older child. Sleeping will then be associated with punishment, and this will make your child even less willing to go to bed.
☐ Never give your baby or child a sedative without your doctor's advice.

S

Sleepwalking

Sleepwalking, when a child wanders about the house while asleep, is a sort of "mobile dreaming." A sleepwalking child does not walk around with his eyes closed and his arms held straight out in front of him as is popularly supposed. His eyes will be open, but he will be asleep. He won't see you and won't understand anything you say to him. Many children go through a short phase of sleepwalking, but it passes. Sleepwalking may be asso-ciated with **nightmares** if your child is unduly troubled about something. If he has had frequent nightmares and you have tried to ignore them, he may be walking in his sleep to find you and seek reassurance.

Is it serious?
Sleepwalking is not serious unless your child is in physical danger, such as from stairways or glass doors.

What should I do first?

1 If you find your child sleepwalking, don't try to waken him. Lead him slowly and gently back to bed.

Should I consult the doctor?

There is no need to consult your doctor unless sleepwalking becomes very frequent and you need reassurance that nothing is seriously wrong.

What might the doctor do?

☐ Your doctor will question you about the frequency and nature of your child's sleepwalking and whether he has had any nightmares.
☐ Your doctor may recommend you and your child see a child psychologist to find the cause of the problem if your child is sleepwalking frequently.

What can I do to help?

☐ Protect your child—for instance, by putting a barrier at the top of the stairs at night and by making sure no windows are left open.
☐ Try to reassure your child if you think you know the underlying cause of the sleepwalking.

S

SEE ALSO:
Nightmares, *page 187*

Words in **bold** are A-Z entries

Snake bite

Any bite from a snake, whether venomous or not, can be extremely frightening for your child. In the United States, there are four poisonous snakes—rattlesnake, copperhead, moccasin and coral snake.

Is it serious?
A snake bite should always be treated as serious. Prompt treatment is necessary in case the bite was from a poisonous snake. However, deaths from snake bites are rare.

Possible symptoms
● Swelling and pain at the site of the bite.

Appearance of bite

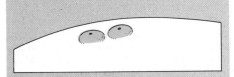

● One or two puncture marks.
● Pain or numbness spreading through the rest of the limb.

What should I do first?

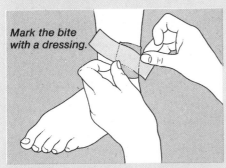

Mark the bite with a dressing.

1 Clean the skin around the puncture mark, and place a dressing over it. This helps mark the wound when you get to the hospital.

2 Take your child to the nearest emergency room. If possible, lay your child down flat on the way. Don't raise the affected part above the level of the heart; this will spread the venom.

3 Keep your child calm and still, and warm, if he seems clammy and pale.

4 Don't apply a tourniquet or suck out the poison.

Should I consult the doctor?
Take your child to the nearest emergency room or call an ambulance.

What might the doctor do?

☐ If bitten by a poisonous snake, your child will be sick and admitted to the hospital.
☐ Your child will be given an antivenom injection if the snake was recognized as, or thought to be, poisonous.
☐ There is always the risk of **tetanus** with a snake bite. Your child will be given a tetanus booster.

What can I do to help?

☐ Teach your child to be cautious around snakes and to identify the poisonous and non-poisonous ones.

SEE ALSO:
Tetanus, *page 238*

Sore throat

A sore throat is usually a symptom of an infection of the respiratory tract. With a baby or young child, he may not be able to tell you about the raw feeling in his throat. But you will notice he has difficulty swallowing. Sore throats most often occur because of a viral infection. Some may occur from inflammation of the tonsils (**tonsillitis**), caused by the *streptococcal bacterium*. Sore throats also occur with the **common cold** or **influenza** virus. If there is inflammation elsewhere, as there is in the larynx when your child has **laryngitis**, this can also give a raw feeling in the throat. If the glands in the neck are swollen, such as with **mumps**, for example, this may be felt by your child as pain in the throat.

Is it serious?
Most sore throats are not serious.

What should I do first?

1 If your child complains of a sore throat or if he has difficulty swallowing and isn't eating, examine his throat in a good light, with his head held back and the tongue depressed gently with the handle of a clean spoon (*see page 243*). Ask him to say a long "aaah." This will open up the throat so you can see if there is any inflammation.

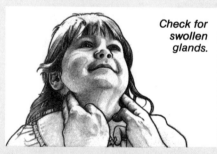

Check for swollen glands.

2 Run your fingers down both sides of your child's neck and under his chin to check for swelling in the glands. Swollen glands will feel like large peas under the skin.

3 Take your child's temperature to see if he has a fever.

4 The sore throat is probably caused by an infection, so keep your child away from school until you have seen your doctor.

Should I consult the doctor?

Consult your doctor if you think it is a streptococcal infection. It should be treated promptly to avoid complications.

What might the doctor do?

☐ Your doctor will take a throat culture to determine the cause of the sore throat. If it is a streptococcal bacterium, your doctor will prescribe antibiotics.

What can I do to help?

☐ Soothe your child's sore throat with cold drinks or hot lemon drinks.
☐ Give your child plenty of liquid. If he isn't eating because it hurts to swallow, purée foods when possible.
☐ Give your child ice cream, jello, Popsicles and milk shakes to keep his fluid level up and because they are easy to swallow.

SEE ALSO:
Appetite, loss of, *page 58*
Common cold, *page 91*
Influenza, *page 165*
Laryngitis, *page 172*
Mumps, *page 184*
Scarlet fever, *page 213*
Tonsillitis, *page 243*

S

Words in **bold** are A-Z entries

Spina bifida

In a child born with spina bifida, the bones of the spine (the vertebrae) that normally protect the spinal column fail to join properly, leaving a gap. In extreme cases the nerves of the spinal column are exposed. The condition most commonly affects the lower region of the spine and can be relatively minor or very serious, such as when the spinal cord is under-developed and the gap in the spine is covered by a large red membrane instead of skin. Symptoms reflect the severity of the condition. These may range from no symptoms at all, except for skin markings, to complete paralysis of the lower limbs and incontinence. With a moderate-to-severe form of spina bifida, the development and function of your child's lower body will never be quite normal. He may be physically stunted or walk with a limp. Nine out of 10 spina bifida babies also have hydrocephalus—a condition in which excessive fluid accumulates in the brain.

Possible symptoms

- Part of the spinal cord exposed.
- Swelling over part of the spine— covered by skin or only a large red membrane.
- Paralysis of the lower body.
- Excessively large head.
- Incontinence.

What can be done to help?

Severe cases of spina bifida are recognized at birth. The degree and extent of paralysis will be assessed as soon as possible by your pediatrician, and a brain scan will be performed to see if excessive fluid is present on the brain. In very severe cases, a child will be paralyzed below the waist, and there could be mental retardation as well. Surgery can be done to correct the skin defect and prevent infection, but this will not restore function to the spinal cord. A drainage-valve operation can also be performed to control the hydrocephalus.

Less severe cases are referred for surgery, then a program of rehabilitation and physiotherapy. Checkups will be made at frequent intervals on bladder control, kidney function and the development of hip joints.

If there is a family history of spina bifida, it is important to make a special search for this during pregnancy. This can be done by ultrasound scanning and measuring the alphafetoprotein levels in the mother's blood. If necessary, amniocentesis can be performed. If the tests are positive, you will be given the option of terminating the pregnancy.

Splinter

A splinter is a tiny piece of material that becomes embedded in or under the skin. It may be wood, metal, glass or a thorn. Usually it is unnecessary to get medical help; most splinters can be removed at home.

Is it serious?
A splinter is rarely serious. However, splinters that cause deep wounds, particularly if they do not bleed much, can be serious because they carry the risk of **tetanus** infection.

What should I do first?

1 Find out from your child what material is embedded in the skin. If it is glass, the entire surface of the splinter is capable of cutting into your child's flesh. Don't try to remove it yourself; seek medical help.

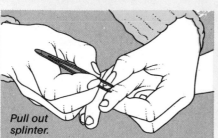

Pull out splinter.

2 If the splinter is not glass and the end is sticking out of the skin, remove it with tweezers. Distract your child so he doesn't flinch too much when you gently pull out the splinter.

3 Splinters often work themselves out in a day or 2 if left alone or covered lightly with a Band-aid.

4 If the splinter doesn't work itself out, use a sharp sewing needle to remove it. Place a piece of ice over the splinter area so the skin is lightly numbed, then use the needle to gently break the skin's surface and expose the splinter. Once the end of the splinter is free, pull it out with a pair of tweezers.

5 Clean the area with soap and water, and apply an antiseptic cream. Don't put a Band-aid on unless your child asks for one.

Should I consult the doctor?

Consult your doctor immediately if the splinter is glass, if it is deep in the skin, if it's contaminated with manure (which increases the risk of tetanus) or if you cannot remove it yourself.

What might the doctor do?

☐ If the splinter is a piece of glass or deep in the skin, your doctor will remove it under a local anesthetic.
☐ If there is any manure in the wound, your doctor may give your child a tetanus booster.

> **SEE ALSO:**
> **Tetanus,** *page 238*

Sprain

A sprain is the tearing of the tough, strap-like structures (ligaments) that support a joint and limit its movement. The sprain usually occurs because of overstretching or a sudden twisting action that wrenches the joint beyond its normal movement. The tearing causes bleeding into the joint, which results in swelling, pain and a bad **bruise**. (If only a few fibers of a ligament tear, it is called a *strain*.)

The most common sites of a sprain are the ankle, knee and wrist. Because ligaments are near the skin's surface in these joints, and there is just hard bone beneath them, swelling shows rapidly. Your child will not be able to take any weight on the sprained joint.

It is rare for young children to suffer a sprain because their joints are so supple. Sprains are common in the 6-to-12 age group.

Is it serious?
A sprain is painful but not serious, though it can be difficult to determine without an X-ray whether the injury is a sprain, a **broken bone** or a dislocated joint.

Possible symptoms
- Swelling and tenderness.
- Pain when the affected joint has to bear any weight.
- Bruising.

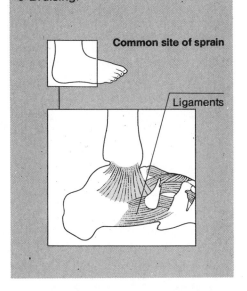

Common site of sprain

Ligaments

What should I do first?

1 If the affected joint or limb is not misshapen (which could indicate a dislocation or fracture), lay your child down and raise the injured part.

2 Apply a cold compress to reduce swelling.

3 Support the joint with a firm elastic bandage. Check the bandage regularly to make sure swelling does not make it too tight.

4 Encourage your child to rest the joint for at least 24 hours.

Should I consult the doctor?

Consult your doctor immediately if there is intense pain and the affected joint or limb is misshapen, suggesting a dislocation or fracture. Consult your doctor if, after 48 hours, the swelling has not subsided or if your child still complains of severe pain and cannot bear any weight on the injured part.

What might the doctor do?

☐ If your doctor suspects a fracture, X-rays will be taken.
☐ If the injury is a sprain, your doctor will wrap the damaged joint with a firm bandage.

S

SEE ALSO:
Broken bone, *page 73*
Bruise, *page 78*

Stammering

Stammering is a speech disorder in which the flow of words is interrupted while the child struggles to start a word. It is perfectly normal in a child who is learning to speak, when excitement, a profusion of ideas and the inability to form sentences properly may result in jerky speech. Nearly all children grow out of this phase by the time they reach school age. If stammering continues beyond this time, there may be an under-lying emotional problem, such as fear, anxiety or tension, usually caused by parental concern. Stammering tends to run in families.

Is it serious?
Stammering is not serious and can be controlled, if not cured. Drawing un-necessary attention to the stammer may make your child feel self-conscious and worsen the problem.

What should I do first?

1 Resist the temptation to give your child the word you think he needs. Give him plenty of time to express himself.

2 Check to see if there is any cause for anxiety or stress in your child's life, and do your best to deal with it.

Should I consult the doctor?

Consult your doctor if your child is obviously embarrassed and upset by the stammering and it causes him to contort his lips, tongue and face when he tries to express himself or if he needs reassurance.

What might the doctor do?

□ Your doctor may reassure you the stammer will soon disappear.
□ Your doctor may refer your child to a speech therapist for assessment and therapy. If therapy is started early, there is a good chance of eliminating the stammer from your child's speech.

What can I do to help?

□ Your child needs your help to prevent losing confidence in himself. Never ridicule or draw attention to your child's stammering. Try to be open and frank about discussing it, and never show embarrassment.
□ If your child is old enough to under-stand, discuss with him the possibility of therapy. Ask him if he would like professional help and see how he responds. He may be quite happy to live with his stammer.
□ Don't push your child or interrupt him when he's talking. !f he asks for help with a word, give it.
□ Suggest your child impose a rhythm when speaking and to speak slowly to accentuate the rhythm of his sentences. Stammerers don't stammer while they are singing or reciting poetry.

Words in **bold** are A-Z entries

Sticky eye

Sticky eye is a mild eye infection that is usually common in the first week of a baby's life. It is due to a foreign substance getting into the baby's eye during delivery, possibly a drop of amniotic fluid or blood. Your baby's eye will ooze pus, and when he wakes from sleep, the eyelashes will be stuck together.

Is it serious?
Sticky eye is not serious. There is no danger to your baby's eyes, but it should be treated promptly to prevent **conjunctivitis** from developing.

Possible symptoms

● Pus coming from the inner corner of one or both of the eyes.
● Eyelashes stuck together after sleep.

What should I do first?

Wipe from the corner of the eye downward.

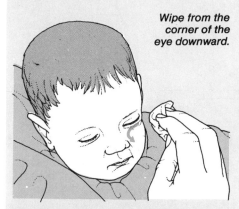

1 Wash both eyes with warm water, using a clean piece of cotton for each eye. Start on the outside corner of the eye and move downward.
2 Put your baby down to sleep with the infected eye up. The other eye may become infected from the crib sheet.

Should I consult the doctor?

Consult your doctor immediately if your baby's eyeball is red. It could be conjunctivitis. Consult your doctor if the sticky eye does not improve within 24 hours.

What might the doctor do?

☐ If there is an infection, your doctor will prescribe eye drops or an eye ointment to apply to the eye 3 or 4 times a day.

What can I do to help?

☐ Bathe your baby's eyes frequently, whenever you notice a discharge.
☐ Change your baby's crib sheet regularly to avoid contaminating his eyes.

S

> **SEE ALSO:**
> **Conjunctivitis,** *page 93*

Stings

Most stings, whether from insects or jellyfish, cause only local irritation, pain and swelling. In rare cases where there is severe allergic reaction to a sting, shock may develop (*see page 293*). This is called *anaphylactic shock*. Bee and wasp stings make a small puncture hole in the skin. Bees leave their stingers behind, but wasps rarely do. Jellyfish stings cause a localized burning sensation.

Is it serious?
A sting is rarely serious. However, treat it as an emergency if it causes an allergic reaction, with severe swelling leading to loss of consciousness; if it is in the mouth or throat, where swelling could lead to breathing problems; if it is caused by a Portuguese man-of-war jellyfish sting or if your child is stung by a number of insects (in which case the amount of poison in his body could be more than he can cope with).

Possible symptoms
- Small puncture mark, with or without the stinger left behind.
- Localized swelling and irritation.
- Red swelling with pieces of jellyfish still adhering to the skin.
- Breathing difficulties.
- Signs of shock—rapid pulse, clammy and pale skin, shortness of breath, sweating and faintness.

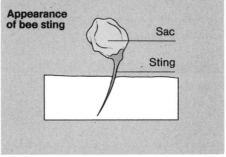

Appearance of bee sting — Sac — Sting

What should I do first?
Calm your child, and keep him as still as possible to slow down the poison's rate of spreading.

If your child is stung by a bee or wasp

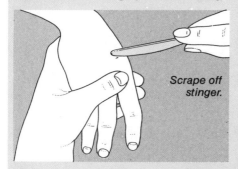

Scrape off stinger.

1 If the stinger is still in the skin, remove it by scraping it out of the skin with a fingernail or knife blade. Avoid squeezing the sac at the top of the stinger because this will force more poison into your child's body.

2 To reduce the pain and swelling, apply a cold compress of diluted vinegar for wasp stings and baking soda-and-water paste for bee stings. Ice packs or a paste of meat tenderizer and water are also helpful. Don't rub the area; just lay the compress on top.

If the sting is in the mouth or throat

1 If the stinger is visible, try to scrape it out. Avoid squeezing the sac at the top of the stinger because this will force more poison into your child's body. Give your child cold water to drink or a cube of ice to suck.

2 If the area swells quickly, place your child in the recovery position (*see page 285*), and get medical help immediately.

Continued on next page ▶

Words in **bold** are A-Z entries

Stings

◀ *Continued from previous page*
If your child is stung by a jellyfish

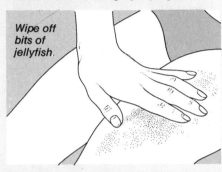

Wipe off bits of jellyfish.

1 Use dry sand to wipe away any bits of the jellyfish.

2 Wash the area with water or soap and water if available.

3 Relieve the pain and irritation with calamine lotion or ice.

4 Make a paste of meat tenderizer and water, and apply it to the sting.

Should I consult the doctor?

Take your child to the nearest emergency room if he has an allergic reaction, if he has been stung numerous times and is having difficulty breathing or swallowing, or if he has been stung by a Portuguese man-of-war jellyfish. Consult your doctor immediately or go to the nearest emergency room if he develops any symptoms of shock (*see page 293*), has breathing difficulties or if your child has been stung in the throat or mouth.

What might the doctor do?

☐ The hospital doctor will treat your child for shock.
☐ If your child has suffered an allergic reaction to a sting, your doctor may prescribe antihistamine tablets or cream, depending on the severity of the reaction. Your doctor may also give your child a series of desensitizing injections to prevent the same reaction in the future.

What can I do to help?

☐ Buy Benedryl over the counter to help control severe itching.
☐ Make up an emergency kit of antihistamine medication if your child suffers an allergic reaction to insect stings. Take it with you on vacations and outings.
☐ Take some aerosol sting reliever with you on picnics and outings. The quick relief of pain and itching reduces any fear your child may have about insects like wasps or bees.
☐ Have a bracelet or medallion engraved for your child to wear stating he is allergic to stings and should be given immediate medical treatment.

S

Strabismus

It is common for eyes of newborn babies to move independently until they are about 8 to 10 weeks old. At about this time, the baby's eyes should become permanently aligned. If this doesn't happen, and one or both eyes wander, this is called a strabismus or crossed eyes. This condition is commonly caused by muscle imbalance of the eye. It may also be associated with other vision defects, such as near- or farsightedness. The brain compensates for the wandering eye by blocking out what it sees.

Is it serious?
Strabismus that persists is serious because the child could lose sight from that eye.

Possible symptoms

Common form of strabismus

● Eyes appear to be looking in different directions.

What should I do first?

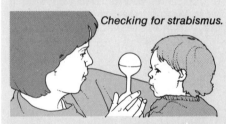
Checking for strabismus.

1 If you think your baby's eyes wander or are out of focus, check it by getting him to follow your finger or a colorful toy. See if both eyes track the object together or if one eye wanders to one side.

Should I consult the doctor?

Consult your doctor if the problem persists after your baby is 3 months old.

What might the doctor do?

☐ Your doctor will treat the condition by blacking out the strong eye with a pad or patch. This forces the muscles of the wandering eye to work and become stronger. The treatment usually corrects the laziness in the eye within 4 or 5 months.
☐ If your child is older, an eye specialist will teach your child a series of simple exercises to help strengthen eye muscles.
☐ If your child's problem is associated with a vision defect and glasses are required, you will be referred to an optician.
☐ If strabismus persists, surgery may be performed to correct muscular imbalance. This will not be contemplated until your child is at least 2 years old.

What can I do to help?

☐ Have your child's eyes checked annually.
☐ If you are concerned about your child's eyes, go to an ophthalmologist for another opinion.

SEE ALSO:
Vision problems, *page 252*

Words in **bold** are A-Z entries

Sty

A sty is a pus-filled swelling on the edge of the eyelid. It is caused by inflammation of one of the hair follicles from which the eyelashes grow. It appears on the lower eyelid and comes to a head and bursts in 4 or 5 days. Rubbing and pulling eyelashes may cause sties, and sties may be associated with a general irritation of the eyelids called **blepharitis**. Sties are not highly infectious, but they can be conveyed from one eye to the other.

Is it serious?
A sty is usually harmless and can be treated at home.

Possible symptoms

Common site

● Swollen, sore red area on the eyelid, which enlarges and becomes pus-filled.

What should I do first?

1 If the spot on the eyelid is red and sore, leave it alone, and discourage your child from touching or rubbing it. You can buy over-the-counter sty medicine which may help clear it up. If the sty is painful and unsightly, keep the eyelid covered with a pad of gauze or a clean handkerchief held loosely in place with adhesive tape.

2 If the sty is pus-filled and painful, apply a warm compress, or a ball of cotton squeezed in hot water, for a few minutes every 2 or 3 hours. This will soothe the pain and bring the sty to a head.

3 Once the sty comes to a head, your aim is to release the pus and ease the pain. If you can see the eyelash at the center of the sty, try to pull it out gently with a pair of tweezers. If it won't come out, leave it, and continue with the warm compresses. As soon as the eyelash comes out, the pus will drain.

4 Note whether eyelids are red-rimmed, with dandifflike flakes clinging to the eyelashes. This may be blepharitis.

Should I consult the doctor?

Consult your doctor if the home treatment does not improve the sty within 4 or 5 days, if the eyelid becomes swollen or if the sty is accompanied by blepharitis.

What might the doctor do?

☐ If there is an infection of the eyelid or the eye itself, your doctor will prescribe an antibiotic ointment or eye drops. If the sty is accompanied by blepharitis, your doctor may prescribe an ointment to clear it up.

What can I do to help?

☐ Keep your child's face cloth and towel separate from the rest of the family's to avoid spreading any infection.
☐ Wash your hands before and after treating the sty. Discourage your child from touching the area.

> **SEE ALSO:**
> **Blepharitis,** *page 69*

S

Sunburn

Sunburn is inflammation of the skin caused by excessive exposure to the ultraviolet rays in sunlight. The best cure is prevention. Even adults should acclimatize themselves to the sun. This must be done gradually, and it is necessary to be strict with children who may not appreciate the dangers. Your child's sunburn can result in tender and damaged skin that may **blister** or peel off. Even in mild sunshine, the effects of the sun can be increased if you are near water, snow or sand where the rays are reflected off the bright surface.

Is it serious?
Sunburn can be serious if a large area of the skin is involved. The skin may lose its ability to regulate body temperature so your child's temperature soars and **heatstroke** results.

Possible symptoms
- Red, hot, tender skin.
- Blisters.
- Itchiness prior to peeling skin.

What should I do first?

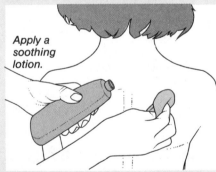

Apply a soothing lotion.

1 Apply a soothing lotion or a cold compress to any tight, red skin to cool it down and reduce irritation.

2 When you're inside, don't put any clothing on the sunburned areas. Leave them exposed to the air. Cover sunburned areas when you are outside.

3 If blisters appear and your child is in pain, give him acetaminophen.

4 Take your child's temperature to see if he has a fever. If his temperature is over 102F (38.9C), consult your doctor. Try to reduce the fever with tepid sponging (*see page 31*).

5 Keep your child out of direct sunlight for at least 48 hours.

Should I consult the doctor?

Consult your doctor if blisters form on your child's sunburned skin and he is feverish and unwell. Consult your doctor immediately if your child has a fever but his skin is dry and he seems confused and drowsy. This could be heatstroke, which should be treated as an emergency.

Continued on next page ▶

S

Words in **bold** are A-Z entries

Sunburn

◀ *Continued from previous page*

What might the doctor do?

☐ In a mild case of sunburn, your doctor may prescribe a soothing cream.
☐ If blisters have formed and your child is feverish, your doctor may prescribe an anti-inflammatory cream to help the skin heal more quickly.
☐ If your child is suffering from heat-stroke, your doctor will treat this accordingly.

What can I do to help?

☐ To prevent sunburn, use a sunscreen with a sun-protection factor (SPF) of at least 8 in darker-skinned children and 15 in lighter-skinned children. Buy the *waterproof* kind if your child will be in the water. Use the sunblock *every* time your child is out in the sun.
☐ Draw the sheets on your child's bed tightly so that nothing scratches his skin.

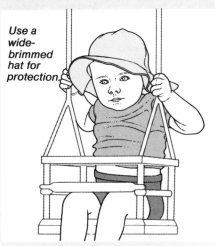

Use a wide-brimmed hat for protection.

☐ Increase exposure to sun by 10-minute increments each day.
☐ Cover your child's lips and nose with a sunblock or zinc oxide, and protect the nape of his neck with a wide-brimmed hat.

☐ Apply the sunblock again after your child has been swimming if the kind you use isn't waterproof.
☐ Watch your child's skin, even after the first few days when he should be acclimatized to the conditions. If his skin starts to get red, cover him up immediately or take him inside.

S

SEE ALSO:
Blister, *page 70*
Heatstroke, *page 156*

Tantrums

Temper tantrums are normal in children between age 2 and 4. They occur because the child hasn't acquired the judgment to match his will nor has he the linguistic skills to argue or explain what he wants. Clashes with parents tend to become frequent toward the end of the second year, leading to the time known as the "terrible twos." Tantrums take many forms, but usually the child throws himself on the floor, kicking and screaming, banging his feet against the walls or perhaps holding his breath with frustration. The child's actions show no regard for his own safety, and he can easily hurt himself on hard objects as he kicks about.

Are they serious?

Temper tantrums are not serious, though they may happen at inconvenient times and in embarrassing situations. Even if your child holds his breath until he turns blue, he won't be able to harm himself. There is an automatic reflex that forces the body to take a breath when it is running short of oxygen, and this cannot be overriden by willpower.

What should I do first?

1 Stay calm. Even if your child's anger affects you, don't let him see you are upset.

2 Ignore your child as much as possible. Walk away. A tantrum loses much of its effect if there is no audience.

3 If this doesn't work, try holding your child on your lap while he calms down. He may fight to get away, or he may realize comfort and sympathy are really what he wants.

4 Put your child in another room. Sometimes removing him from the situation helps a great deal.

Should I consult the doctor?

There is no need to consult your doctor about temper tantrums. If your child continues to throw tantrums after age 5 or if you find them difficult to cope with, ask your doctor for advice.

What might the doctor do?

☐ Your doctor will ask you about the frequency and nature of the tantrums and whether they are accompanied by other behavioral problems. Your doctor may refer you and your child to a child psychologist for assessment.

What can I do to help?

☐ Tantrums are directed against you. Your child is trying to gain your attention. Tantrums can be difficult to deal with in a public place when your child may sense that he will succeed. But if you show tantrums never succeed, they should stop.

☐ Try to anticipate problems and forestall clashes with distraction tactics. As your child grows up, he will be better able to tolerate delays and accept compromises.

☐ Don't ask your child why he is angry during a tantrum. He won't be able to reason with you.

☐ Don't slap your child to bring him out of a breath-holding attack. Just leave him alone, and it will end naturally.

Words in **bold** are A-Z entries

Teething

Teething is the term used to describe the eruption of a baby's first teeth. It usually begins at about age 6 to 7 months, with most of the first teeth breaking through before your baby is 18 months old. Your baby will produce more saliva than usual and will drool. He may try to cram his fingers into his mouth and chew on his fingers or any other object that he can get. He may be clingy and irritable, have difficulty sleeping and cry and fret more than usual. Most of these symptoms occur just before the teeth erupt. It is important to realize that the symptoms of teething do not include bronchitis, diaper rash, vomiting, fever, diarrhea or loss of appetite. These are symptoms of an underlying illness, *not* teething.

Is it serious?

Teething and the symptoms associated with teething are never serious.

Possible symptoms

- Increased saliva and drooling.
- Desire to bite on any hard object.
- Irritability and increased clinginess.
- Sleeplessness.
- Swollen red area where the tooth is being cut.

Order of appearance

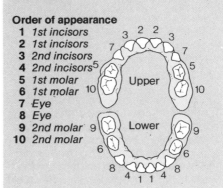

1	1st incisors
2	1st incisors
3	2nd incisors
4	2nd incisors
5	1st molar
6	1st molar
7	Eye
8	Eye
9	2nd molar
10	2nd molar

What should I do first?

Feel your baby's gums.

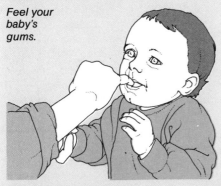

1 If you can't work out why your baby is so irritable, and he has no other symptoms of illness, feel his gums. If a tooth is coming through, the gum area will be swollen and red.

Should I consult the doctor?

You shouldn't need to consult your doctor unless your baby has other symptoms that can't be attributed to teething or you are unduly worried.

What might the doctor do?

☐ Your doctor will give you advice on how to cope with the symptoms of teething and may prescribe a mild analgesic to be used for a short time to relieve the irritation.

What can I do to help?

☐ Nurse your baby often. A teething baby needs your comfort and closeness. Don't think the arrival of teeth means a speeding-up of the weaning process. Babies with teeth can still be breast-fed with no discomfort to the mother.

Continued on next page ▶

Teething

◀ Continued from previous page

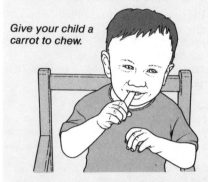

Give your child a carrot to chew.

☐ Distract your child with a chilled teething ring or a piece of carrot or apple—something with a firm texture. Stay with your baby while he chews on it so he doesn't choke on the food.

☐ Try not to resort to acetaminophen unless your baby is very uncomfortable.

☐ Rub the swollen gum with your finger. Try to avoid teething jellies that contain local anesthetics because these have only a temporary effect, and they can cause an allergy.

☐ If your child refuses food, encourage him with cold, smooth foods, such as yogurt, ice cream or Jello.

☐ It is *not* advisable to rub whiskey on gums.

T

SEE ALSO:
Crying, *page 102*
Sleeplessness, *page 219*

Words in **bold** are A-Z entries

Testes, undescended

The testes grow and develop inside the abdomen, near the kidneys. Shortly before a baby boy is born, they move down or "descend" into their normal position in the bag of skin called the

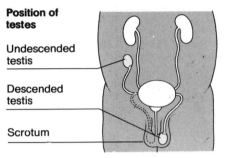

Position of testes

Undescended testis

Descended testis

Scrotum

scrotum. For testes to develop normally at adolescence and produce sperm, it is necessary for them to hang outside

the body. This is because sperm production can proceed only at a temperature that is slightly below the body's internal temperature. If one or both of the testes fails to descend, sperm and testosterone (which produces male characteristics, such as a deeper voice and body hair) will not be produced normally. Theoretically, one descended testis could be sufficient to produce sperm and male hormones. But if your son's testes have failed to descend by age 1, the problem should probably be corrected surgically.

Are they serious?
Undescended testes are not serious under 1 year, and they cause no health problems in childhood.

What should I do first?

When a baby boy is born, your pediatrician will examine his testes to see if they have descended. If not, you will be told and reassured they may descend naturally. If your baby's testes did not descend at birth, feel for them occasionally in the scrotum. If they have descended, they will feel small—each about the size of a pea. Warm your hands before you do this, otherwise the testes may temporarily retract into the abdomen.

Should I consult the doctor?

Your doctor will be aware of your baby's problem and will check the scrotum regularly.

What might the doctor do?

☐ Your doctor will probably advise to wait until your son is 1 year old before taking action. If by this time the testes have failed to descend, your doctor will refer you to a surgeon for an operation to lower the testes.

What can I do to help?

☐ Try to stay with your baby in the hospital when he has the operation to lower his testes.
☐ Keep your son quiet and calm when he returns home after the operation.

Tetanus

Tetanus is a rare, serious bacterial infection caused by the bacterium *Clostridium tetani.* The bacterium is commonly found in farm and garden dirt, gravel and rusty metal. It usually enters the body through a cut that could be caused by anything from a rose thorn to a sharp piece of metal. The bacterium, which thrives in the low-oxygen environment created by a deep cut, makes a poison or toxin that causes the muscles of the body to go into spasm (uncontrollable contraction). The jaw muscles are often affected first, hence the common name for the illness, *lockjaw.* This is followed by spasm of muscles throughout the rest of the body. Symptoms of tetanus can occur any time from a week to several months after the wound was sustained.

Possible symptoms
- Muscle stiffness and cramps, at first around the jaw and mouth.
- Sore throat.
- Difficulty in swallowing or breathing.

Tetanus is entirely preventable if your child has a course of injections within the first 5 years of life, updated every 5 years. Because of this program, tetanus is very rare.

Is it serious?
Tetanus is very serious. Sometimes the breathing muscles go into spasm, and even with intensive care this can result in death.

What should I do first?

1 Always examine any wound your child receives to see if it is deep and dirty. Clean the wound thoroughly with an antiseptic solution or soap and water, removing the dirt where you can.

2 Take your child to your doctor or the emergency room for a tetanus booster if it's been more than 5 years since his last booster.

3 If your child complains of muscle stiffness, especially of the jaw and neck, get medical attention at once.

Should I consult the doctor?

Consult your doctor immediately or take your child to the emergency room if your child has a deep cut from a possibly contaminated source, if 5 years have elapsed since his last tetanus injection or if he develops symptoms of tetanus.

What might the doctor do?

☐ The doctor will clean a deep or dirty wound and give your child a booster if he is already immunized. If your child is not immune, an injection of anti-tetanus globulin will be given to provide immediate protection against the poison.

☐ If tetanus develops, treatment includes a course of antibiotics and nursing in an intensive-care unit. The child's breathing is supported by a respirator for the time it takes the disease to run its course, which may be several weeks.

What can I do to help?

☐ All babies should receive a course of three tetanus injections (usually as part of DTP) in the first year. This provides good immunization against the toxin. Booster injections are needed at 18 months and five years of age, then every 5 years to maintain protection.

T

Words in **bold** are A-Z entries

Thrush

Thrush is an infection caused by the yeast *candida albicans*, also called *monilia*. Under normal circumstances, this yeast is kept under control by other bacteria that also live in the intestines. If the balance is disturbed—for example, when your child is on antibiotics or his natural resistance is low because of illness — the yeast can overgrow, causing infection in any part of the gastrointestinal tract. Thrush most often affects the mouth, causing white patches to appear on the tongue, roof of the mouth and inside the cheeks.

The monilia can also cause **diaper rash**, which does not respond to the usual self-help treatments. Oral thrush is rare after infancy.

Is it serious?
It is rare for thrush to cause serious symptoms, but it does not respond to self-help treatment, so you should get medical advice.

Possible symptoms

● Creamy yellow or white patches inside the cheeks, on the tongue and the roof of the mouth that become raw or bleed when wiped off.
● A pimply red rash around the anus or elsewhere on the diaper area.

What should I do first?

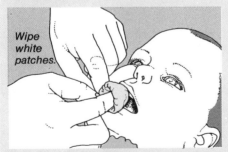

Wipe white patches.

1 If your baby refuses to eat, check his mouth for any white patches. Try to wipe them off with a clean handkerchief. If they don't come away easily or if they leave raw patches underneath, your baby probably has oral thrush.

2 Avoid giving your child spicy foods, and cool all cooked food to lukewarm. Yogurt is the best food to give until you have consulted your doctor.

3 Change your baby's diapers frequently. The yeast is in his stools, and this could cause thrush on the diaper area.

Should I consult the doctor?

Consult your doctor as soon as possible if you suspect your child has thrush.

Continued on next page ▶

Thrush

◄ Continued from previous page

What might the doctor do?

☐ Your doctor will prescribe a liquid anti-fungal medication to be put on the affected area in your child's mouth if he has oral thrush.
☐ Your doctor will prescribe an anti-fungal cream if there is a monilia diaper rash present.

What can I do to help?

☐ Feed your child with bland, puréed foods if he has oral thrush.
☐ Leave your baby's bottom exposed to the air as much as possible if he has monilia diaper rash.

Leave your baby's bottom exposed.

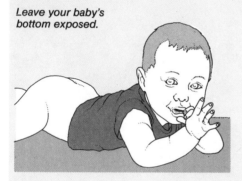

T

SEE ALSO:
Diaper rash, *page 112*

Words in **bold** are A-Z entries

Thumb sucking

Thumb sucking is a comfort habit that many babies adopt from an early age. There is clear evidence that babies suck their thumbs in the womb. Sucking fingers or a thumb can be soothing for a baby and is probably more hygienic than a pacifier. When a baby is weaned, the thumb may replace the breast or bottle as something to suck on for comfort. However, thumb sucking may put enough pressure on front teeth to move them forward eventually, if it persists until age 6 or 7, though most children have outgrown the habit by this age. Some psychiatrists believe thumb sucking provides a mother substitute. Others believe it is instinctive behavior that becomes habitual.

Is it serious?

If a child sucks his thumb, it won't cause serious damage to his teeth until permanent teeth begin cutting through his gums.

What should I do first?

1 Don't worry if your baby sucks his thumb. This is normal. If you can't ignore it, try providing another comfort mechanism, such as a pacifier.

2 If your child is age 6 or over and still sucks his thumb, and this bothers him, help him try to change the habit. Give him extra attention, and explore whether he is under stress. Once he decides to try to stop sucking, set him goals. Give rewards for any progress toward the goal.

Should I consult the doctor?

You should not need to consult your doctor unless your child wishes to stop the habit and the reward system has not helped.

What might the doctor do?

☐ Your doctor will probably refer you to a dentist who may fit a training device in your child's mouth to prevent the thumb from touching the roof of his mouth. This is only satisfactory if your child is willing to cooperate.

What can I do to help?

☐ Don't make your child anxious about the thumb sucking. Don't let him see that it irritates you, just believe he will eventually outgrow the habit.

T

Tics

A tic in a child is a jerky movement of the body or face that can become a mannerism. It is not the result of neuralgia, as are facial tics seen in elderly people. The most common tics in children are slight twitching of the eye or the corner of the mouth, wiggling the nose or blinking. Other habits include tossing the hair back off the forehead, fiddling with the hair, clearing the throat and sniffing. Some believe head banging is a form of tic. Tics of all kinds are usually transient; they often appear when a child is particularly stressed or fatigued and disappear when the child settles back to normal. In young children, some sort of tic is fairly common and is not usually indicative of any problem.

Is it serious?
A tic is not serious, although it can be irritating.

Possible symptoms
● Habitual, jerky movement of parts of the face or body.

What should I do first?

1 Don't overreact to a tic; you may increase your child's anxiety and make it worse. Play it down, and pretend not to notice, even though it may be irritating to you.

Should I consult the doctor?

Unless the tic interferes with everyday life or causes a problem at school, you don't need to consult a doctor.

What might the doctor do?

☐ If you seek advice, your doctor will reassure you there is no long-term problem.

What can I do to help?

☐ A tic is usually worse when a child gets tired, so make sure he has plenty of rest.
☐ Learn to control your irritation so you don't increase your child's tension.
☐ If your baby is a head banger, make sure he isn't left alone to get bored. Put bumper pads around his crib so he can't hurt himself.

Words in **bold** are A-Z entries

Tonsillitis

Tonsillitis is an acute infection of the tonsils usually caused by the *streptococcus bacterium* but sometimes by a virus. Positioned on either side of the back of the throat, the tonsils form the body's first line of defense by trapping and killing bacteria and keeping them from entering the respiratory tract. In the process, the tonsils themselves can become infected and inflamed, causing the symptoms of a **sore throat**, **fever** and swollen glands. The adenoids, positioned at the back of the nose, may be affected as well. Babies under age 1 rarely suffer from tonsillitis. The infection occurs mainly among school-age children, when the relatively large tonsils and adenoids are exposed to infectious microbes. As resistance to infection increases and adenoids become smaller, attacks of tonsillitis should lessen. Most children stop suffering from tonsillitis around age 10.

Is it serious?
Tonsillitis is not serious. Tonsillar abscess is serious. The symptoms include severe sore throat, fever, only one side of the throat enlarged (one tonsil) and fullness in the neck.

Possible symptoms
● Sore throat, possibly bad enough to cause difficulty swallowing.

Area affected

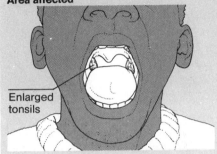

Enlarged tonsils

● Red, enlarged tonsils, possibly covered with yellow spots.
● A temperature of over 100F (37.5C).
● Swollen glands in the neck.
● Mouth-breathing, snoring and a nasal voice when the adenoids are affected.
● Unpleasant breath.

What should I do first?

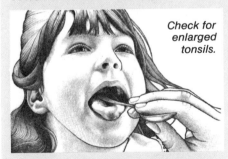

Check for enlarged tonsils.

1 If your child complains of a sore throat or you notice he has difficulty eating, examine his throat in a good light, with his head held back and the tongue depressed gently with the handle of a clean spoon. Ask him to say a long "aaah." This will open up the throat, and a second or 2 should be enough for you to see whether his tonsils are red, enlarged or covered with yellow spots.

2 Take your child's temperature to see if he has a fever.

Continued on next page ▶

T

Tonsillitis

◀ Continued from previous page

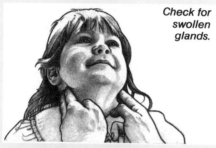

Check for swollen glands.

3 See if your child's glands are swollen by running your fingers down the sides of his neck and under his chin—swollen glands will feel like large peas under the skin.

4 If your child is old enough, ask him if he has **earache**. In a young child, note whether he pulls or rubs one of his ears. Check the ear to see if there is any discharge.

5 Give him plenty of cool drinks, Popsicles and ice cream to sooth his throat.

Should I consult the doctor?

Consult your doctor if you suspect tonsillitis.

What might the doctor do?

☐ Your doctor may take a throat culture (it is painless), to be sent to a laboratory for identification of the organism that is causing the infection. Your doctor may prescribe antibiotics if a bacterial infection seems likely.

☐ Your doctor will examine your child's ear and eardrum to check for any ear infection. If there is any sign of infection, antibiotics will be prescribed.

☐ If your child suffers from frequent attacks of tonsillitis, you may be referred to a specialist to see whether the tonsils and adenoids should be removed. The circumstances under which the operation might be performed would take the following into account:

a *Age*. The operation is seldom performed before a child is 4 years old.

b *The onset of tonsillitis*. The length of time that your child has been suffering from recurrent attacks of tonsillitis or earache is important. Most doctors wait 2 years before deciding to operate.

c *Effect on the child*. Tonsillectomy is advisable if the attacks are so frequent that they affect your child's education because he is absent from school so often or if his health is deteriorating because he cannot eat well.

What can I do to help?

☐ Treat your child the same way you would for a fever. Bed rest is not necessary.

☐ Keep your child's fluid intake up by offering regular drinks.

☐ Purée your child's foods if he finds swallowing difficult, but don't force him to eat. Offer him his favorite foods, especially those that slip down easily like ice cream or yogurt.

SEE ALSO:
Earache, *page 124*
Fever, *page 138*
Sore throat, *page 222*

T

Words in **bold** are A-Z entries

Toothache

Toothache is the pain that results when a tooth is decaying. The decaying process erodes the outer protective coatings of the tooth and bores through to the nerves in the soft center, causing pain particularly when anything cold, hot or sweet touches the tooth. Tooth decay, also called *dental caries* and gum disease are caused by plaque. This is a thin film of saliva and food residue in which bacteria grow. The bacteria thrive in the presence of sugar in the mouth—for example, in the form of refined white sugar or the sugar in dried fruits and even honey—which is one reason why sugar in the diet is so harmful to teeth.

Teeth can become resistant to the action of bacteria and sugar if they are painted or coated with fluoride as they would be if regularly brushed with a fluoride-containing toothpaste. This is one of the main ways to prevent tooth decay, along with good oral hygiene and regular dental checkups. It's important that children do not lose their first teeth through tooth decay or as a complication of tooth decay—a gum boil—in which the root of the tooth also decays. The permanent tooth may come through misaligned if a gap is left for too long while the new tooth is developing.

Is it serious?

Toothache is not serious as long as it is treated immediately. If untreated, a gum boil may erupt, causing damage to or loss of a second tooth.

What should I do first?

1 If your child complains of pain in the jaw, **earache** or throbbing, stabbing pains in the mouth, tap his teeth gently with a small metal spoon to see if this identifies the source of the pain.

2 Give your child acetaminophen to relieve the pain, then call the dentist.

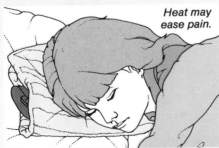

Heat may ease pain.

3 Put a hot-water bottle covered with a cloth or towel against your child's cheek to relieve the pain.

4 Do not apply oil of cloves or anesthetic jellies because it may cause damage to the gum around the tooth.

Should I consult the doctor?

You don't need to consult a doctor, but you should consult your child's dentist immediately for an appointment.

What might the dentist do?

☐ Your dentist will examine the tooth to determine the extent of damage. The tooth may only need to be drilled and filled. If there is a gum boil, the dentist will drain the pus from the abscess. If there is no possibility of saving the tooth, it will be extracted (maybe under general anesthetic), depending on the age of your child.

T

Continued on next page ▶

Toothache

◀ Continued from previous page

What can I do to help?

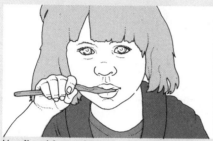

Use fluoride toothpaste.

☐ Prevent tooth decay. Use fluoride toothpastes and, depending on the level of fluoride in your local water supply, use fluoride tablets or drops in your child's drinks. Ask your dentist to give you information on this subject.

☐ Limit your child's intake of foods that are high in sugar.

☐ Brush your child's teeth yourself once a day and supervise the tooth brushing up until age 6 or 7.

☐ Once your child gets his 2-year molars, take him for a dental checkup every 6 months. Get him used to the dentist from an early age so the prospect holds no mystery or terror for him.

☐ Encourage your child to drink plenty of water after eating sweet foods. The water will immediately wash much of the sugar off his teeth.

☐ Ask your dentist about fissure sealing. When your child is about 4 or 5, his permanent back teeth can be sealed with a plastic coating to prevent plaque from getting into the biting surfaces.

> **SEE ALSO:**
> **Earache,** *page 124*

Toxocara

Toxocara is a rare infection caused by the *toxocara* **worm** that lives in the intestines of some cats and dogs. The eggs of the worm are passed out in the animal's feces; if a child plays on ground contaminated with the feces then puts his hands into his mouth, he may ingest the eggs. The eggs hatch, and the worms burrow through the intestinal wall into the body and are carried in the blood-stream to the lungs and other parts of the body. They are then coughed up from the lungs. If swallowed, they develop in the child's intestines and set up a rein-festation cycle. Children show few specific symptoms of the disease.

Is it serious?
Toxocara is rarely serious in children, although in rare cases a worm may lodge in the eyes, causing blindness.

Possible symptoms
- Loss of appetite.
- Slight fever.
- Attacks of abdominal pain.
- Loss of sight.

What should I do first?

1 If your child has a mild infestation, you may not even be aware of it. If he suffers from unexplained fever and abdominal pain, it's wise to seek medical advice.

Should I consult the doctor?

Consult your doctor if you suspect that there is something wrong with your child, particularly if you have a pet or if your child has played in areas where animals defecate regularly.

What might the doctor do?

☐ Your doctor will examine your child and take a sample of his stools or blood.
☐ If evidence of worms is found, your doctor may prescribe a special anti-parasite drug, or he may advise you to keep your child away from all animals or possibly contaminated areas for 6 months while the worms die off.

What can I do to help?

☐ Encourage your child to wash his hands after playing with animals.
☐ Worm your dog or cat regularly.
☐ Train your pet to use its own toilet area away from places frequented by the family.
☐ Disinfect any area where your children play if the dog or cat has fouled it.

SEE ALSO:
Worms, *page 261*

Tuberculosis

Tuberculosis (TB) is caused by bacteria. If left untreated, it can destroy large areas of an affected organ. It most commonly affects the lungs, but can also affect the kidneys and membranes covering the brain and spine (*meninges*). The disease can take many forms because it is capable of traveling through the bloodstream and affecting any organ in the body. This makes it difficult to diagnose. Tuberculosis has been almost completely eradicated by means of a pasteurization program for milk and tuberculin testing of the dairy herds, skin testing and improved drug treatment.

If a healthy child becomes infected by an adult, this first infection (the primary lesion) hardly ever progresses to anything serious because the body forms a strong resistance to the tuberculous organism and prohibits its spread by walling it off within a chalky coating. If the child remains healthy and doesn't become

Possible symptoms

- Tiredness.
- Weight loss through loss of appetite.
- Persistent, dry cough with blood and pus in the sputum if the lungs are affected.
- Headache, fever and coma if the meninges are affected.

reinfected with tuberculosis, there may never be any effects of the disease. If there is a period of malnourishment and illness, the primary lesion may break out of its chalky coating and spread to other organs. The symptoms of this secondary phase of the disease depend on the organ that is affected.

Is it serious?
Tuberculosis is a serious disease if left untreated.

What should I do first?

1 It is extremely unlikely that you would suspect that your child had tuberculosis from any of the symptoms.

Should I consult the doctor?

Consult your doctor if you are worried about your child's general health or a persistent, dry cough.

What might the doctor do?

☐ Your doctor will give your child a skin test to see if there is an active TB infection or not. If there is, your child will have an X-ray and sputum and urine tests to find out which organs are affected. Most TB cases can be adequately managed at home. Antibiotics will be prescribed, but rest and a good diet are also essential. Your child will need to be away from school for many months. There will be periodic

checkups after the treatment is finished to make sure the TB does not flare up again. At the end of 2 years, your child should be cured.

What can I do to help?

☐ Administer drugs regularly.
☐ Keep your child happy and as involved in normal life as possible.
☐ Arrange for a friend to play with your child regularly. After the drug treatment is started, your child will no longer be contagious and can safely play with friends.

Words in **bold** are A-Z entries

Umbilical–cord infection

After birth, the umbilical cord, which joins the baby to the placenta, is clamped and cut close to the baby's body. It withers, and the remaining stump drops off, usually within 10 days of birth. You will be advised to clean the navel area and umbilical stump daily because it may become wet with urine. The stump is infected if it weeps, crusts over, discharges pus or appears red or swollen.

Is it serious?
Infection of the umbilical cord is rarely serious and is easily treated.

Possible symptoms
- Redness and swelling in the umbilical area.
- Umbilical stump weeps fluid, which then crusts over.
- Pussy discharge.
- Foul odor.

What should I do first?

1 Check the stump at every diaper change for signs of infection. If the area seems to be getting red, contact your doctor.

Should I consult the doctor?

Consult your doctor if the stump shows any signs of infection. Consult your doctor if you are worried about the umbilical cord.

What might the doctor do?

☐ Your doctor will probably prescribe an antibiotic cream or powder to apply to the cord several times a day. He will also give you advice on daily hygiene.
☐ If your doctor thinks the infection is spreading along the cord and into your baby's body, your baby will need to be admitted to the hospital for treatment with antibiotics.

What can I do to help?

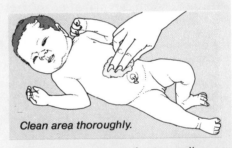
Clean area thoroughly.

☐ Clean the stump and surrounding area thoroughly at every diaper change. Gently wipe around the stump with a piece of cotton soaked in alcohol.
☐ Allow the stump to fall off naturally. Never pull or twist it in an attempt to remove it.

U

249

Urinary–tract infection

A urinary-tract infection can infect any part of the urinary tract. This includes the kidneys, bladder and urethra (the tube leading from the bladder to the outside of the body). In most cases, the part infected is the lining of the bladder, and the condition is called *cystitis*.

Girls suffer from these infections more often than boys because the female urethra is shorter, making it easier for infecting microbes to reach the bladder. Young girls sometimes do not clean themselves thoroughly after going to the bathroom. If they wipe their bottom from back to front, it may bring fecal material near the urethral opening, which could cause infection. Rarely, a minor structural abnormality of the urinary tract is to blame for urinary-tract infections. The most common symptoms of infection are pain on passing urine and the need to pass urine frequntly.

Is it serious?
A urinary-tract infection is serious.

Possible symptoms
- Pain or burning sensation on passing urine.
- Fever.
- Frequent urination, which can lead to bedwetting where previously the child was dry at night, or a feeling of urgency for the child.
- Unpleasant-smelling and/or cloudy urine.
- Low abdominal pain.
- Low back pain.

The urinary system

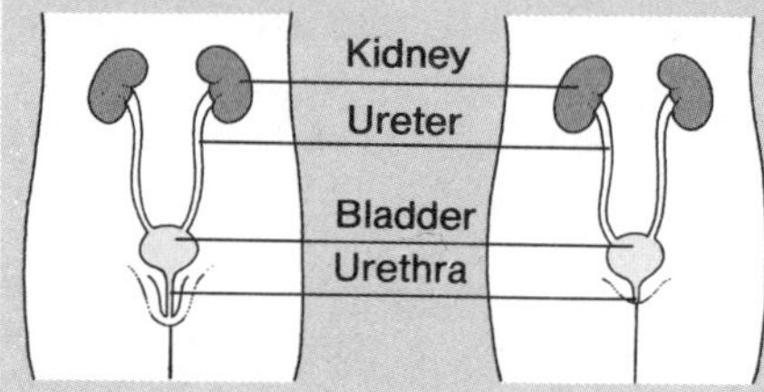

The urinary system, Male and Female, with labels: Kidney, Ureter, Bladder, Urethra.

What should I do first?

1 If your child complains of pain when passing urine, check his temperature to see if he has a fever.

2 Check his urine to see if it is cloudy or unpleasant smelling.

3 Give your child plenty of fluid to keep his kidneys flushed out.

4 Place a hot-water bottle against his back if he is suffering from low back pain.

Should I consult the doctor?

Consult your doctor immediately if your child complains of pain on urinating.

What might the doctor do?

☐ Your doctor will examine your child and take a sample of his urine for laboratory examination to identify the type of organism causing the infection. Your doctor will then prescribe the appropriate treatment, usually a course of antibiotics.

☐ If the infection recurs, your doctor may perform a series of special X-ray tests. If there is any abnormality, your child may be referred to a urologist.

What can I do to help?

☐ Show your daughter how to wipe herself from the front backward after going to the bathroom so her urethra is not contaminated by her feces.

SEE ALSO:
Bedwetting, page 66
Fever, *page 138*

Words in **bold** are A-Z entries

Vagina, foreign body in

A little girl is naturally curious about her vagina, and she will investigate it with her fingers or perhaps something else. Fortunately, it is rare for a foreign body to become lodged in a child's vagina, despite such exploration. However, if there is a foreign body in your child's vagina, there may be symptoms of local soreness and tenderness. After a day or 2, an unpleasant-smelling, blood-stained discharge from the vagina may occur. A discharge with itchiness, especially around the anus, may be an infestation of **worms**.

Is it serious?
Discharge from the vagina or soreness of the genital area, sometimes called **vulvovaginitis**, is rarely serious.

Possible symptoms
● Soreness or tenderness around the vagina.
● Unpleasant-smelling or blood-stained discharge.

What should I do first?
1 Ask your child if she has tried to push anything into her vagina.
2 Check your child's stools for tiny, threadlike worms.

Should I consult the doctor?
Consult your doctor if you notice any inflammation or discharge.

What might the doctor do?
☐ Your doctor will examine your child to try to determine whether the vulvovaginitis is the result of a foreign body being pushed into the vagina. If he thinks there is something there, he may refer you to a gynecological specialist who will perform an internal examination. The specialist will remove the foreign body, treat any infection with antibiotics and prescribe an ointment to relieve soreness or itching.

What can I do to help?
☐ Don't make too much fuss about the incident.
☐ Discourage your child from using any instruments when playing "doctors and nurses."

SEE ALSO:
Vulvovaginitis, *page 256*
Worms, *page 261*

Vision problems

Most vision defects are due to a fault in the eye itself and are not the result of disease or injury. Babies are rarely born totally blind, and routine checkups during a child's preschool years should detect any defect that could later lead to problems with vision.

Cross section of eye

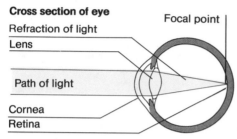

Refraction of light

Lens

Focal point

Path of light

Cornea

Retina

Many defects are caused when the light entering the eye does not focus properly on the retina. If the eyeball is too long from front to back, the images of distant objects will be focused in front of the retina and will appear blurred. Near objects will be seen clearly. This is called *nearsightedness*. If the eyeball is too short from front to back, the images of both near and far objects will focus behind the retina. All images will be blurred, but near objects will be the worst. This is called *farsightedness*. Nearsightedness usually develops in late childhood and tends to run in families. A child with a parent who is nearsighted should be regularly tested. Farsightedness is generally present at birth and can cause eye fatigue as your child strains to focus on objects close to him. Both near- and farsightedness can be easily corrected with glasses.

Color blindness is another common condition, especially in boys, and it tends to run in families. True color blindness, when everything appears gray, is rare. What most people refer to as color blindness really is an inability to distinguish between reds and greens. There is no treatment for this condition, but it does not interfere greatly with everyday life.

Strabismus is the other common eye problem. If your baby is under 3 months old and one or both eyes seem to wander slightly, there is no need to worry. However, if the problem persists, you should seek medical advice.

Are they serious?
Vision problems can be serious if they go untreated. Eyes need constant exercise and stimulation to keep them healthy, and a disused eye, as occurs in strabismus, will deteriorate rapidly. However, early treatment, generally with glasses, occasionally with an operation, should correct most problems.

What should I do first?

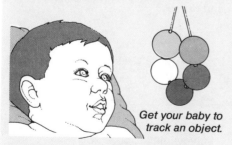

Get your baby to track an object.

1 Although your baby will have regular sight tests, you can check his vision yourself when he's about 3 months old. Dangle a familiar object about 8 inches (20cm) from your baby's face. Move it slowly to one side. Your baby's eyes should track the object.

2 Be on the alert for any changes in the appearance of your child's eyes, such as the development of strabismus.

3 Be responsive to signs that your child cannot see clearly—if, for example, he is always bumping into
Continued on next page ▶

Words in **bold** are A-Z entries

Vision problems

◀ *Continued from previous page*
furniture or is not able to follow the trajectory of a ball that is thrown to him.

4 Get another eye test done if your child does not cooperate with the doctor at a regular checkup and the test is not carried out thoroughly. A child who is unable to do the test may cover up the disability with bad behavior.

Should I consult the doctor?

Consult your doctor if you suspect any defect in your child's vision or notice any change in the appearance of his eyes, if your child complains of sore eyes and rubs his eyes a lot for no apparent reason or if your child's school performance is poor for no obvious reason. Your child may be having difficulty following his teachers because of some vision problem and may be misbehaving or not concentrating during his lessons because of it.

What might the doctor do?

☐ Your doctor will check your child for sharpness of vision. Your child will be asked to read the letters on a card placed 20 feet (6m) away from him. Each eye will be tested separately. A child under 3 years old will be asked to match figures or pictures placed in front of him with the same object held up for him by the doctor.

☐ Your doctor will check the general condition of your child's eyes with an ophthalmoscope to see if there is any internal eye disorder. If treatment is necessary, your child will be referred to an optician or an ophthalmologist. In most cases, suitable glasses will be prescribed and fitted.

What can I do to help?

☐ Get glasses with plastic lenses—they are lighter to wear and don't break as easily.

☐ Keep a spare pair of glasses because children tend to break frames often.

☐ Teach your child how to keep the lenses clean, and encourage him to clean them daily.

☐ Be firm with your child to make sure he wears his glasses as often as the doctor instructs him to, particularly in the early weeks when he is still getting used to them.

☐ Help your child cope with any teasing from his playmates by emphasizing the benefits of being able to see clearly.

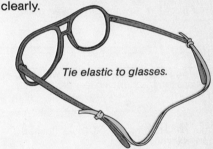

Tie elastic to glasses.

☐ Tie a piece of elastic around the back of your child's glasses so they stay on during active play.

SEE ALSO:
Strabismus, *page 230*

Vomiting

Consult your doctor if vomiting is accompanied by diarrhea or a fever, or if the vomiting is accompanied by any other symptoms, such as earache.

Accompanying symptoms	Common causes
Your baby often spits up a little milk during or after a feeding, but seems contented, eats well and is gaining weight.	This regurgitation of a little milk is normal and harmless.
Your baby is less than 10 weeks old and has more than once vomited forcibly during, or immediately after, a feeding.	He could have **Pyloric stenosis**, *page 205*.
Your baby seems well and hungry but vomits during, or immediately after, his feeding.	Solids given before he can chew properly may be the cause. Until your baby is 6 or 7 months, give him puréed foods only.
Your baby has a runny or blocked nose, congestion or a cough.	A **Common cold**, *page 91*, can make your baby vomit if he swallows a lot of the mucus it produces. A **Cough**, *page 98*, may also make him vomit.
Your bottle-fed baby, seems unwell and has passed frequent, watery stools.	**CONSULT YOUR DOCTOR IMMEDIATELY** Your baby may have **Gastroenteritis**, *page 144*.
Your child seems unwell, looks flushed and feels hot.	An infection is the most likely cause. See **Fever**, *page 138*.
When traveling, your child becomes pale and quiet.	**Motion sickness**, *page 181*, is the most likely cause.
Your child has abdominal pain around the navel and to the lower right side of his groin.	**CONSULT YOUR DOCTOR IMMEDIATELY** Your child could have **Appendicitis**, *page 56*.
Your baby is in severe pain and is passing stools that contain blood and mucus, resembling red jelly.	**CONSULT YOUR DOCTOR IMMEDIATELY** Your baby could have bowel blockage called **Intussusception**, *page 168*.
Your child cannot bend his neck forward without pain and turns away from bright light.	**CONSULT YOUR DOCTOR IMMEDIATELY** Your child may have **Meningitis**, *page 177*.

Words in **bold** are A-Z entries

Vomiting

Vomiting is the violent expulsion of the contents of the stomach through the mouth. A baby may spit up small quantities of curdled milk after a feeding, but this should not be confused with vomiting. Vomiting has many causes (*see page 254*), but in the majority of cases there is little warning; after a single bout your child should be comfortable and back to normal. Vomiting can be a symptom of a specific disorder of the stomach, such as **pyloric stenosis**, or a symptom of an infection, such as an ear infection. It frequently accompanies a **fever**. Even a **common cold** can cause vomiting if your child swallows enough mucus to irritate his stomach. If your child has a bad cough, it may cause him to vomit up food that he has recently eaten. Other causes of vomiting include **appendicitis**, **meningitis**, **food poisoning** and **motion sickness**. Some children vomit because of excitement and anticipation, but this is usually limited to toddlers and they frequently grow out of it.

Is it serious?

Vomiting should always be taken seriously because it can rapidly cause **dehydration**, particularly in a baby or young child.

What should I do first?

1 Put your child to bed, and place a pan for him to vomit into within easy reach.

2 Give your child frequent, small amounts of liquid, preferably cold water, every 10 to 15 minutes.

3 Check your child's temperature to see if he has a fever.

4 Keep your child cool by wiping his face with a cool, damp cloth.

5 Get him to brush his teeth to take away the taste.

Should I consult the doctor?

Consult your doctor immediately if your child continues to vomit over a 6-hour period; if vomiting is accompanied by diarrhea or a fever over 100F (37.5C); or if the vomiting is accompanied by any other worrying symptoms, such as **earache**.

What might the doctor do?

☐ Your doctor will diagnose the cause of the vomiting and treat your child accordingly. He will also make sure there is no danger of your child becoming dehydrated.

☐ Your child may be admitted to the hospital to be given fluids intravenously if he is in danger of becoming dehydrated.

What can I do to help?

☐ Give your child plenty of his favorite drinks, but dilute any fruit juices. Don't give him milk.

☐ Feed your child bland foods when the nausea and vomiting have passed. Reintroduce solid foods slowly.

SEE ALSO:
Appendicitis, *page 56*
Common cold, *page 91*
Dehydration, *page 109*
Earache, *page 124*
Fever, *page 139*
Food poisoning, *page 141*
Meningitis, *page 177*
Motion sickness, *page 181*
Pyloric stenosis, *page 205*

Vulvovaginitis

Vulvovaginitis in girls is an irritation of the vulva, the area around the opening of the vagina. It is fairly common in young girls. The irritation is made worse because the lack of female sex hormones in the vagina of a prepubescent girl means there are no protective acid secretions. When urinating, the acid in the urine may sting the sore, itchy skin. Painful urination can also mean a **urinary-tract infection.**

The condition can be triggered by a number of things: fecel bacteria, introduced into the vagina by wiping from the rectum forward; irritation from bubble baths; poor air circulation from nylon panties; masturbation; sensitivity to the chemicals in laundry detergents or soaps; a threadworm infestation or a foreign body in the vagina.

Possible symptoms

- Sore, red, itchy vulva.
- Foul-smelling, bloody vaginal discharge.
- Pain when urinating.

What should I do first?

1 If there is a smelly vaginal discharge, see if your child has pushed a foreign body into her vagina. Check for a blood-stained discharge on her panties.

2 Give your child a warm sitz bath, and dry the area carefully. You can add 1 cup of white vinegar to the bath water. Have your child open her legs and splash water on her vulva.

3 Apply a barrier cream, such as petroleum jelly, to prevent urine stinging and reduce irritation until you can get to the doctor.

4 Allow your child to wear only cotton panties. Have her sleep without panties.

5 Don't let your child have bubble baths or hang around in a wet bathing suit.

6 If your child is scratching around her anus, check her stools for **worms.**

Should I consult the doctor?

Consult your doctor if your child has irritation of the skin around her vagina and the above-mentioned methods do not alleviate the problem, or if you notice a blood-stained discharge.

What might the doctor do?

□ Your doctor will not give your child a vaginal examination unless there is a possibility of a foreign body. If there is, he may refer you to a surgeon or gynecologist for its removal.

□ Your doctor will prescribe a cream to apply to the vulva to reduce irritation and clear up any skin condition caused by an allergic reaction.

□ If your child has an infestation of worms, your doctor will prescribe medication to kill the worms.

□ Your doctor will ask for a urine specimen to check for infection.

What can I do to help?

□ Teach your child to wipe her bottom from the front backward.

□ Dry the area after bathing. Do *not* use soap in the genital area.

□ Make sure your child has a clean pair of cotton panties each day.

□ No bubble baths.

SEE ALSO:
Urinary-tract infection, *page 250*
Vagina, foreign body in, *page 251*
Worms, *page 261*

Words in **bold** are A-Z entries

Warts

Warts are small, benign lumps caused by the wart virus. They are made up of an excess of dead cells that protrude above the surface of the skin. They can appear singly or in large numbers over all parts of the body, including the face and genitals. If they occur on the soles of the feet, they are called **plantar warts**. It takes about 2 years for the body to build up a resistance to the wart virus. After that time, warts usually disappear spontaneously. Warts are spread by direct contact with an infected person.

Are they serious?
Warts are neither serious nor painful.

Possible symptoms

● Hard lumps of dried skin that appear spontaneously and grow singly or in clusters anywhere on the body.
● Small black dots in the lumps. (These are blood vessels, not dirt.)

What should I do first?

1 Try ignoring the warts. They will go away on their own.

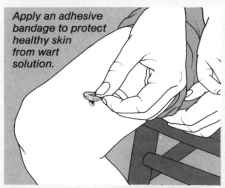
Apply an adhesive bandage to protect healthy skin from wart solution.

2 If your child wants the warts removed or they appear on a part of the body where they would easily infect other people, try over-the-counter wart cures from the drugstore. These work by the application of a weak acid solution to the wart and the daily removal of the resulting burnt skin. Follow the manufacturer's instructions carefully, and avoid applying the solution to healthy skin. Don't use wart cures on the face or genitals. You may cause scarring.

Should I consult the doctor?

Consult your doctor if you're unsure whether the lumps are warts. Any growth or lump on your child's skin that you're uncertain about should be checked by a doctor. Consult your doctor if the warts continue to multiply or appear on the face or genitals and you want them removed.

What might the doctor do?

☐ Your doctor may advise you to ignore the warts or refer you to a dermatologist. Methods of wart removal include cauterization and surgical removal.

What can I do to help?

☐ Try not to draw attention to your child's warts.

SEE ALSO:
Plantar warts, *page 253.*

257

Wax in the ears

Some wax in the external ear canal is normal. It is produced by glands in the skin of the canal to protect the ear from dust, foreign bodies and infections. Wax appears as golden-brown or rust-colored waxy crumbs. The wax is usually moved along and out of the canal by chewing movements of the jaw, but in some children excess wax is produced. Very occasionally wax may collect, dry and block the ear canal, leading to a temporary reduction in hearing.

Is it serious?
Excess wax is not serious, although it may affect the hearing temporarily until the plug of wax is removed.

Possible symptoms
- Visible buildup of wax in the ear canal.
- Partial deafness.
- Feeling of fullness in the ear or a ringing sound.

What should I do first?

1 Check your child's ears regularly for wax buildup. Dislodge the wax only if it is at the opening of the ear canal and can be lifted out easily. Never poke anything, such as a cotton swab, into the ear canal.

Should I consult the doctor?

Consult your doctor if you cannot remove the wax easily and your child seems to be having trouble hearing.

What might the doctor do?

☐ After examining your child's ears with an otoscope, your doctor may wash his ears with warm water to wash out the wax. This is a painless, though perhaps uncomfortable, procedure.
☐ If the wax is hard and compacted, your doctor may prescribe ear drops to soften and dissolve the wax. You may have to return to have your child's ears washed a few days later if the drops have not dislodged the wax.

What can I do to help?

☐ Insert the ear drops just before your child's bedtime. Lay your child across your lap or on his side on a bed, and drop the required amount into the ear canal. Be sure he lies still for 2 minutes so the drops don't drain out of the ear.
☐ After inserting the ear drops, make an ear plug from cotton, and leave it in your child's ear overnight. The wax may come out with the ear plug in the morning. If it doesn't, you may have to return to the doctor to have the ear washed.
☐ Be on the alert for a possible blockage in the future. The tendency to produce excess wax is inherited, and a blockage may recur.

> **SEE ALSO:**
> **Deafness,** *page 108*

Words in **bold** are A-Z entries

Whooping cough

Whooping cough is one of the most dangerous childhood diseases, especially in babies under 12 months of age. It is caused by the bacterium *bordatella pertussis*, which causes the airways to become clogged with mucus.

Whooping cough begins as an ordinary cold with a cough. The coughing becomes severe, with spasmodic coughing attacks that make it difficult to breathe. When your child does manage to draw breath during a coughing attack (which can last up to a minute), there is a characteristic whooping sound as air is drawn in past the swollen larynx. The breathing difficulties are even greater for babies, who may never develop the technique of whooping to get air into their lungs, an inability that can prove fatal.

Sometimes **vomiting** occurs after a coughing attack. The coughing phase of whooping cough can last up to 10 weeks. The risk of developing a secondary infection, such as **pneumonia** or **bronchitis**, is high after this illness.

There is some controversy surrounding the vaccine for whooping cough. However, doctors believe it is better for your child and for the community if *all* children are vaccinated. A few babies should be placed in a special category and not immunized (for example, those with epilepsy in the family). Ask your doctor's advice.

Possible symptoms

- Cold symptoms of a fever, runny nose, aches and pains.
- Excessive coughing, with a characteristic "whoop" as the child struggles to draw breath.
- Vomiting after a coughing bout.
- Sleeplessness because of the coughing.

Is it serious?

Whooping cough is a serious disease, especially in babies who may become dangerously short of oxygen during a coughing attack. If vomiting is severe, there is also the danger of **dehydration**. A severe attack of whooping cough can damage the lungs and cause recurrent bronchial infections.

What should I do first?

1 If your child's cold fails to improve and his cough worsens, put him to bed. Call your doctor immediately.

2 If you suspect your baby has whooping cough, call your doctor immediately.

3 If you suspect your child has whooping cough, do not send him to school or nursery school until you have seen your doctor.

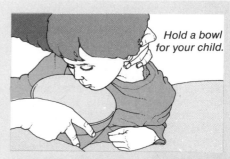

Hold a bowl for your child.

4 If your child is having a long coughing attack, sit him up and hold him so he is leaning slightly forward. Hold a bowl nearby so he can spit up any phlegm into it.

Continued on next page ▶

Whooping cough

◀ Continued from previous page

Should I consult the doctor?

Consult your doctor immediately if you suspect whooping cough.

What might the doctor do?

☐ Your doctor may prescribe antibiotics to reduce the severity of the cough and limit the infectiousness of the child. However, whooping cough is difficult to diagnose during the preliminary stage of the disease. Medication must be taken early to do any good. Your doctor may need to take a throat culture from your baby to diagnose whooping cough because babies rarely whoop.

☐ Your doctor will keep a close check on a baby with whooping cough, and if the disease is severe, he will probably recommend hospital admission to prevent dehydration and to administer oxygen quickly if this should become necessary.

☐ Your doctor will make sure you know how to hold your child during a coughing attack and will show you how if you are unsure. He may advise you to raise the foot of your baby's crib and put your baby to sleep on his stomach.

What can I do to help?

☐ During a coughing attack hold your child as described on the previous page, and keep him calm. Panic will make the breathlessness worse. Hold a bowl under his chin and encourage him to spit the phlegm into it. This helps clear the airways.

☐ If your child vomits after a coughing attack, give him small meals and drinks afterward. This gives him a better chance to keep some food and liquids down and keep his strength up.

☐ Don't let your child play boisterously while he's recuperating. Exertion will bring on a coughing attack quickly and leave him exhausted.

☐ Keep your child away from cigarette smoke.

☐ Sleep in the room with him so he is never alone during a coughing attack.

☐ Don't give your child any cough medicine without your doctor's advice.

☐ After the whooping cough has cleared up, if your child seems unwell and is breathing with difficulty, contact your doctor immediately in case of a secondary infection, such as pneumonia or bronchitis.

☐ Don't worry if your child "whoops" when he catches another cold. This is not a return of the disease; your child is simply repeating a habit learned during all those coughing attacks.

☐ Immunize your other children against whooping cough.

W

> **SEE ALSO:**
> **Bronchitis,** *page 76*
> **Dehydration,** *page 109*
> **Pneumonia,** *page 201*
> **Vomiting,** *page 255*

Words in **bold** are A-Z entries

Worms

There are a number of worms that can live in the human body, but the most common in temperate climates is the pinworm. The worm usually enters the body as an egg in contaminated food. It hatches in the intestine and develops into an adult in 15 to 28 days. The female worms lay more eggs around the host's anus, which causes **itching**, especially at night. If your child scratches himself, he can easily pick up the eggs and start the whole cycle again by putting them into his mouth. Pinworms, which are 1/16 to 1/2 inch (2 to 13mm) long, are harmless, but they can produce unpleasant symptoms, like itching around the anus. Pinworms are highly infectious, and the entire family should be treated simultaneously.

Roundworms are rare but are most likely to infect children in areas where sanitary conditions are poor. They are more common in tropical climates. These parasites are long—4 to 6 inches (10 to 15cm)—and resemble a white earth worm. They are swallowed in contaminated food or drink. After hatching in the intestine, the worms lay eggs that are sometimes excreted in stools. Your child will appear undernourished, and he will fail to thrive.

Are they serious?
Worms are not usually serious and are easily treated.

Possible symptoms

Pinworms
● Itching around the anus, usually at night.

Appearance of worms

● White threadlike worms in the stools.
● Sleeplessness caused by intense itchiness.

Roundworms
● Failure to thrive.

Appearance of worm

● White worms in the stools.

What should I do first?

1 If your child scratches his bottom, inspect the area about an hour after he goes to bed. This is when the adult female usually comes out to lay eggs. The worm will look like a tiny piece of white thread.

2 Inspect your child's stools. If your child has pinworms you should be able to see many worms.

3 If you have recently been traveling in areas where infections of round-worm are common and your child seems unwell and malnourished, inspect his stools for the larger roundworm

Should I consult the doctor?

Consult your doctor if you find any worms. Consult your doctor if you've been in an area where the roundworm is common and your child is not thriving.
Continued on next page ▶

Worms

◀ Continued from previous page

What might the doctor do?

☐ Your doctor will prescribe medication; he may wish to prescribe for the whole family. Inform him if any family member is pregnant.

☐ If your child has roundworms, your doctor will prescribe a drug to be taken by mouth that will paralyze the worm. He will also prescribe a laxative so your child can pass the worm easily in his stools.

What can I do to help?

☐ Carefully follow the instructions for the medication. Bowel movements may be loose for 12 hours afterward, so you may be advised to give the medication early in the morning.

☐ Repeat the dosage for all the family after 2 weeks, as directed. One dose of medication usually kills the worms, but a follow-up dose will kill off any eggs that were not yet hatched when the first dose was taken.

☐ Be meticulous about hygiene. The eggs can be picked up under the fingernails and reingested.

☐ Make sure your child wears pajamas or pants at night so when he scratches, his hands don't come into direct contact with his anus and any eggs that might be there.

W

SEE ALSO:
Failure to thrive, *page 137*
Itching, *page 169*
Toxocara, *page 247*

Words in **bold** are A-Z entries

Safety

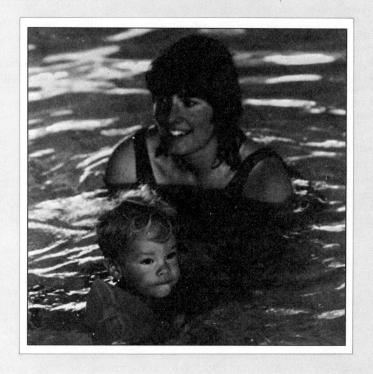

Safety around the home

Most accidents occur at home, and over half happen to children under age 5. Many accidents are preventable, so look around your home to minimize the chances of an accident occuring by altering the layout and position of items in your home and by training your child. Teach your child self-protection from an early age by making him aware of dangers. He won't fully understand your instructions at first, and he'll probably forget them, but with persistence, the message will get through. As your child gets older, he'll begin to understand the logic of your advice and will start to do as you say.

However, when your child is young and can't understand reasoning, there are certain simple, strict rules that should be observed at all times. These rules include never touching electric sockets and never playing with sharp objects.

General safety tips

- Never leave your child alone for long. No matter how busy you are, always check on what your child is doing and know where he is. Be especially cautious at the end of the day when you are tired and possibly preoccupied with other members of the family.
- Check all electrical cords. They are dangerous if frayed or split. Replace any dangerous ones immediately.
- Teach your child that radiators and heaters are hot to the touch. Arrange furniture so the heaters cannot be reached by your child, or use them in areas where they cannot be touched by your child.
- If you keep a gun in the house, *never* leave it loaded. Lock it away, and lock bullets in a separate container. Television has made guns more familiar to children, and a child is now much more likely to use a gun as part of his play.
- When you give your child medicine, make sure you administer the correct dose.
- Make all upper-storey windows safe by fitting bars or safety catches, depending on the style of window. Don't leave any furniture beneath a window—your child may climb up and attempt to open or lean out of the window.
- If you have smooth-tiled or wood floors, use a special polish to make the surface non-slip. Don't let your child run around in stocking feet.
- Fit safety film to large areas of glass that your child could fall against, such as picture windows and patio doors.
- Put safety covers on *all* unused electric sockets throughout the house.
- Keep emergency numbers by the telephone, especially if you are out and your child has a baby sitter.
- When visiting friends who have no children, check the house for possible problems, especially if children don't visit often. Breakable items or sharp objects may have been left in accessible places, and cleaning chemicals may not have been put out of reach. Never be complacent; always presume your child will find trouble if he tries.

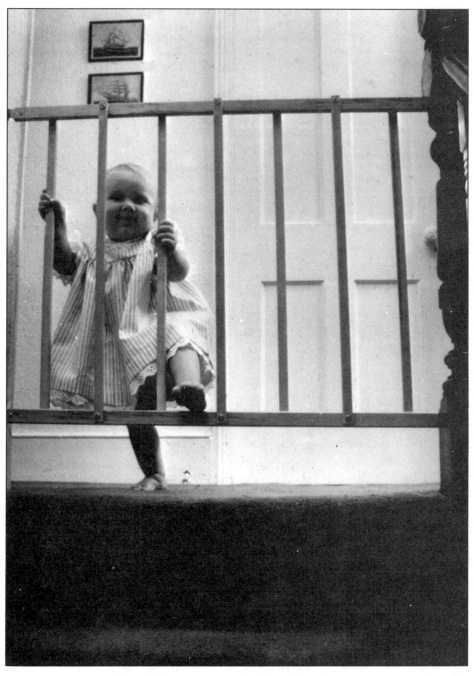

Kitchen

The kitchen may be a focal room for the entire household and is often full of the bustle of the family. It is potentially dangerous for many reasons—from cooking (boiling water and hot fat); from cooking utensils (knives and hot pans) and from the fact that you are preoccupied with food preparation and may not pay full attention to what your child is getting in to.

Point saucepan handles away from the front of the range so your child can't grab the handle and pull the contents down on himself. When possible, use back burners.

Keep your iron in a safe place, out of your child's reach. A wall-mounted iron rest is ideal.

Never leave objects near the edges of work surfaces. Push them well back.

Attach locks or childproof catches to all cupboards and drawers.

Clean out your pet's bowls after use, or keep them out of reach.

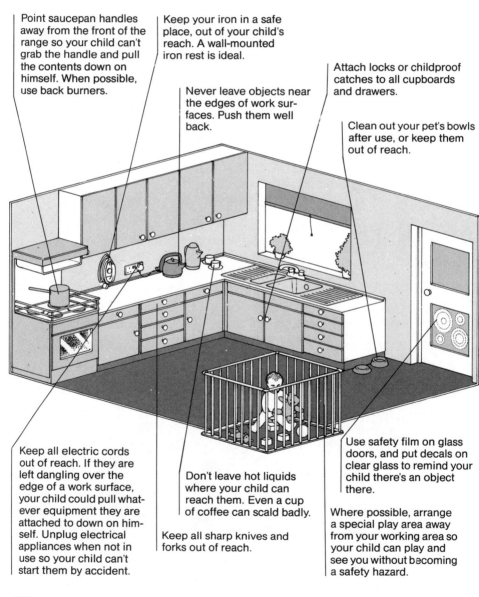

Keep all electric cords out of reach. If they are left dangling over the edge of a work surface, your child could pull whatever equipment they are attached to down on himself. Unplug electrical appliances when not in use so your child can't start them by accident.

Don't leave hot liquids where your child can reach them. Even a cup of coffee can scald badly.

Keep all sharp knives and forks out of reach.

Use safety film on glass doors, and put decals on clear glass to remind your child there's an object there.

Where possible, arrange a special play area away from your working area so your child can play and see you without becoming a safety hazard.

266

Kitchen

Highchairs

Until your child is old enough to sit at the table, a highchair is the most suitable and comfortable way of feeding him. Highchairs are available in a variety of designs, but there are certain safety features you should look for, no matter what style you choose. Choose a chair that is stable,

with widely spaced legs. If the tray is removable, it should have a strong lock or clasp to hold it in position while the chair is being used. There should be special clips at either side for attaching a safety belt; this should always be used when your child is in the highchair. Never leave your child unattended in a highchair.

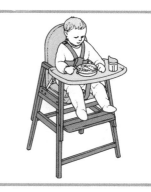

Make sure your floor is non-slip and free of grease. Clean up any spills.

Don't store uncooked meat next to cooked meat—one can contaminate the other. Don't store open cans in the refrigerator. Put the remainder into a clean container.

Gastroenteritis can be a risk for a bottle-fed baby, so clean all equipment carefully. Milk is a favorite breeding ground for bacteria. Never leave prepared formula standing at room temperature. Don't keep the remains of the last feeding for the next.

Secure a swinging or self-closing door when your child is around. He could easily catch his fingers in the door or be knocked over.

Keep a fire extinguisher and fire blanket in the kitchen in case of fire.

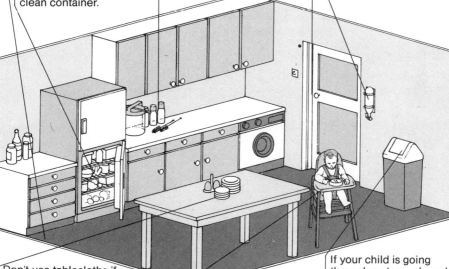

Don't use tablecloths if you have a toddler. Even a crawling baby can pull on a cloth and bring the table's contents down on his head. Keep all items in the center of the table.

Place the highchair out of the way of doors and thoroughfares, well away from work surfaces.

If your child is going through a stage where he digs in the trash, be very careful with sharp-edged cans or broken glass. Always put a can lid inside the can, and squeeze the sides together

Bedroom

An awareness of safety in the bedroom is especially important in the first year of your baby's life because this is probably the room where your child will spend a lot of his time—either sleeping being nursed or being changed.

Buy a crib with rounded edges. If the crib has a movable side rail, make sure it has strong clasps so your child cannot release it and get his fingers caught. Buy a crib with rails spaced no farther than 2⅜ inches apart; This is a federal regulation. It will decrease the risk of your baby's head becoming trapped.

Don't leave open electric or gas heaters in your child's room when he's asleep or unattended.

Have your baby's changing equipment close to the changing table but never above it, in case something falls on the baby. Never leave your baby alone on the table because he could roll off.

Use wall-mounted or ceiling lights to avoid trailing cords.

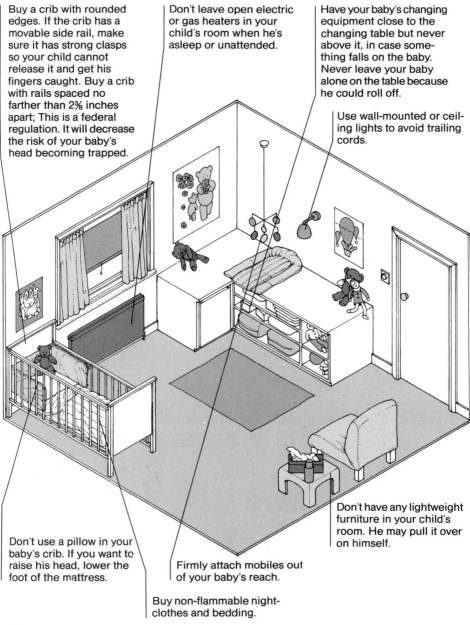

Don't use a pillow in your baby's crib. If you want to raise his head, lower the foot of the mattress.

Firmly attach mobiles out of your baby's reach.

Buy non-flammable night-clothes and bedding.

Don't have any lightweight furniture in your child's room. He may pull it over on himself.

Bathroom

Your child is at risk from falls, poisoning and electrocution in the bathroom. Be sure no one touches *any* plugged-in electrical appliances while they are wet or if their hands are wet. Only wall-mounted heaters should be used, and these should be positioned high, out of reach. Portable electric heaters should *never* be taken into the bathroom. Never leave a child under age 3 alone in the bath; he could drown.

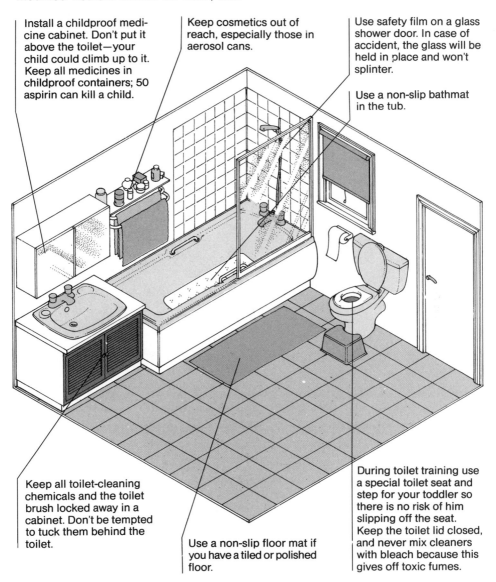

Install a childproof medicine cabinet. Don't put it above the toilet—your child could climb up to it. Keep all medicines in childproof containers; 50 aspirin can kill a child.

Keep cosmetics out of reach, especially those in aerosol cans.

Use safety film on a glass shower door. In case of accident, the glass will be held in place and won't splinter.

Use a non-slip bathmat in the tub.

Keep all toilet-cleaning chemicals and the toilet brush locked away in a cabinet. Don't be tempted to tuck them behind the toilet.

Use a non-slip floor mat if you have a tiled or polished floor.

During toilet training use a special toilet seat and step for your toddler so there is no risk of him slipping off the seat. Keep the toilet lid closed, and never mix cleaners with bleach because this gives off toxic fumes.

Living room

Much day-to-day living goes on in the living room or den, as well as the kitchen. One of the problems for parents trying to childproof these areas is how to make it safe for their child and how to preserve valuable and much-loved objects. It may be easier to keep breakables out of reach, but, with time, repeated warnings should work.

If you have an open fire, always use a screen when the fire is lit to prevent your child from falling into the flames.

Keep the television turned so the back cannot be touched. It's also advisable to keep any recording, video or stereo equipment out of reach.

Make sure carpets and rugs are in good condition, with no holes or turned up edges that could trip your child.

Keep all breakable items out of reach.

Use safety film on picture windows or patio doors

Don't leave anything belonging to your child above the fireplace or on a window sill. He may try to climb up to get at it.

Make sure none of your houseplants is poisonous.

Don't leave hot drinks, alcohol, cigarettes, matches or lighters where your child can get them. Don't place heavy objects on low tables.

Pin electric cords along the floor, and position long cords where they cannot be tripped over or played with by putting them behind furniture or under carpets.

If you have sharp-edged table tops and there is a risk that your child could run into them, fit edges with plastic safety corners.

Hall and stairs

The two major dangers in halls and stairways are the stairs and the possibility your child could run out the front door, into the street. Until your child has the balance to come down a step at a time holding onto the banister, train him to come down the stairs on his bottom. Always stop him from going outside unless he is accompanied by you.

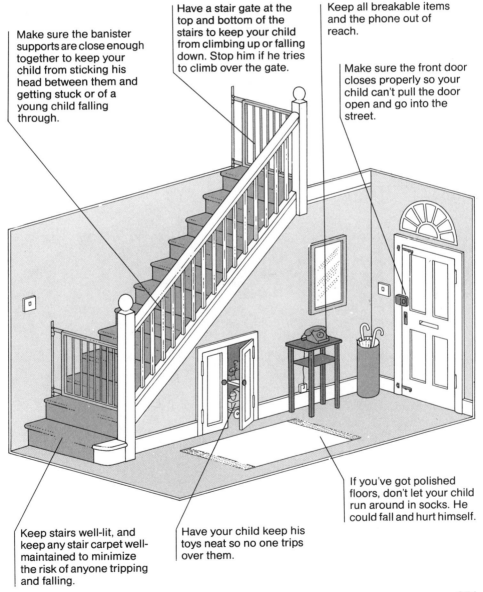

Have a stair gate at the top and bottom of the stairs to keep your child from climbing up or falling down. Stop him if he tries to climb over the gate.

Keep all breakable items and the phone out of reach.

Make sure the banister supports are close enough together to keep your child from sticking his head between them and getting stuck or of a young child falling through.

Make sure the front door closes properly so your child can't pull the door open and go into the street.

Keep stairs well-lit, and keep any stair carpet well-maintained to minimize the risk of anyone tripping and falling.

Have your child keep his toys neat so no one trips over them.

If you've got polished floors, don't let your child run around in socks. He could fall and hurt himself.

The yard

The yard can be a dangerous place for a child because it may provide the means of escape onto roads and because of the machinery used to maintain it. There is the added danger, especially for toddlers, that some plants are poisonous but look like candy. Although rarely fatal if eaten, they can produce unpleasant effects, ranging from skin to stomach irritation. Never let your child play unattended— keep him away from sharp or prickly plants like roses and cactuses, and don't let him play in dirt. It may be contaminated with chemicals or have bits of glass and animal dirt in it. If you have an area in the yard where you keep your car, make sure you know *exactly* where your child is before you start up the engine and drive away.

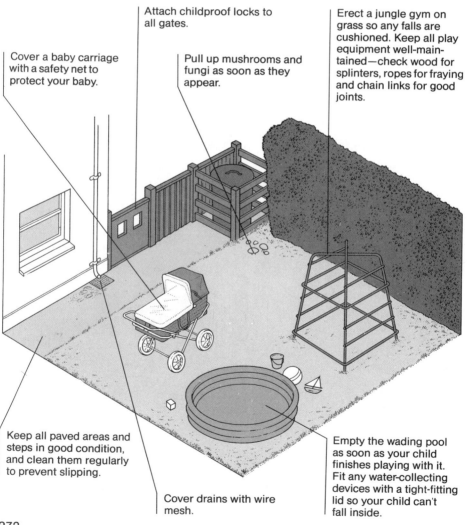

Attach childproof locks to all gates.

Cover a baby carriage with a safety net to protect your baby.

Pull up mushrooms and fungi as soon as they appear.

Erect a jungle gym on grass so any falls are cushioned. Keep all play equipment well-maintained—check wood for splinters, ropes for fraying and chain links for good joints.

Keep all paved areas and steps in good condition, and clean them regularly to prevent slipping.

Cover drains with wire mesh.

Empty the wading pool as soon as your child finishes playing with it. Fit any water-collecting devices with a tight-fitting lid so your child can't fall inside.

The yard

Poisonous plants

Skin irritation
Bleeding heart
Poison ivy
Poison oak
Poison sumac
Christmas rose
Foxglove

Mouth and throat irritation
Daphne

Jack-in-the-pulpit
Buttercups
White bryony

Stomach irritation
Daphne
Ivy
Wisteria
Belladonna lily
Christmas rose
Daffodil

Hyacinth
Iris
Sweetpea

General poisoning
Rhododendron
Crocus
Hydrangea
Oleander
Lily of the valley
Laburnum

Keep all chemicals in a locked room or shed, and never put any poisonous substances into unmarked containers.

Make sure staked plants have sticks that are at least 4 feet high. Put a plastic container over the top of them to make them obvious and to avoid accidents.

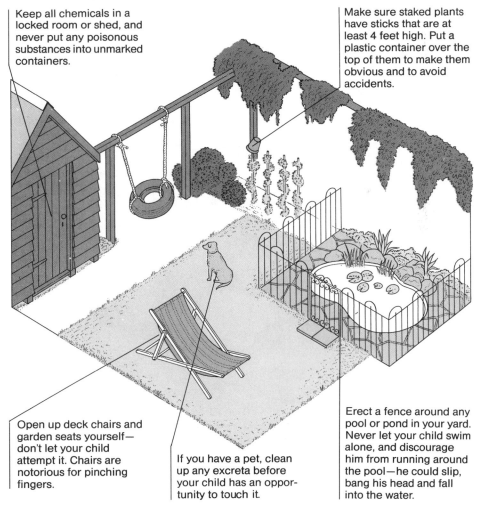

Open up deck chairs and garden seats yourself— don't let your child attempt it. Chairs are notorious for pinching fingers.

If you have a pet, clean up any excreta before your child has an opportunity to touch it.

Erect a fence around any pool or pond in your yard. Never let your child swim alone, and discourage him from running around the pool—he could slip, bang his head and fall into the water.

273

Road safety

Outside the home, most accident's to children occur on the street. It's important that, from an early age, your child is taught the rules of the road where it's safe to cross, how to judge distances and where to play safely. Road codes may differ slightly between busy city streets and quiet country roads, but wherever you are, talk to your child while walking or driving, and explain what you're doing and why.

Never be complacent about your child's road sense; keep reminding him of the rules. Even up to age 12 children may have difficulty interpreting road safety. They may always regard a pedestrian crossing as safe, even with fast-approaching traffic. They may be distracted and not think before stepping out onto the road. They won't be able to judge the speed of on-coming traffic or may not be able to hear an unseen car.

A safety code

● Teach your child road safety.
● Find a safe place to cross, such as a pedestrian crossing or a light.
● Stop at the curb, look in both directions and listen for traffic.
● If traffic is coming, let it pass.
● Look in both directions again and, when no traffic is coming, walk across the road. Keep looking and listening while you cross.

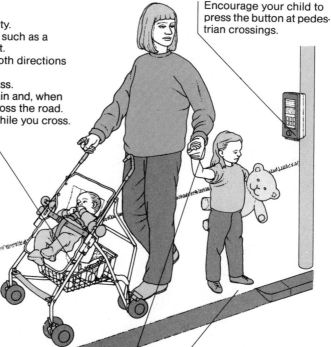

Encourage your child to press the button at pedestrian crossings.

Never push a stroller into traffic without first checking to see if there is traffic coming. Some parents forget the stroller sticks out in front of them by at least 3 feet. Make the curb the safety line, and make it clear to your child that he's not to cross it without holding your hand.

Teach your child to wait at pedestrian crossings until the traffic stops for him.

Beware of strangers

At frequent intervals, remind your child of the dangers of talking to strangers, of accepting candy and of taking a ride in a stranger's car. Be sure your child understands what a "stranger" is. Make up your own code word so if you have to send a friend or neighbor to pick up your child, this word can be used.

When crossing with a stroller and an older child, make sure you hold the hand of the walking child. When you know you can trust him not to run away, he can hold onto the side of the stroller.

Road safety

Points to remember

Never allow your child to play or cycle on the sidewalk near a busy street. Unless you live on a very quiet road with few parked cars, don't let your child play in the street. Instead, encourage him to play in a yard or park.

Never let your child play on the sidewalk near a blind curb.

Stress to your child that he must never chase a ball, pet or friend out into the road without stopping to look and listen.

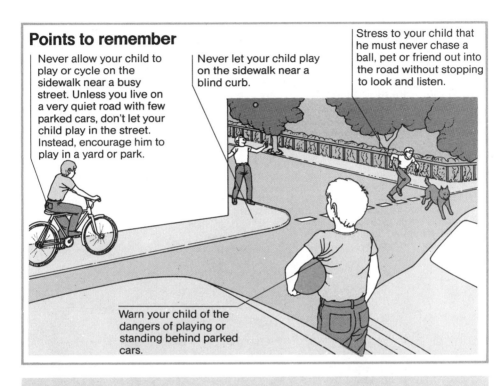

Warn your child of the dangers of playing or standing behind parked cars.

Stroller safety

When you go out with a stroller, never put heavy shopping bags over the handles—they could easily tip the stroller backward. Instead, buy a stroller with a basket underneath it. When you park a stroller, put on the brakes, but also point the stroller so it won't roll into the road. Never leave a child unattended in a stroller, and never tie a dog to the stroller.

If the stroller is collapsible, make sure it has a safety lock to prevent it from collapsing suddenly.

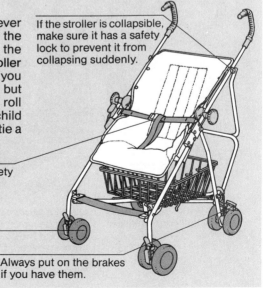

There should be a safety strap so you can strap your child in.

Make sure the stroller is stable, with a base wide enough and sturdy enough so it doesn't tip over easily.

Always put on the brakes if you have them.

Car safety

The safety laws for children traveling in cars differ from state to state, but whatever they are, never allow a child to travel without wearing a seat belt. Parents should also wear seat belts. Children are often more vulnerable than adults in cars because in a collision, a child who is not secured by a belt or in a special seat will be thrown forcefully against the seat or passengers in front or through the windshield. Apart from this basic feature of car safety, there are certain rules that you should observe to make traveling with your child as safe as possible. These are discussed below. Even after you have stopped the car, you should be vigilant—for example, never leave your child unattended, even briefly.

Be careful when closing car doors. Children often leave their fingers in the way, and if you've already locked the door, the effort to release trapped fingers will be even more frantic.

Teach your child to get out of the car on the sidewalk side. Never open the door on the traffic side, even on the quietest street.

When you're driving, never turn around to talk to your child. Keep your eyes on the road.

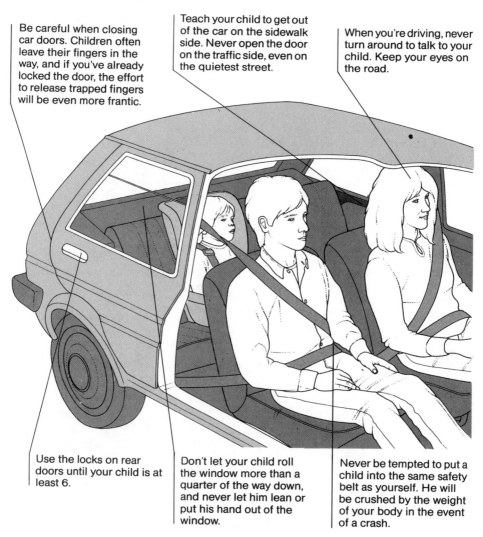

Use the locks on rear doors until your child is at least 6.

Don't let your child roll the window more than a quarter of the way down, and never let him lean or put his hand out of the window.

Never be tempted to put a child into the same safety belt as yourself. He will be crushed by the weight of your body in the event of a crash.

Car safety

If your child is under age 4 or weighs less than 40 pounds (18kg), a regular seat belt is not the correct device for him. His pelvic bones are not sufficiently developed to protect the internal organs from the pressure of the belt in case of a crash. Your child should be restrained in a special car seat or safety harness. Whatever design you select, make sure it is federally approved, and be sure you have it properly installed before use.

A baby in an infant seat should be put in a *car* seat with restraining straps, and straps should be bolted to the car frame or secured by the seat belt. Car seats may also need to be bolted to the frame. Check manufacturer's instructions. When your child outgrows his infant car seat, he can be strapped in with a safety harness and raised on a booster seat to see out of the window.

Safety for babies
Until your baby is old enough to sit up and support his own weight, he will have to travel in a special near-facing baby seat that is buckled into an adult safety belt. It faces backward so in an accident, any force is exerted against the baby's back, not his pelvis.

Safety for older babies and toddlers
Once your child can support his head and can sit well on his own, he can sit in a forward-facing seat. Some infant car seats can be converted to forward-facing car seats. As he gets older, you

may choose a safety harness and booster seat arrangement. These come in several styles and sizes. It's important to find the one that best suits your child by shopping around and trying your child out in the ones available.

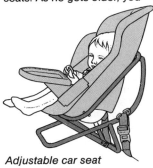

Adjustable car seat

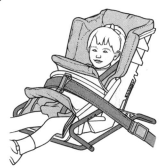

Car seat with protective shield

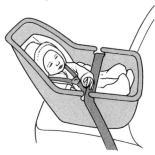

Rear-facing car seat

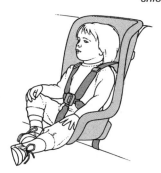

Molded car seat

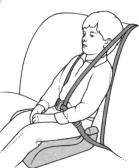

Booster seat with safety harness

Toys and play equipment

Although there are now strict rules governing safe production of toys and the awareness of manufacturers is greatly improving, every year children are hurt and even killed by toys they play with. When buying toys or equipment for your child, try to buy those approved by the Consumer Product Safety Commission (this may be indicated on the item). If in doubt, contact a local consumer association.

Any household is potentially dangerous for a child because there is so much to explore—a couple of minutes away from your child and he could find that shirt button you lost, swallow it and choke. *Never* give your young child anything to play with that is so small that he might swallow it by accident or push it up his nose or in his ear. Make sure there are no sharp edges or projections on any toys. Avoid those made of thin, rigid plastic. On soft toys and animals, be sure eyes and nose, bells and ribbons are well-secured and cannot be pulled off. Toys are often marked suitable for a certain age—follow these guidelines, and always supervise your child while he's playing if he's under 1.

Toys and objects
Examine toys carefully *before* you buy or give them to your child. Smooth-edged, hand-sized or larger toys, are safest until your child is old enough to know not to put objects into his mouth. Before giving him household objects to play with, check them for cracks, sharp parts and splinters. Don't let your child play with pens or other long objects that he could accidentally poke into his eye.

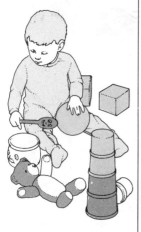

Baby walker
Select a walker with a wide base for stability. Avoid the X-type walker—these collapse easily and can trap fingers. Keep an eye on where your child moves in his walker. If you have any steps or ledges, be sure they are fenced off with a gate. Babies can build up speed in a walker, and if they hit a raised threshold, even a carpet edge, they can tip over or be catapulted out of it.

Baby swing
Make sure your child is secured properly in the swing seat.

Baby swing

Paints and pencils
Always give your child non-toxic, edible paints, pencils and crayons to play with. (For your own peace of mind, use non-spill paint jars.)

Baby walker

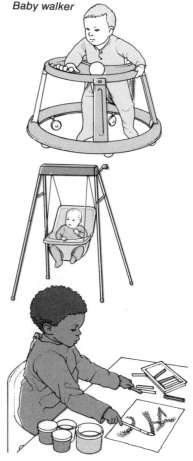

Toys and play equipment

Whatever sport or pastime your child takes up, be sure he is properly equipped for it and he is taught basic rules for safety. For example, if he's skateboarding or BMX bike-riding, make sure he goes to any specially set-up areas rather than on the road and that he wears as much protective equipment as necessary. For example, get him to wear the helmet, knee pads and gloves that are necessary. Almost every child learns to swim and ride a bike, and safety tips for these pastimes are given below.

Bicycle safety

Children under 10 should only ride their bikes in the yard, parks or special areas. They should *never* ride on the road, not even when crossing it. They shouldn't be allowed to ride on the sidewalk because they are a hazard to pedestrians, especially when going around corners. When you buy your child's first bike, buy one with training wheels. This allows him to gain confidence and general bike sense without having to worry about falling off.

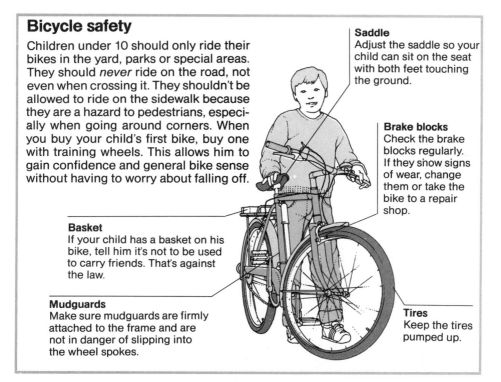

Saddle
Adjust the saddle so your child can sit on the seat with both feet touching the ground.

Brake blocks
Check the brake blocks regularly. If they show signs of wear, change them or take the bike to a repair shop.

Basket
If your child has a basket on his bike, tell him it's not to be used to carry friends. That's against the law.

Mudguards
Make sure mudguards are firmly attached to the frame and are not in danger of slipping into the wheel spokes.

Tires
Keep the tires pumped up.

Water safety

The most important element in water safety is your child's ability to swim. Ask at your local swimming pool about mother and baby groups. Take your child to the nearest pool as often as possible to get him accustomed to the water and to encourage him to learn to swim. Never let your child play in or near water without supervision. When you are at the beach, heed local advice about swimming conditions. Never swim when you are advised not to, no matter how competent family members are at swimming. At the beach always keep a close eye on your child, no matter how old he is, and don't let your child play alone with a raft. It's very easy for the currents or wind to pull your child out from the shore. Children get cold quickly so keep swimming times short.

Playgrounds

All children get bored playing in their own or a friend's yard. If there's a playground in your area, children are bound to want to visit it, especially if it has a lot of equipment. Try to help your child to understand his limitations and be cautious. The bravado that comes from being with friends who act like daredevils can easily lead to accidents. Playgrounds may have special areas for younger children and toddlers. Keep young children in these areas because older children play more roughly. Be sure you accompany your child to the playground. Warn older children to be wary of strangers at a park or playground.

Check that merry-go-rounds have smooth surfaces and move around easily. Tell your child never to put his feet underneath the merry-go-round.

Make sure your child has non-slip soles on his shoes and that he is wearing sturdy jeans.

Jungle gyms should be built on grass or sand to break falls, and they should be completely stable.

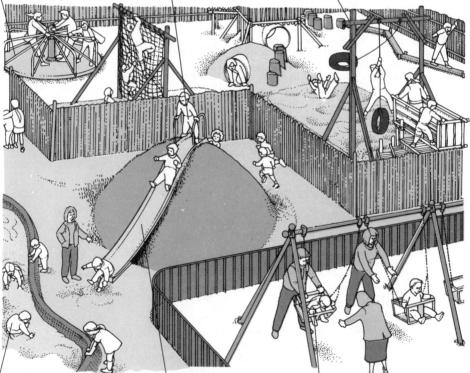

Discourage your child from throwing sand in the sandpit. Sand can scratch the surface of the eye and cause an injury. Make sure the sandpit is too shallow for your child to bury himself.

Slides should be no higher than 8 feet, probably on an earth mound so any fall is broken. The slide should be of a smooth, continuous piece, not jointed panels.

Swings should be surrounded by a fence to keep children from running in front of, or behind, them and being knocked over. Until your child can hold on properly, always use the box-type swing.

First aid

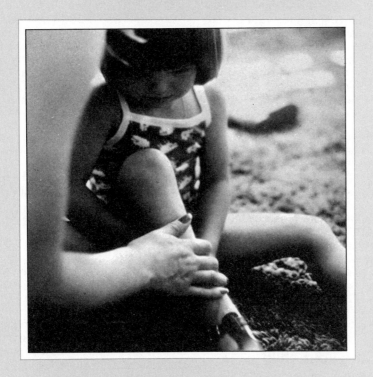

Dealing with an accident

Children are prone to accidents because they are naturally inquisitive and often unaware of danger. Although most accidents are relatively minor, it is important that you are familiar with life-saving first-aid techniques so you know what to do in case of a serious accident. Knowing the right way to deal with the situation will enable you to act quickly and efficiently and help you stay calm. The calmer you are, the more you can comfort your child and the more you will be able to help him.

On pages 290 to 300, I have described the immediate action and treatment for several emergencies, such as choking, unconsciousness, electric shock, serious bleeding, shock, drowning and burns. Other injuries are covered in the A-Z section beginning on page 52.

Priorities

Whatever injury your child has sustained, if he is unconscious do the following:

1 Make sure he is breathing (*see opposite and page 284*). If he is not, begin mouth-to-mouth resuscitation (*see page 286*) before you take care of any other injury.
Note: *If your child is breathing, his heart will also be beating.*

2 Stop any severe bleeding (*see page 292*).

3 After steps 1 and 2 have been dealt with, treat any other injuries.

Examining your child

1 If your child is unconscious, but breathing, and his injury is not immediately obvious, examine him carefully from head to foot. Keep his head tilted back to keep his airway open (*see opposite page*). If possible, get someone else to support his head while you examine him.

2 Compare one side of his body to the other side or one limb to the other. Move him as little as possible. Slide your hand under his back or his head to make sure there is no sign of bleeding. Treat any injury you find.

Multiple injuries

Your child may have suffered several injuries, and the treatment of one may interfere with the treatment of another. If this is the case, treat the injury you consider the most serious, then treat the others as correctly as you can.

Calling for help

Your child will need to be taken to the nearest emergency room following any accident resulting in unconsciousness, difficulty in breathing or other injuries, such as bleeding, broken bones or burns. Always call an ambulance if your child needs a stretcher or if you are on your own and first aid needs to be continued on the way to the hospital. However, if there is another adult available who can drive you to the hospital, it may be faster if you sit in the back of the car with your child and continue first aid.

Many communities have a special emergency number (911). Dial this number instead of the operator or an ambulance company.

Resuscitation

Everyone needs a constant supply of oxygen to survive—permanent brain damage can result after only 3 minutes without oxygen. If your child is unconscious and not breathing, you may be able to save his life by taking over his breathing and blood circulation. Cardiopulmonary resuscitation (CPR) is the term used to describe the techniques used to revive someone who is unconscious and not breathing. These techniques include: opening the airway (*see below*), breathing for your child (*mouth-to-mouth resuscitation*, see page 286) and circulating his blood (*external chest compression, see page 288*).

It is *always* worth starting cardiopulmonary resuscitation; keep going until a doctor arrives or your child starts to breathe again on his own.

OPENING THE AIRWAY

The airway consists of the passages between your child's mouth and nose and his lungs. If your child is unconscious, particularly if he is lying face upward, breathing may be difficult. Air may not be able to get through to his lungs because: the tongue has fallen back and blocked the windpipe; the head has tilted forward, narrowing the top of the windpipe; fluid or vomit has collected at the back of the throat and is unable to drain.

> **IMPORTANT**
> **Keep your fingers and hand away from the soft tissues under your child's chin and along his neck.**

What should I do?

1 Lay your child on a firm surface. Place one hand on the child's forehead and one hand under the back of his neck. Press very gently on the forehead, and tilt the head back. It is in the right position when you can see straight down his nostrils.

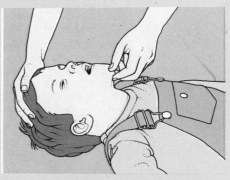

2 Place two fingers of one hand on your child's chin, and lift his jaw up so his chin juts forward. The tongue will come forward with the jaw, thus opening the airway. Check breathing (*see following page*).

Opening the airway for babies and small children

Babies have very short necks and soft windpipes, and if you tilt the head back too far, you can easily block the airway.

1 Lay your child on a firm surface. Place one hand on the child's forehead, and press very gently to tilt his head slightly.

2 Support the jaw by placing two fingers of the other hand on the *bony* part of the chin. Check breathing (*see following page*).

> **IMPORTANT**
> **I urge all parents to take a cardiopulmonary (CPR) course through the Red Cross or American Heart Association. This will prepare you to administer CPR if it is ever needed.**

Resuscitation

CHECKING BREATHING

If your child is unconscious, before you do anything else, make sure he is breathing. Open the airway as described on the previous page, in case the tongue has fallen back and blocked the air passages. Then check his breathing as described below.

What should I do?

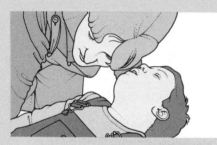

1 With his head tilted back, place your ear as near to his mouth and nose as possible, and look along his chest at the same time.

2 If he is breathing, you will see his chest moving, and you will hear and feel his breath against your face.

3 If he is not breathing, try to clear the airway, as shown at right.

IMPORTANT
If your child is breathing, even slightly, leave him alone. Do not try to give him mouth-to-mouth resuscitation to try to increase the breathing rate. Just put him in the recovery position, and keep checking his breathing.

CLEARING THE AIRWAY

If your child is not breathing after you have tilted his head back, take a look inside his mouth to see if there is something blocking the airway.

What should I do?

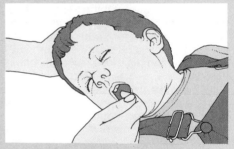

1 Turn your child's head to one side. Quickly, but carefully, run your index finger around the inside of his mouth. Remove anything you find.

2 Be very careful not to push anything farther down his throat. If you think your child has choked on something, *see page 294.*

3 Check your child's breathing again (*see left*).

IMPORTANT
With a young baby, don't put your finger in his mouth unless you can see the foreign body clearly and you are sure there is no risk of pushing it down his throat. It's better to hold him upside down and slap his back (*see page 294*).

What should I do next?

● If your child is now breathing, place him in the recovery position (*see opposite*). Remember, if he is breathing, his heart will be beating.

● If your child is still not breathing, immediately begin mouth-to-mouth resuscitation (*see page 286*).

Resuscitation

THE RECOVERY POSITION

If your child is unconscious but breathing, place him in this position while you are waiting for an ambulance. It keeps your child's tongue forward and allows any fluid or vomit to drain from his mouth, allowing him to breathe without choking. Immobilize any broken bones (*see page 73*) before turning him.

The method shown below assumes your child is lying on his back. If he is lying on his side or his front, you may only need to move his head back and move his uppermost leg and arm up, as shown in the last step, to keep him from rolling onto his face.

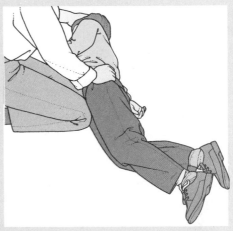

Positioning your child

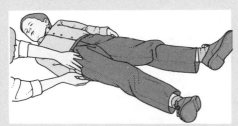

1 Turn your child's head toward you and tilt it back slightly to open the airway. Place the arm nearest you by his side and, keeping his fingers flat, slide his hand under his buttock.

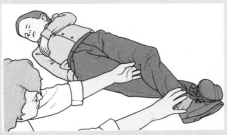

2 Lay your child's other arm across his chest, and bring his farther leg across the near one at the ankle.

3 Kneel beside your child, level with his chest. Grab his clothing at the hip; while supporting his head with the other hand, pull him toward you until he is resting against your knees. Readjust the position of his head to make sure it is back and he can breathe easily.

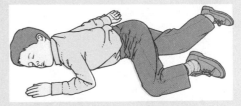

4 Bend the upper arm and leg up to support the child and keep him from rolling onto his face. Make sure that your child's other arm is free. Leave it lying parallel to his back to keep him from rolling onto his back.

IMPORTANT
Never leave an unconscious child alone, even when he has been placed in the recovery position. Try to get someone else to call an ambulance while you stay with him.

Resuscitation

MOUTH-TO-MOUTH RESUSCITATION

This is the resuscitation technique to use if you find your child unconscious with no signs of breathing (*see pages 283-84*). Start this wherever you find your child. If he is in the water, start mouth-to-mouth resuscitation there. If for any reason you can't put your mouth over your child's mouth, close off his mouth and breathe into his nose. If he is very small, it may be easier to place your mouth over his mouth and nose together (*see opposite*).

What should I do?

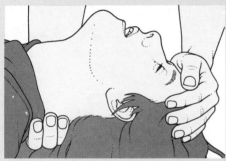

1 Tilt your child's head back to open the airway. If necessary clear the airway (*see pages 283-84*).

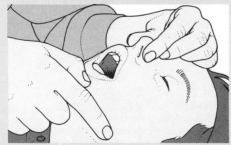

2 Support your child's jaw with one hand. Be careful not to rest your hand on his neck because you can close

off the windpipe. Pinch your child's nostrils shut with two fingers of the other hand.

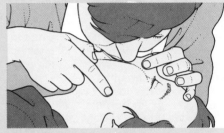

3 Take a deep breath. Open your mouth wide, and seal your lips around your child's mouth.

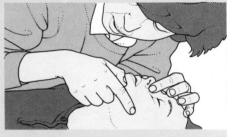

4 Breathe gently, but firmly, into his mouth. Blow from your lungs, not just your mouth, until you see his chest rise. Look along your child's chest—you should see the chest fall again if you have been successful.

IMPORTANT
If your child's chest has not risen, check to see if:
1. The head is in the correct position (*see page 283*). You should be able to see straight down his nostrils.
2. You are pinching the nostrils shut and your mouth is forming an air-tight seal around his mouth.
3. Try again; if you're still unsuccessful, give him back slaps as described for choking (*see page 294*).

Resuscitation

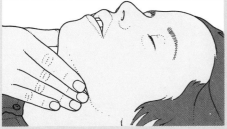

5 Repeat the breathing procedure 3 more times, as quickly as possible. Wait for the chest to fall between each breath. Then check your child's heartbeat (*see following page*).

6 If your child's heart is beating, continue rescue breathing at a rate of 15 to 20 breaths per minute until he can breathe by himself. As soon as he is breathing on his own, place him in the recovery position (*see page 285*) while you wait for the ambulance.

7 If your child's heart is not beating, START EXTERNAL CHEST COMPRESSION NOW (*see page 288*).

Mouth-to-mouth for babies and small children

Although the basic breathing techniques are the same, you have to take the baby's smaller size into account when giving mouth-to-mouth resuscitation. The gap between the nose and mouth is small, so you may find it easier to place your mouth over his mouth and nose together. You'll only have to breathe a small amount of air into his lungs, at a slightly faster rate of 20 breaths per minute; don't breathe too hard.

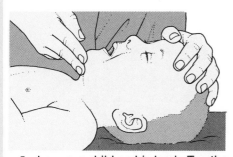

1 Lay your child on his back. Tap the soles of his feet to make sure he really is unconscious. If there is no reaction, tilt his head back slightly by pressing on his forehead and support-ing his chin with your fingers (*see page 283*). Do not tilt the head too far.

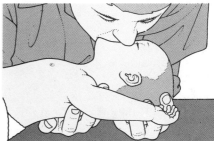

2 Slide one hand under his back to support him and keep his head back. Put your mouth over his mouth and nose together. Breathe out gently until his chest rises. Repeat 3 more times, as quickly as possible, then check heartbeat (*see following page*).

> **IMPORTANT**
> **If you cannot inflate the lungs, check and see if the airway is open. If you still cannot force air in, hold him upside down and give him back slaps (*see page 294*).**

Resuscitation

EXTERNAL CHEST COMPRESSION

This resuscitation technique is used in conjunction with mouth-to-mouth resuscitation when a child is unconscious and not breathing and his heart is not beating after you have started mouth-to-mouth. Chest compression is important because if the heart is not beating, the oxygen you breathe into your child will not get to the body tissues. Permanent brain damage can occur after only *3 minutes* without oxygen.

Checking for the heartbeat

To find out whether your child's heart is beating, check the pulse in the carotid arteries—the arteries that supply blood to the brain.

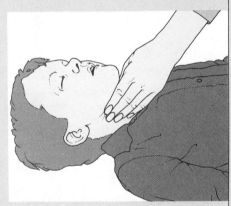

1 Find the front of your child's windpipe (*see page 18*), and slide the pads of three fingers across into the groove between it and the large muscle in the neck, just below the jaw and in line with the ear lobe. Don't use your fingertips because they have a pulse of their own.

2 Feel for about 5 seconds. If you can't feel anything, the heart has stopped beating.

What should I do?

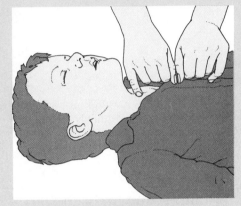

1 If your child's heart has stopped beating, lay him on a hard surface, and kneel beside him facing his chest. Find his breastbone (the bone that runs down the center of his chest, *see page 13*). Feel for the top in the groove between the two collarbones at the top of your child's chest, then find the center of the breastbone by measuring as shown.

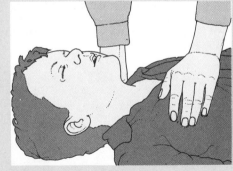

2 Place the heel of one hand over the lower half of the child's breastbone. Keep your fingers off his ribs. Position yourself so your shoulders are directly over the child's breastbone. Depress it 1 to 1½ inches (2.5 to 3.5 cm), then release the pressure.

Resuscitation

3 Complete 5 compressions at a rate of about 80 to 100 compressions per minute (count "1-and-2-and-" as you go). Then stop and give your child one breath of mouth-to-mouth resuscitation (*see page 286*).

IMPORTANT
It is important to follow these instructions very carefully because if you press too hard, you could crush your child's chest.

---

4 Continue giving 5 compressions followed by one breath of mouth-to-mouth for about a minute, then stop and check the carotid pulse again.

5 If the heart is still not beating, continue giving him 5 compressions followed by one breath of mouth-to-mouth, but stop to check the pulse at least every 3 minutes.

6 As soon as you can feel a pulse again STOP PUMPING. Continue giving your child mouth-to-mouth until the ambulance arrives or he starts breathing again.

External chest compression for babies and small children

The sequence of steps for giving chest compression to babies and small children under age 2 is the same as for large children, but you must use less pressure.

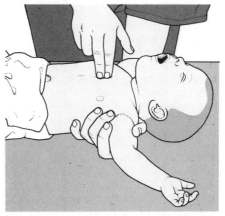

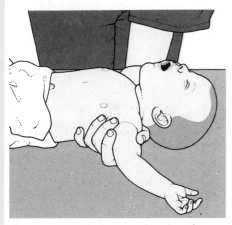

1 Lay your baby on a hard surface, such as a table, and support the head and back by placing one hand under his back and grasping the top of his arm.

2 Imagine a straight line across the child's chest between his nipples and place two fingers of the other hand on the center of the line. Depress the breastbone ½ to 1 inch (1.5 to 2.5 cm), then release the pressure.

3 If your baby is too large for you to depress the breastbone easily with your fingers, don't put your hand under his back. Use the heel of one hand to depress the breastbone.

4 Give 5 compressions to one breath of mouth-to-mouth, the same as for large children. Check the pulse after 1 minute and again every 3 minutes.

Dealing with unconsciousness

The danger of unconsciousness is that the normal reflexes, such as coughing that prevents a child choking while he is asleep, do not work properly or do not even work at all.

Head injury (*see page 151*), shock (*see page 293*), electric shock (*see page 298*), choking (*see page 294*), convulsions (*see page 96*) and diabetes (*see page 111*) can all result in unconsciousness.

If your child regains consciousness or has been unconscious only for a very short time, he must still be seen by a doctor, even if he appears to be all right.

Levels of unconsciousness

Your child may pass through various stages of unconsciousness before becoming completely unconscious. The same will apply as he regains consciousness. At first he may appear very confused. He may then lapse into a stupor, when he will behave as if he is drunk, and then a coma, when he will become completely unconscious. Because of this, it is essential that you remain with the child at all times. If possible, send another adult to call for an ambulance. Watch your child carefully, and note any changes in his state of awareness. This information may help the doctor decide what treatment to give him later.

What should I do?

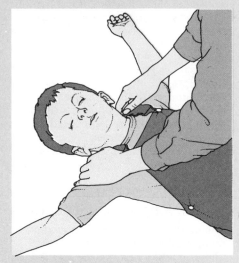

1 Shake your child gently by his shoulders, or pinch his ear lobe. Question him, asking him if he is all right. Give him about 10 seconds to respond.

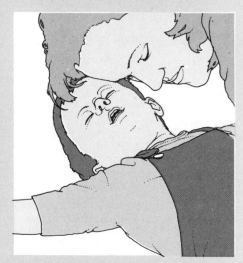

2 If your child does not respond, tilt his head back (*see page 283*), and check to see if he is breathing (*see page 284*).

Dealing with unconsciousness

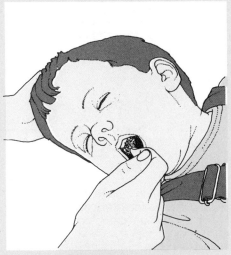

3 If he is breathing but is making snoring or gurgling sounds, there may be something blocking the airway. Clear the airway (*see page 284*).

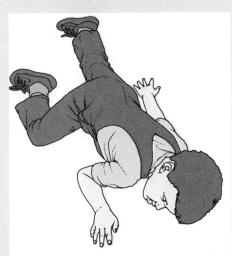

4 If he is breathing, keep his head tilted, and examine him from head to foot. Turn him into the recovery position (*see page 285*). If there is any fluid coming from your child's ear, position him so he is lying on the affected ear and it can drain away.

Place a pad or a clean rag under the ear.

5 If your child is still not breathing, start mouth-to-mouth resuscitation (*see page 286*) and external chest compression, if necessary (*see page 288*).

IMPORTANT
Any child who has been unconscious must be seen by a doctor. Do not give a child who has been unconscious anything to eat or drink before he is seen by a doctor.

Dealing with an unconscious baby

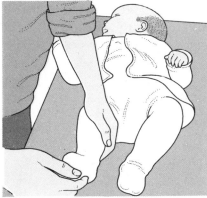

The procedure for treating an unconscious baby is the same as for an older child, except you should tap his feet to establish whether he is unconscious. He is unconscious if there is no response.

When opening the airway, don't tilt a baby's head back as far as for an older child. Blow gently into the mouth when giving mouth-to-mouth. Apply only gentle pressure when giving external chest compression (*see page 288*).

Dealing with bleeding

Bleeding happens when any of the vessels that carry blood around the body are cut or torn. It can be external and visible or internal and not visible (*see opposite*). Serious bleeding should be treated as an emergency because if too much blood is lost from the child's circulatory system, there will not be enough left to supply the body cells with oxygen. Shock can result (*see opposite*). Treat the child as described below, and constantly reassure him.

What should I do for minor injuries?

Most small cuts and scrapes can easily be dealt with at home. Apply pressure if necessary to stop bleeding. Hold the affected area under running cold water, wash, then protect the injury with an adhesive bandage (*see page 104*).

What should I do for severe bleeding?

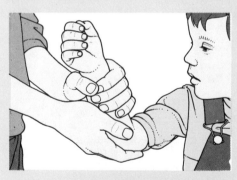

1 As soon as you see your child is injured, apply pressure directly on the wound to compress the ends of the damaged blood vessels. At the same time, raise the affected area above the level of his chest (heart). This slows down the flow of blood to the injured area by making it flow uphill and keeps the vital organs supplied with blood.

2 If your child is not already lying down, help him lie down. Keep the affected area raised, and maintain pressure on the wound.

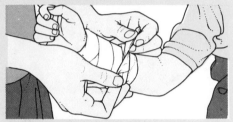

3 If you have a first-aid box near you, place a wound dressing (*see page 35*) or a pad and bandage over the wound. If not, use any clean *non-fluffy* material near at hand, and secure it with a scarf, tie or similar material. Tie the ends in a knot directly over the pad on the wound to maintain pressure.

4 Get your child to the emergency room as soon as possible because he may need stitches. Call an ambulance, or get another adult to drive you there while you sit with your child, continuing first aid if necessary.

Dealing with a foreign body or broken bone

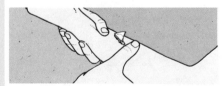

1 If there is something sticking out of your child's wound, do not press directly on it. Raise the affected part, and press the area above and below the object or bone end.

2 Never remove a foreign body from your child's wound because it may be plugging it and preventing bleeding. You may cause more damage by pulling it out.

Dealing with shock

Shock in this context does not mean your child is suffering from fright. Medical shock is a potentially fatal condition that can occur if blood pressure becomes severely lowered after a loss of body fluids, such as blood, or if the heart is not working properly. None of the vital organs can function if they don't get enough blood.

Shock can be caused by serious bleeding, severe burns, electric shock or dehydration following profuse vomiting or diarrhea. Shock can also be caused by a severe reaction to an insect bite, such as a bee sting, or some medicines, when it is called *anaphylactic shock*.

Even if your child is not suffering from any of the symptoms listed below, but he is bleeding or badly burnt, for example, there is a possibility of shock developing. Treat him as described, and get him to the hospital as quickly as possible.

Possible symptoms

If your child is suffering from shock, he may show some or all of the following symptoms:
- Pale, blue/gray skin. (This is particularly noticeable just inside his lips and under his fingernails).
- Rapid, weak pulse.
- Shallow, fast breathing.
- Cold, clammy skin.
- Sweating.
- Dizziness.
- Blurred vision.
- Restlessness.
- Thirst.
- Unconsciousness.

What should I do?

1 Reassure your child. Take care of bleeding, and move him as little as possible.

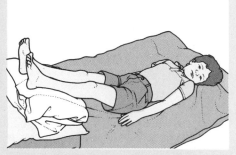

2 Lay him down on a blanket on a flat surface. Raise his legs so they are higher than his chest (heart), and support them on cushions or pillows. Loosen any tight clothing, particularly around his neck, chest and waist, and turn his head to one side.

3 Keep your child comfortably warm. Cover him with a blanket if he is cold, but don't let him get too hot. Never use a hot-water bottle or heating pad to warm him because they cause blood to come to the surface of the body, taking it away from the vital organs.

If your child is unconscious

Turn your child into the recovery position immediately (*see page 285*). Watch his level of consciousness (*see page 290*), and check his breathing rate (*see page 284*) every few minutes until the ambulance arrives or you can get to a doctor.

Internal bleeding

This can happen if, for example, an internal organ is damaged in an accident or a large bone, such as the thigh bone or pelvis, is broken. If your child develops any of the symptoms listed at left, without obvious injury, if he complains of severe pain in the chest or is unusually quiet after an accident, treat as above and get him to the hospital quickly.

Dealing with choking

Small children are liable to choke because they may eat something they cannot chew properly and because they have a habit of putting small objects in their mouths. You must act quickly because, if the object is not removed, breathing could stop.

Possible symptoms

● Coughing.
● Grasping the throat.
● Blueness in the face—the blood vessels in the neck and face may stand out.
● Inability to talk.

What should I do?

1 If your child is coughing, encourage him to keep coughing hard, and do not interfere.

2 If he is not coughing, quickly lay him head-down across your thigh.

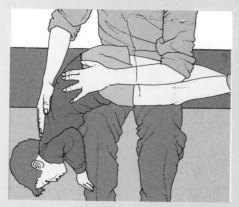

3 Support him so his head is lower than his chest. Give him four slaps on the upper part of his back between his shoulder blades.

4 Continue the back slaps until the object is cleared. Then either hook the object out with your finger—be very careful not to push it back down his throat—or ask your child to spit it out.

Dealing with a choking baby

If your baby is choking on something you must act very quickly.

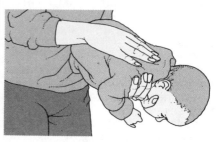

1 Pick him up immediately, and place him face down on your forearm. Support his head and neck.

2 Hold your baby so his head is lower than his chest. Give him quick slaps between his shoulder blades. Continue slapping his back until the blockage is cleared.

3 If you can see the foreign body in his mouth, try to remove it. Never probe his mouth (*see page 284*).

The Heimlich maneuver

The use of the abdominal thrust, called the *Heimlich maneuver*, is controversial in pediatrics. But there are many well-documented reports of its success in individual cases of choking.

To perform, put your arms around the child's stomach. Place your fist with thumb toward the child. Grasp your fist with your other hand between the child's navel and sternum (breastbone). Make sure your hands are not too high or too low. Give four quick thrusts by squeezing and pulling your fist inward and upward into the child's abdomen. Usually the object will fly out. If breathing does not start immediately, begin artificial respiration (*see page 283*).

Dealing with drowning

You can help your child *only* if you are safe. Don't jump into the water if you can throw him a life belt or reach him with your arm or a pole. If your child is not breathing, start mouth-to-mouth resuscitation immediately, even if you're in the water. To do this while dragging a child to safety can be quite difficult. You need to be a strong swimmer.

Very young children can go into a state of "underwater hibernation" and hold their breath for amazingly long periods of time, so never give up mouth-to-mouth resuscitation. Keep going until help arrives. Do not try to drain water from your child's lungs if he is not breathing — he will cough it up when he starts to breathe again.

Water does not have to be deep to drown a child. He can be drowned in only 2 inches (5cm) of water, so never leave a young child unattended when he is outside near water or when he is in the bath. If you have a pool, fence it. If your child is immersed in cold water for any length of time, there is a danger of hypothermia (*see page 300*).

What should I do?

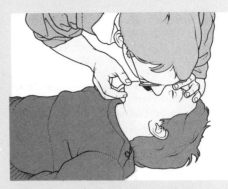

2 *If your child is unconscious,* check to see if he is breathing. If he is not breathing, start mouth-to-mouth resuscitation (*see page 286*) even while he is still in the water. Get him out of the water, and continue mouth-to-mouth until help arrives, even if your child has been submerged for a long time.

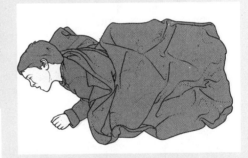

3 If your child is unconscious but breathing, get him out of the water. Place him in the recovery position (*see page 285*), and cover him with anything readily available to keep him warm, but don't take off his wet clothes. Keep checking his breathing and level of consciousness. Be prepared to start mouth-to-mouth if his breathing stops.

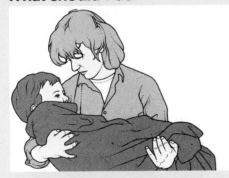

1 *If your child is conscious,* get him out of the water as quickly as possible. Cover him with dry clothing while you get him into the house or the nearest shelter. Replace his wet clothes with dry ones to prevent hypothermia.

4 Wait for the ambulance to arrive. If you know it will take quite awhile to arrive (because of distance or other problems), it may be quicker to go to the nearest emergency room.

Dealing with burns

Severe burns need urgent treatment because of the risk of infection and because of the risk of shock (*see page 293*) following the loss of body fluid.

Burns can be divided into two main types—superficial and deep. *Superficial burns* involve damage to the surface of the skin. *Deep burns* involve the entire thickness of the skin. If more than $\frac{1}{10}$ of the body's surface—an area roughly the size of the child's abdomen—is burned, even superficially, shock will occur.

The most important thing to remember is that only small, superficial burns can safely be treated at home (*see page 79*). If you are in doubt consult the doctor.

IMPORTANT
If burns are extensive or severe, call an ambulance immediately. Treat your child as described for shock, (see page 293) and prevent the burned area from coming into contact with the ground by laying him on a sheet of *non-fluffy* material.

What to do if clothing is on fire

If your child's clothing is on fire, stop him from running around in a panic—this will fan the flames. Get him down on to the floor with the flames on top. Put the flames out as quickly as possible, then treat any burns.

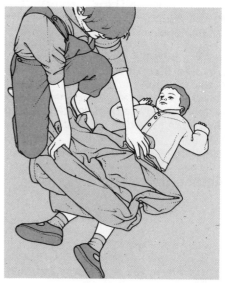

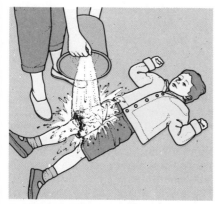

1 If there is a bucket of water nearby, douse the flames with water. Don't use water if the clothes have been set on fire by an electric heater and the child is still near the heater—you will electrocute yourself (*see page 298*).

2 If you have no water, smother the flames by covering your child with a coat or blanket made of a NON-flammable material. A synthetic material will melt, intensifying the burn.

3 As a last resort, lie on top of your child, but be sure you lie right down on top of him. A tunnel of air will develop in the smallest gap and fan the flames, setting your clothes on fire.

4 Rolling your child on the floor also works to smother flames.

Dealing with burns

What should I do?

1 Remove your child from the source of danger. Break any electrical contact if necessary (*see page 298*). Reassure him; burns are very painful, and your child will be frightened.

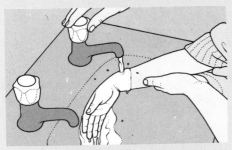

2 Cool the affected area immediately. This stops the heat from damaging your child's skin any more. Hold the affected area under cold running water for as long as the child can stand it—at least 10 to 20 minutes. If a large area is burned, put the child in a cool bath, or cover him with a cold, wet cotton or linen sheet. (It must not be fluffy.)

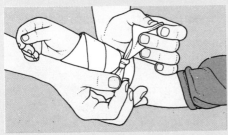

3 Cover the injury with a gauze dressing that is larger than the area of the burn. If you have no suitable dressings in your first-aid box, protect a large burn on a hand or foot by placing a clean plastic bag over it.

4 While you are waiting for the ambulance or are taking your child to the hospital, treat your child, as described on page 293, to prevent shock.

IMPORTANT
1. Never put any fats, ointments or lotions on a burn.
2. Never break a blister caused by a burn.
3. Do not use bandages to cover a burn or cover it with anything fluffy, such as cotton, because it may stick to the injury.
4. Be very careful about immersing very young children in cold water for too long; it can cause hypothermia (*see page 300*).

Dealing with chemical burns

1 Put the affected part under cold running water as quickly as possible and for as long as your child can stand it—about 10 to 20 minutes— to wash the chemicals off. Hold your child so the contaminated water can drain away without touching any other part of his skin or your own.

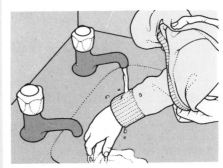

2 While you're washing off the chemicals, very carefully remove any contaminated clothing, then treat as for burns, above.

Dealing with electric shock

Contact with household electricity can cause burns, and the shock from electricity may cause unconsciousness or even stop your child's breathing and heartbeat. If your child is still in contact with the electricity switch off the power source or break the electrical contact (see below) *before* touching him, or you will electrocute yourself.

Contact with electricity can also result in burns. Although these burns look small, they are often deep. In addition, there may be a burn not only where the electricity enters your child's body but also where it leaves the body. There is a serious risk of infection, so it is essential that all electrical burns, however small, are seen by a doctor.

Breaking electrical contact

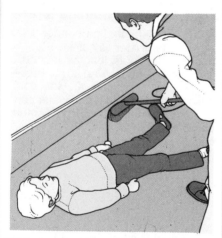

If it isn't possible to switch off the source of power, break the contact immediately. Find something that will not conduct electricity, such as a broom handle or plastic tube, and push your child's limb away from the electricity. Make sure your hands and whatever you use are dry and you are not standing on anything wet or metal.

What should I do?

1 When the contact is broken, examine your child carefully—if you find a burn, check to see if there is another burn on the other side of the limb.

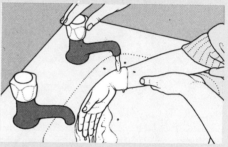

2 Cool any burns by placing the affected area under a cold tap for 10 to 15 minutes (*see page 297*). Cover the burns with dressings, and get your child to the nearest emergency room.

3 Treat your child for shock (*see page 293*) while you are waiting for the ambulance or being driven to the hospital.

If your child is unconscious

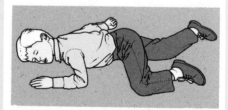

When you have broken the electrical contact, check your child's breathing, and begin resuscitation if necessary (*see Dealing with unconsciousness, page 290*). If your child is unconscious but breathing, turn him into the recovery position to keep his airway open (*see page 285*). Treat any burns or other injuries.

Dealing with poisoning

If your child has eaten something poisonous or something you think may be poisonous, find the container if there is one, and read the list of ingredients. Call your local poison control center, your doctor or the nearest emergency room immediately, and tell them what you think your child has swallowed. They will probably be able to tell you whether the substance is poisonous and what you can do while waiting for the ambulance or being driven to the hospital.

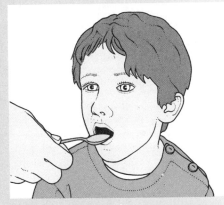

Possible symptoms

● Vomiting and diarrhea.
● Burns around his mouth if he has taken corrosive poison.
● Convulsions for no apparent reason.
● Empty or open container known to have held poison or medicine lying near your child.
● Poisonous plant or berries in his hand or near him if he is unconscious.

What should I do?

1 Quickly ask him to tell you, or point to, what he has taken because he may lose consciousness.

2 Keep a sample of what you think your child has taken, for example a few leaves or berries or the empty bottle or can. If he has eaten some pills, keep the container even if it is empty because it will help the doctor decide what treatment to give him.

3 If your child has taken some form of corrosive poison, such as bleach, lye or weed-killer, NEVER try to make him vomit. Anything that burns the throat and esophagus going down will burn them again coming up. Get him to the emergency room immediately.

4 If you are absolutely positive that your child has NOT TAKEN A CORROSIVE POISON, you can try to make him vomit after being told to by your doctor or by poison control. Give him syrup of ipecac or a glass of salty water. However, do not make him sick if he is unconscious, having a convulsion or is very confused.

If your child is unconscious

Call an ambulance immediately or get another adult to drive you to the nearest emergency room while you give first aid in the back of the car.

1 Place your child in the recovery position, and treat him for unconsciousness (*see Dealing with unconsciousness, page 290*).

2 Keep checking his breathing. Watch for any change in his level of consciousness.

3 If it becomes necessary to give your child mouth-to-mouth resuscitation (*see page 286*), be careful not to get any of the poison in your mouth. Try to wash the poison off his face before you start and, if necessary, hold your child's lips together and breathe into his nose.

Dealing with hypothermia

Hypothermia is a dangerous condition that can develop if your child's body temperature drops below 95F (35C). It is potentially fatal because the functions of vital organs, such as the heart, liver, lungs and intestines, will slow down and eventually stop.

The symptoms are not always easy to see so you have to be on the lookout. A child's body can lose heat just as quickly through wet clothing as through being in water if the surrounding temperature is very low.

3 An older child can be put in a bath that feels warm to the inside of your wrist or your elbow.

4 If your child is conscious, give warm, NOT HOT, sweet drinks.

5 Take your child's temperature every ½ hour or feel the temperature of his skin. Continue these warming procedures until you are sure your child's body temperature is back to normal.

6 If your child's temperature does not begin to rise, get him to an emergency room as soon as possible.

Possible symptoms
- Severe shivering.
- Very cold skin, particularly areas that are usually warm.
- Skin may look pale, even blue.
- Drowsiness and loss of strength.
- Slurred speech.
- Confusion.
- Temperature below 95F (35C).

What should I do?

1 If your child is outdoors, put something dry on top of his wet clothes, and carry him to the nearest shelter or into the house.

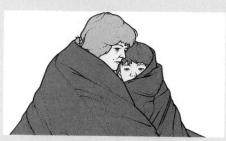

2 Remove his wet clothing as soon as he is in a warm room, and put some dry clothes on him. Wrap him in a blanket next to someone else. Call your doctor immediately.

IMPORTANT
You must warm your child *gradually.* *Never* **use a hot-water bottle or a heating pad because it will take blood away from the body core to the surface. More heat is lost, and this can result in shock (***see page 293***).**

Hypothermia in babies

Very young babies lose heat relatively quickly when sleeping in a room that is not warm enough or if outside without adequate clothing when it is cold.

Possible symptoms
- Cold skin—don't be misled into thinking your baby's all right if his skin looks bright pink and healthy.
- Drowsiness and lethargy—these are danger signs.

What should I do?
Call your doctor immediately. While you are waiting, get into bed or a sleeping bag with your baby to rewarm him gradually with your body heat.

Bandaging techniques

Try to get your child to help because it will take his mind off his injury. When applying an elastic bandage to secure a dressing or support a muscle or joint injury, always start *below* the injury. Work up the limb because the bandage will lie flatter and provide more support (*see following page*). Always leave your child's fingertips or toes exposed so you can check the circulation in the affected area after applying the bandage.

Checking circulation

1 Press one of the exposed fingernails until it turns white, then release the pressure. The nail should become pink again immediately.

2 If color does not return quickly, or the fingers look blue or feel cold, remove the bandage immediately and start again.

SLINGS

Slings are used to support an injured arm or the arm on the injured side if your child has a chest injury. Use a triangular bandage as described below. If you do not have one in your medicine chest, use a piece of material or a large scarf about 1 yard (1m) square, folded in half diagonally.

Applying a sling

1 Sit your child down, and place his arm across his chest so his wrist is slightly higher than his elbow.

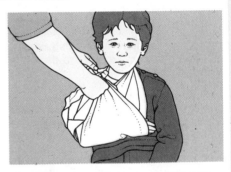

3 Still supporting your child's arm, carry the lower end up over his arm. Tie the ends together in the hollow above his collarbone using a reef knot.

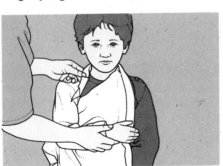

2 Fold up the long edge (base) of a triangular bandage to make a hem, and slide the bandage up through the gap between your child's elbow and his chest. Keep the base parallel to his side, and carry the top end over his shoulder and around to the front on the injured side.

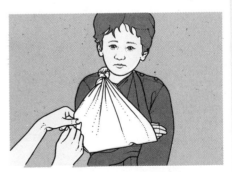

4 Fold the corner of the bandage at the elbow back and bring the point forward. Pin it to the front of the sling.

5 Check the circulation in your child's fingers and, if necessary, adjust or reapply the sling.

Bandaging techniques

LEG/ARM BANDAGES

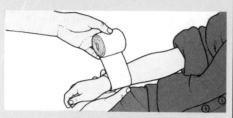

1 Unroll the bandage slightly, and hold it so the rolled part is on top. Working outward from the inside of the leg or arm, place the end of the bandage on the limb below the injury. Make a straight turn around the limb to secure the end of the bandage.

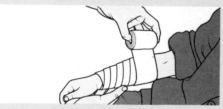

2 Work up the limb, making spiral turns so each layer covers about ⅔ of the previous turn. Finish with a straight turn, and secure the end with a safety pin or butterfly clips.

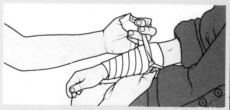

3 If you don't have a safety pin or butterfly clips, leave about 6 inches (15cm) hanging free—enough to wind once around the limb. Cut the center of the piece of bandage, and tie a knot at the bottom of the split. Wrap the ends around the limb, and tie on the other side.

ANKLE/HAND BANDAGES

1 Raise and support your child's foot. Unroll a few inches of the bandage. Holding it in one hand so the rolled part is on top, work from the inside of his leg outward. Make one straight turn around his ankle.

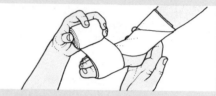

2 Wrap the bandage diagonally across your child's foot to his big toe, around under the ball of his foot and up at the base of his little toe. Make two straight turns around the ball of the foot.

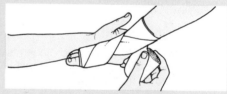

3 Take the bandage up and across his foot to his ankle, around the ankle and diagonally across his foot to the toes. Continue these figure-8 turns so each layer covers ⅔ of the previous layer until his foot is covered.

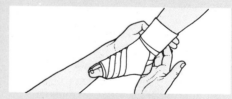

4 Finish with one straight turn around the ankle, and secure the bandage with a safety pin or tie the ends, as described at left.

5 To bandage a hand, support the affected hand injured side on top, and bandage as above.

Personal records

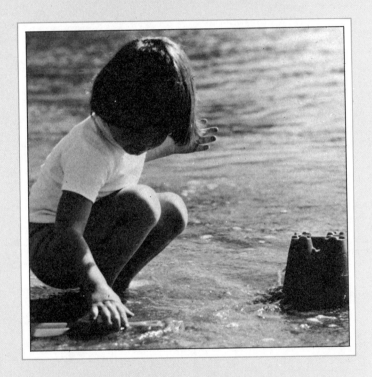

Growth charts

Your child will grow and put on weight at his own rate, so while it is interesting to plot his development, don't become obsessive or anxious about it. It is only in the first few months of a baby's life that weight gain should be watched closely, and it will be monitored by your doctor. After this stage, it is regularity of weight gain, that is most important.

To use the chart, first weigh your baby. Then go along the bottom axis until you find his age. Look up the vertical axis until you reach your baby's weight. The point where the two axes meet will give you an idea of your baby's progress in comparison to an average figure.

KEY

Large baby	Medium baby	Small baby
••••••••••	——————	- - - - - - -

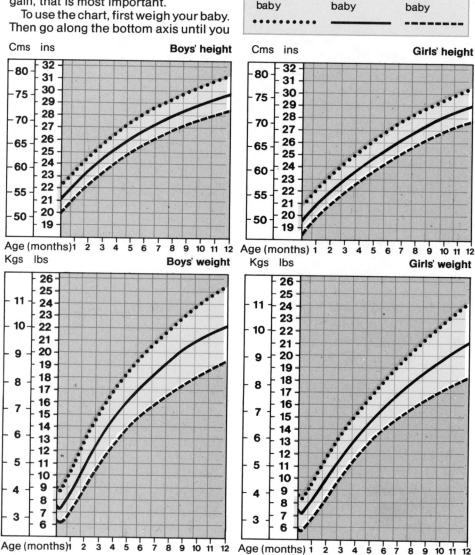

Immunization

The aim of immunization is to protect individuals and communities from infectious diseases. Every parent should take steps to have their child properly immunized. Even if a disease seems to have been eradicated, it is still necessary to continue immunizing against it to prevent its re-emergence.

Immunization works by preparing the body to repel infection. The body usually has to have an infection once before its defenses are capable of responding against it. Immunization does this for us—by means of injection, drops in the mouth or scratching the skin. The substance introduced into the body is called a *vaccine*, and the method for doing so is known as vaccination or inoculation.

Most vaccination programs start when your baby is 2 months old. Your doctor will give you a card to record dates and types of vaccination.

Your doctor will also ask about family medical history. This is necessary to help determine whether or not your child should have a particular vaccination. For instance, children who suffer from convulsions, who have a family history of epilepsy or who have a heart or lung disease may be advised not to have a measles or whooping cough vaccination.

It is quite common for a small red bump to develop at the site of an inoculation. However, if your child becomes irritable or develops a fever, or if he develops a high pitched scream or if your baby has a convulsion, get in touch with your doctor immediately.

The chart below outlines commonly recommended immunizations of childhood. The guide to infectious fevers (see page 306) lists the symptoms and treatment for some of the most common childhood illnesses. It also lists preventive measures, where applicable. If you think your child has contracted an infectious fever, always contact your doctor to confirm the diagnosis.

Disease	Time	Reaction	Protection
Diphtheria, whooping cough (pertussis), tetanus Also known as DTP or triple vaccine	Injections at 2, 4 and 6 months; repeat diphtheria and tetanus at 18 months and 5 years.	Child may become feverish; the site of the injection may be sore	Tetanus must be repeated every five years to provide continuing protection
Polio	Oral vaccine at 2, 4 and 6 months, repeat at 18 months and 5 years	None	Has to be repeated to provide continuing protection
Measles	Injection at 15 months	Child may become feverish and have a slight rash	Not known how long protection from vaccination lasts
German measles (Rubella)	Injection at 15 months	Child may complain of sore joints	Not known how long protection from vaccination lasts
Tuberculosis In some areas, tuberculosis skin-test screening is repeated annually	Test at 12 months	None	—

Infectious fevers chart

Disease	Incubation Period	Symptoms
Chickenpox (see page 83)	7-21 days	Groups of spots that quickly develop into intensely itchy blisters. These appear in crops every 3 or 4 days, usually starting on the trunk, then spreading to the face, arms and legs. The spots are usually accompanied by headache and fever.
German measles (see page 146)	14-21 days	Slightly raised temperature, a rash of tiny pink or red spots that starts behind the ears, spreads to the forehead, then to the rest of the body, and enlarged glands at the back of the neck.
Measles (see page 176)	8-14 days	The first signs are a runny nose, dry cough, headache, fever with a temperature as high as 104F (40C), and white spots inside the mouth and on the linings of the cheeks (Koplik's spots). Also, the eyes may be red and sore. These symptoms are followed by a brown-red rash that starts behind the ears and spreads to the face and torso.
Mumps (see page 184).	17-28 days	Swelling and soreness of the glands at the sides of the face, just below the ears and beneath the chin, painful swallowing, dry mouth, fever and a headache. In boys, the testes may be swollen and painful; girls may experience lower abdominal pains.
Roseola infantum (see page 211)	7-14 days	A fever with a temperature of 102-104F (38.7-40C) for 3 days, with no other symptoms. As the fever subsides, a rash of separate, flat, red or pink spots appears, first on the trunk, then spreading to the limbs and neck.
Scarlet fever (see page 213)	1-5 days	Sore throat, inflamed tonsils, fever with a temperature as high as 104F (40C), vomiting, abdominal pains, rash of small spots starting in the chest and neck, then merging over the body, except the area around the mouth, and strawberry-red patches on a furry tongue.
Whooping cough (see page 259)	5-14 days	Slight temperature, runny nose, slight cough that develops into a compulsive cough accompanied by whooping breath

Treatment	Complications	Immunity	Prevention
Relieve itching with calamine lotion. If your child develops a fever, reduce it by tepid sponging (see page 31), and acetaminophen. *Never use aspirin because of the possible complications of Reye's syndrome (see page 208).*	In rare cases, chickenpox may cause encephalitis (see page 128) or be complicated by Reye's syndrome.	Lifelong	None
If the child's temperature rises above 100F (37.8C), give him acetaminophen.	None to your child, but fetal damage could occur in a pregnant woman who comes into contact with your contagious child.	Lifelong	Inoculation at 15 months of age.
Try to reduce your child's temperature with tepid sponging (see page 31) and acetaminophen.	In rare cases, otitis media (see page 195), pneumonia (see page 201) and encephalitis (see page 128).	Lifelong	Inoculation at 15 months of age.
Try to reduce your child's temperature with tepid sponging (see page 31) and acetaminophen. Purée food if eating is painful, and give your child plenty to drink.	In rare cases, encephalitis (see page 128) and meningitis (see page 177).	Usually lifelong	None
Try to reduce your child's temperature with tepid sponging (see page 31) and acetaminophen.	Possible febrile convulsions.	Usually lifelong	None
Try to reduce your child's temperature with tepid sponging (see page 31) and acetaminophen.	Rare, though scarlet fever can cause inflammation of the kidneys or of the joints and heart (rheumatic fever, see page 209).	Lifelong	None
Antibiotics must be given early to be effective.	Very rare today, although there's a possibility of bronchitis (see page 76) or pneumonia (see page 201).	Lifelong	Inoculation at 2, 4 and 6 months.

Records

The charts below are designed to help you keep track of any events concerning your family's health. It is important to keep records to ensure that you stay up to date with immunizations and to provide reliable information in the future.

Birth record

	First baby	Second baby
Baby's name		
Date of birth		
Time of birth		
Place of birth		
Height		
Weight		
Blood group		
Problems during pregnancy		
Type of delivery		
Problems with delivery		
Post partum problems		

Family medical history

Mother's birth date

Illnesses

Father's birth date

Illnesses

Family allergies and chronic conditions

Records

Illness, injury and allergy record

First child

Illnesses	Injuries	Allergies

Second child

Illnesses	Injuries	Allergies

Immunization record

	First child Date/Age	**Second child** Date/Age
Diphtheria, whooping cough, tetanus (DPT)		
DT boosters		
Polio		
Polio boosters		
Measles		
German measles		
Tuberculosis		

Telephone numbers

Pediatrician	Dentist
Family doctor	Police
Hospital	Fire department
Drugstore	Poison control center

Glossary

Words in **_bold italic_** denote glossary entries

Abscess
Localized collection of *pus* that collects as part of the body's way of fighting *infection.*

Acetaminophen see *Analgesic*

Acute
Term applied to short, severe attacks of a disease or pain.

Allergen
Substance—often as common as house dust, grass pollen, animal fur or a particular food—which is harmless to most people, but which provokes an allergic reaction in certain individuals. Such substances are also called antigens.

Allergy
Abnormal reaction of the body to substances called *allergens.* These are harmless to most people, but certain individuals develop a sensitivity to them. *Antibodies,* usually produced by the body's defense system to fight infection, react to the allergen causing an allergy, resulting in a variety of symptoms.

Analgesic
Pain-relieving drug. The two most frequently given to children are children's aspirin and acetaminophen. Aspirin is a stomach irritant and can cause vomiting, so it is probably best to use acetaminophen. *Never* give aspirin to children with influenza or chickenpox because of the danger of Reye's syndrome.

Anaphylaxis
Very severe, general allergic reaction (see *allergy*). Symptoms can range from asthma attacks and flushing, to collapse and unconsciousness. When a severe allergic reaction results, caused by a sting for instance, shock may develop. This is called anaphylactic shock.

Anemia
Type of blood disorder in which the oxygen-carrying power or number of mature, healthy blood cells is diminished. Lack of *hemoglobin*, the oxygen-carrying agent in the blood, brings about a shortage of oxygen in the body's tissue. Characteristic symptoms of anemia are pale skin, especially at the tips of the fingers, on the lips and tongue and around the eyes.

Anesthetic
Drug used to bring about temporary loss of sensation to remove pain. General anesthesia induces unconsciousness and is usually administered by an anesthetist by injection or through inhalation. Local anesthetics are usually given as injections and remove sensation from only a limited area.

Antibiotic
Drug used to fight bacterial infection. A prescribed course of antibiotics should always be completed, even if the illness is cured. Future treatment with the drug may face greater bacterial resistance if the course is not finished.

Antibodies
Agents of the body's defense system, produced by white blood cells to combat an *infection* or foreign agent, such as grass pollen (see *allergy*).

Anti-coagulant
Drug used to stop the blood clotting.

Anti-convulsant
Drug used to prevent or stop convulsions, often in the treatment of epilepsy. Sudden withdrawal from the drug may itself precipitate a convulsion.

Anti-fungal
Drug used to treat fungal infections, such as those that affect hair, skin, nails or mucous membranes.

Antigen see *Allergen*

Antihistamine
Drug used to counter the effect of a *histamine,* a chemical produced by the body as a result of an inflammatory and allergic reaction (see *allergy*).

Antiserum
Serum prepared from the blood of a person (or animal) whose defense system has been stimulated to fight an infecting agent or foreign protein, such as snake venom. When administered, the antiserum protects against the infecting agent or foreign protein through the *antibodies* contained within it.

Antitoxin
Substance, produced by the body or injected into it, that nullifies the effects of a *toxin,* a poisonous substance produced by *bacteria* and some plants and animals.

Aspirin see *Analgesic*

Glossary

Autoimmune
Term used for a defect in the body's defense system against disease. This defect causes the body to manufacture *antibodies*, normally produced to combat infection, which attack and harm the body's own healthy tissue.

Bacteria
Group of organisms; some are harmless, some are only harmful when they multiply too quickly and some are even beneficial. Certain bacterial infections can be controlled by *antibiotics*.

Benign
Term used to describe unnatural growth that is harmless to surrounding tissue and that will not return, once removed.

Biopsy
Process by which a small piece of body tissue is removed for analysis. It is often used to determine if an unnatural growth is *malignant* (cancerous) or *benign* (harmless).

Bolus
Ball of chewed food, as it passes from the mouth to the stomach.

Bronchodilator
Drug that widens bronchial passages and is used in the treatment of asthma. The drug is taken orally.

Carcinogen
Substance that causes or promotes cancer.

Cauterization
Process by which tissue is destroyed, using a hot instrument or a chemical. Nosebleeds, warts and other skin growths are often treated with this method.

Cerebral
Relating to the structure and workings of the brain.

Chromosomes
Microscopic strands that are present within the nucleus of every cell. They carry the genetic information needed to determine the characteristics of an individual. There are normally 46 chromosomes in each cell. Abnormal numbers or formations of chromosomes are found in sufferers of certain diseases, such as Down's syndrome.

Chronic
Term describing a condition that has lasted, or is expected to last, for some time, while not necessarily being life-threatening. Chronic conditions tend to get better or deteriorate slowly.

Cilia
Minute hairs lining the surface of mucous membranes, for example, in the nose. Their waving movement serves a cleaning purpose, clearing dust particles, mucus and *bacteria*.

Congenital
Term applied to a disease or condition present at birth.

Cyanosis
Blueness of the skin, caused by lack of oxygen.

Cyst
Abnormal, fluid-filled swelling.

Dermatologist
Doctor who specializes in treating diseases of the skin.

Dialysis
Treatment for kidney failure. Waste products, usually excreted by the kidney, are removed by cleansing the blood on a dialysis machine (hemodialysis) or by cleaning the peritoneal cavity (peritoneal dialysis) in the abdomen.

Diuretic
Any substance that increases water excretion and therefore urine production, thus lowering the body's fluid content.

Edema
Swelling of the body tissue caused by excess fluid content. The condition most commonly affects the ankles.

Electroencephalogram (EEG)
Recording of the electrical impulses of the brain, using a painless process called electroencephalography. It involves placing metal tabs on the head that record the impulses graphically.

Embolism
Sudden blockage of a blood vessel, caused by a blood clot or other foreign solid called an embolus.

Endocrinologist
Doctor who specializes in the study of *hormones* and the diseases caused by their disorders.

Endoscope
Instrument enabling a doctor to look into a body cavity, usually the esophagus, stomach or duodenum. Photographs and tissue samples can also be taken, and some small growths can be removed, with an endoscope.

Glossary

Endoscopy
Procedure in which an *endoscope* is used.

Enema
Liquid forced into the rectum, usually to produce a bowel movement or for diagnostic purposes; also the name for this process. An enema should be given only on doctor's orders (see also *suppository*).

Excretion
Removal of the body's internal waste matter by natural processes, such as urination, sweating and exhalation.

Febrile
Characterized by fever and a quickly rising, high tempera-ture, as in a febrile convulsion.

Follicle
Most commonly, a tiny cavity on the body's surface.

Gammaglobulin
Type of blood protein that includes *antibodies*. Obtained from donated blood, gammaglobulin can be used in the prevention of infections, such as hepatitis.

Hematologist
Doctor who specializes in the treatment of diseases of the blood, bone marrow and lymph glands.

Hematoma
Collection of blood under the skin or deep in the tissues.

Hematuria
Blood in the urine, either visible to the naked eye or under a microscope.

Hemoglobin
Oxygen-carrying agent in the blood. It is present only in red blood cells, giving the blood its color.

Hemorrhage
Bleeding, either externally (from the skin or an orifice) or internally (within a body cavity).

Histamine
Chemical released into the body when an allergic or inflammatory reaction takes place (see *allergy*). The most common results are redness, swelling and itching.

Hormone
Chemical released by special (endrocrine) glands into the bloodstream. It regulates the activities of certain body organs and tissues.

Hyper-
Prefix meaning "high" or "above" an expected norm. For example, hyperactive means active above the expected norm.

Immune system
Body's defense system against disease, enabling it to recognize and destroy invading *microbes* (minute *bacteria*, viruses or fungi invisible to the naked eye) or foreign tissues, through the white blood cell's production of *antibodies*.

Immunity
Resistance to disease, developed either by the body's *immune system* when an infection is contracted or through purposeful inter-vention, as in vaccination.

Immunization
Process by which the body is prepared, by inoculation, to repel infection.

Incubation period
Interval (usually measured in days) between the time germs of a disease enter the body and when symptoms begin to appear.

Infection
Type of illness caused by *microbes*—minute *bacteria*, viruses or fungi invisible to the naked eye—invading the body and multiplying within it. The microbes may produce harmful waste products.

Inflammation
Painful, red swelling that is warm to the touch. Inflammation is the body tissue's reaction to a variety of injuries (physical blows, infection, autoimmune disease).

Inoculation
The introduction of a *vaccine* into the body.

Intravenous
Within, or inserted into, a vein. An intravenous (I.V.) drip is used to pass liquid substance, whether blood, saline or *plasma*, from an elevated sterile container, through a vein, into the body. The rate of flow is controlled by the rate of dripping through a transparent container.

Laxative
Type of drug used to ease and increase the frequency of bowel movements. Laxatives should be given to a child *only* on doctor's orders.

Lumbar puncture
Procedure for taking a sample of fluid from the base of the spine by inserting a needle. This is done under

Glossary

local anesthetic. The fluid is analyzed to diagnose certain diseases, particularly those affecting the nervous system, such as meningitis.

Lymph
Colorless liquid that contains white blood cells. Lymph flows in channels, taking nutrients to, and removing waste products from, local cells. The white blood cells in lymph are an important part of the body's defense system against infection.

Malignant
Term applied to a cancerous growth that is likely to spread, and recur, even after removal. A malignant growth is sometimes impossible to eradicate totally.

Membrane
Thin lining or covering tissue of various organs and cavities of the body.

Meninges
Three layers of *membrane* protecting the brain and spinal cord. Meningitis is an inflammation of the meninges.

Metabolism
Body's physical and chemical reactions. Any series of, or single, reactions may be described as metabolic.

Microbes
Minute *bacteria*, viruses or fungi invisible to the naked eye.

Mucous membrane
Membrane lining part of the body, such as the mouth or vagina, which secretes a watery or slimy material.

Neuro-
Pertaining to the body's nervous system. For example, a neurosurgeon specializes in surgery of the nervous system.

Neurologist
Doctor who specializes in treating diseases of the brain and those related to the nervous system. Neurologists often work closely with neurosurgeons, who specialize in surgery of the nervous system, principally the brain and spinal cord.

Obstetrician
Doctor who specializes in looking after women during pregnancy and immediately after childbirth.

Oncology
Study of tumors, closely connected with research into *malignant* (cancerous) growths.

Ophthalmologist
Doctor who specializes in treating eye injury or disease. An optician prepares and dispenses eyeglasses and contact lenses. An optometrist examines eyes and prescribes corrective lenses.

Ophthalmoscope
Instrument for examining the tissues of the interior of the eye by shining a light through the pupil.

Orthodontist
Dentist who specializes in treating teeth abnormalities and jaw disorders.

Orthopedics
Process of curing deformities arising from disease of, or injury to, bones and joints.

Otoscope
Instrument for examining the middle and inner ear, viewed through the semitransparent eardrum, in order to diagnose disease.

Pediatrician
Doctor who specializes in treating children, usually until the age of puberty.

Penicillin
Antibiotic used in the treatment of many infections including strep throat and otitis media. Penicillin may, like any antibiotic, provoke an allergic reaction (see *allergy*). If your child is allergic to penicillin, be sure this is entered on his medical records and he wears a medic-alert bracelet or necklace so he isn't given the drug.

Physiotherapist
Person trained to give treatment through the use of physical exercise and manipulation. Physiotherapy is often used to help children suffering from arthritis, cerebral palsy, muscular dystrophy and other neuromuscular diseases.

Plasma
Liquid (as opposed to cellular) part of the blood, which can be used as replacement fluid in the treatment of shock and burns.

Post-partum
Literally, after birth. Refers to the health of the baby and his mother in the first weeks after birth.

Prenatal
Literally, before birth. Refers to a condition or event during pregnancy.

Glossary

Prophylactic
Substance or procedure that helps to prevent disease (immunization, for example).

Psychiatrist
Medically qualified specialist in mental illness.

Psychologist
Non-medically qualified person trained to assess behavioral problems, measure intelligence quotients (IQ) and development quotients (DQ).

Pus
Yellow-green semiliquid substance, made up of decomposed tissue, *bacteria* and dead white blood cells. The production of pus is a sign of the body's fight against *infection*.

Sebum
Oily substance produced by the sebaceous glands just below the skin's surface. Sebum is the body's own skin moistener, spreading over the skin from the pores. Acne can be caused through a buildup of sebum under the skin's surface.

Secretion
Body's production of substances from special glands or cells. For instance, *sebum*.

Serum
Clear, liquid content of the blood when separated from other blood components, such as clotting substances, that are found in *plasma*.

Spasm
Involuntary, uncontrollable contraction of one or more muscles.

Spitting up
In babies, the harmless habit of regurgitating milk soon after, or during, a feeding.

Stools
Waste matter left over from food, expelled from the rectum.

Suppository
Small piece of medicated substance, placed in the rectum or vagina, to be slowly absorbed into the body.

Swab
Cotton-tipped stick or piece of soft fabric, used for cleaning or sampling.

Tinnitus
Intermittent or continuous ringing, buzzing or roaring sound in the ear, heard only by the sufferer.

Toxin
Poisonous substance produced by *bacteria*, other *microbes* and some plants and animals.

Tracheotomy
Surgical procedure to restore normal breathing when the throat or larynx is blocked. An incision is made in the neck, and a tube is inserted below the blockage to provide an air passage.

Traction
Means "pulling apart" and is used as a treatment for broken bones, crushed vertebrae, prolapsed discs and other problems. Damaged and compressed parts of the body are held apart and in the correct position (often for some time) until healed.

Tumor
Swelling; usually denotes one caused by abnormal cell multiplication within the body.

Ulcer
Open sore affecting either an internal or external body surface.

Vaccination see *Immunization*

Vaccine
Solution made up of an altered, weakened or killed strain of a disease. Usually injected into the body, a vaccine is designed to stimulate the body's resistance to the disease that has been introduced into it.

Vasoconstrictor
Any substance, whether a chemical produced by the body or a drug, that causes blood vessels to narrow.

Vasodilator
Any substance, whether a chemical produced by the body or a drug, that causes blood vessels to widen.

Virus
Smallest type of *microbe* that invades the body's cells and multiplies inside them, giving rise to contagious viral infections, such as influenza.

Index

Page numbers in *italic* refer to the illustrations and captions; * denotes a main reference

Index

Index

Index

Index

Index